MKSAP® for Students

Medical Knowledge
Self-Assessment Program®

Developed by
American College of Physicians–American Society of Internal Medicine
Clerkship Directors in Internal Medicine

American College of Physicians–American Society of Internal Medicine
190 North Independence Mall West
Philadelphia, PA 19106-1572
215-351-2400

Library of Congress Cataloging-in-Publication Data

MKSAP for Students: Medical Knowledge Self-Assessment Program/developed by American College of Physicians–American Society of Internal Medicine.
    p.;cm.
  Chief editor: Patrick C. Alguire, MD
  Includes bibliographical references.
  ISBN: 0-943126-90-8
    1. Internal medicine–Case studies. I. Alguire, Patrick C. (Patrick Craig), 1950-II. American College of Physicians–American Society of Internal Medicine.
    [DNLM: 1. Clinical Medicine—Problems and Exercises. WB 18.2 M6848 2000]
RC66 .M57 2000
616'.0076—dc21

00-022810

Printed in the United States of America

Contributors

MKSAP for Students Development Team

Jeremy S. Abramson, medical student
Mt. Sinai School of Medicine of New York University
New York, New York

Eric J. Alper, MD
Assistant Professor of Medicine
University of Massachusetts Medical School
Worcester, Massachusetts

John W. Caruso, MD
Clerkship Director and Assistant Program Director
Thomas Jefferson Medical School
Philadelphia, Pennsylvania

Richard H. Esham, MD, FACP
Director of General Medicine and Geriatrics
University of South Alabama
Mobile, Alabama

Erica Friedman, MD
Associate Professor of Medicine
Director of Medical Clerkship
Mount Sinai University School of Medicine
  of New York University
New York, New York

Jeanne K. Heard, MD, PhD, FACP
Associate Professor of Medicine
Dean for Graduate Medical Education
University of Arkansas College of Medicine
Little Rock, Arkansas

David R. Lambert, MD
Assistant Professor of Medicine
University of Rochester School of Medicine
  and Dentistry
Rochester, New York

Douglas S. Paauw, MD, FACP
Associate Professor of Medicine
Coordinator of Student Teaching
University of Washington School of Medicine
Seattle, Washington

Andrea M. Tom, medical student
Brown University
Providence, Rhode Island

Glenda C. Wickstrom, MD
Director, Medical Center
Summa Health System
Akron, Ohio

Review Team

David B. Neely, MD, FACP
Director of Undergraduate Medical Education
Department of Medicine
Northwestern University Medical School
Chicago, Illinois

Louis J. O'Boyle, DO
Associate Program Director
Scranton-Temple Residency Program
Scranton, Pennsylvania

Stephen M. Salerno, MD, FACP
Assistant Professor of Medicine
Department of Medicine-EDP
Uniform Services University of the Health Sciences
Bethesda, Maryland

James L. Sebastian, MD, FACP
Director of Student Teaching Programs
Department of Medicine
Medical College of Wisconsin
Milwaukee, Wisconsin

Principal ACP-ASIM Staff
Editor-in-Chief
Patrick C. Alguire, MD, FACP
Director, Education and Career Development

Editors
Karen McFadden
Charles Rossi

Editorial Assistants
Wynne Curry
Sheila O'Steen

Acknowledgments
The American College of Physicians–American Society of Internal Medicine gratefully acknowledges the special contribution to *MKSAP for Students* of Michael Ripca (graphic designer) and Francine Martin (administrator). The College also wishes to acknowledge that many other persons, too numerous to mention, have contributed to the production of this book. Without their dedicated efforts, this publication would not have been possible.

FOREWORD

Dear Student:

An essential part of the practice of medicine is the science and art of problem solving. The enormous body of factual material that must be mastered will, in the final analysis, be of value only if intelligently applied to the care of patients.

As a consequence, medical educators have sought to ensure that problem-solving skills are learned and retained throughout the long professional lifetime of the practicing physician.

More than 30 years ago, the American College of Physicians launched a new program to enable practicing internists to measure how well they have kept abreast of new information and how well they are applying it to the care of patients. The Medical Knowledge Self-Assessment Program (MKSAP) was an instant success, and the current 11th edition has almost 40,000 subscribers, who are glowing in their feedback about the impact the program has had on their professional lives.

During the past year, the leadership of the College and the Clerkship Directors of Internal Medicine have enthusiastically planned for a self-assessment product focused on the needs of medical students during their third and fourth years. Modeled after Internal Medicine MKSAP, the student MKSAP was designed to include case-based multiple-choice questions for self-assessment. Each question has a critique, providing information about the topic of the question and why the various options are either correct or incorrect.

We hope that MKSAP for Students will be a valuable adjunct to your studies and your clerkship experience. If the experiences of hundreds of thousands of internists are a guide, this product will reinforce your learning and help ensure that it is applied in a fashion that will make you the best physician you can be, for your patients will deserve no less!

Good luck in your studies and in your future careers.

Sincerely,

Herbert S. Waxman, MD, FACP
Senior Vice President, Education
American College of Physicians–
American Society of Internal Medicine

PREFACE

The goal of *MKSAP for Students* is to help define and assess mastery of the core knowledge base requisite to internal medicine education in medical school. This study aid is intended primarily for third-year students participating in their required internal medicine clerkship. Other audiences include fourth-year students on an advanced medicine clerkship, second-year students who are developing an understanding of pathophysiology, clinical problem-solving, and problem-based learning, and physician assistant students. In creating this product, we have chosen to model it after the highly successful *Medical Knowledge Self-Assessment Program* (MKSAP) program for internal medicine physicians.

MKSAP for Students consists of a collection of patient-centered self-assessment questions and their answers. The questions begin with a clinical vignette, and the vignettes are organized into 28 different categories that correspond to the "Training Problems" in the *Core Medicine Clerkship Curriculum Guide*. The *Clerkship Curriculum Guide* is a nationally recognized curriculum for the required third-year internal medicine clerkship created and published by the Clerkship Directors in Internal Medicine (CDIM) and the Society for General Internal Medicine (SGIM). It defines the competencies, knowledge, attitudes, and skills that medical students are expected to master by the end of the clerkship. The "Training Problems" categorize the learning content in the areas of health maintenance and disease screening, disease manifestations, specific diseases, abnormal laboratory findings, and risky lifestyles or behaviors.

Each question has a critique that supplies the correct answer, an explanation of why the correct answer is correct and why the incorrect options are not, and a short bibliography. We recommend that students read the clinical vignette, select an answer, and then read the associated critique.

We would like to emphasize that the questions in *MKSAP for Students* are very difficult and are not to be used as a formal evaluation of students. However, we also believe that the questions do reflect the many real management dilemmas faced daily by internal medicine physicians and therefore provide a focused, concise review of important content. In short, *MKSAP for Students* is a learning text, not an evaluation instrument.

MKSAP for Students would have been impossible without the valuable, and entirely voluntary, contributions of many people, some of whom are named in the acknowledgments section. Others, not specifically named, were representatives of a wide spectrum of constituencies and organizations such as the Executive Committee of the Clerkship Directors of Internal Medicine and various committees within the American College of Physicians–American Society of Internal Medicine, including the Education Committee, the Counsel of Associates, the Counsel of Student Members, the Medical Student and Resident Activities Subcommittee, Committee of Young Physicians, and the Board of Governors.

Patrick C. Alguire, MD, FACP
Editor-in-Chief

Contents

Questions

ABDOMINAL PAIN

Abdominal Pain Question 1

An 81-year-old man presents to the emergency department with abdominal and testicular pain that has been present for 2 hours. He is in moderate distress. He denies recent symptoms of nausea, vomiting, diarrhea, constipation, urinary frequency, or dysuria. He had a myocardial infarction 6 years ago and subsequently underwent coronary artery bypass surgery. His medications include aspirin, 325 mg every day, and oral nifedipine XL, 60 mg every day.

On physical examination, his pulse rate is 105/min, blood pressure is 180/110 mm Hg, and lungs are clear to auscultation. Cardiac examination discloses an S_4 and no murmurs. He has an obese abdomen. There is periumbilical tenderness. Bowel sounds are present. Peripheral pulses are all present.

Laboratory studies:

Hematocrit	30%
Leukocyte count	10,100/μL
Platelet count	145,000/μL
Blood urea nitrogen	45 mg/dL
Serum creatinine	1.8 mg/dL

Electrocardiogram shows sinus rhythm and 2 mm of ST-segment depression in leads V_4 through V_6. Abdominal computed tomography (CT) shows an abdominal aortic aneurysm measuring 7.1 cm. Retroperitoneal blood is evident contiguous to the aneurysm.

The most appropriate treatment for this patient is:

(A) Emergent repair of a ruptured abdominal aortic aneurysm
(B) Urgent transfer to the catheterization laboratory for percutaneous transluminal coronary angioplasty (PTCA)
(C) Urologic consultation for treatment of scrotal hemorrhage
(D) Intravenous metoprolol and nitroglycerin
(E) Angiotensin-converting enzyme (ACE) inhibitor and analgesics

Abdominal Pain Question 2

You are asked to evaluate a 75-year-old man for progressive abdominal symptoms. He has been in the hospital for 5 days being treated for an exacerbation of chronic congestive heart failure complicated by atrial fibrillation. He has undergone diuresis for pulmonary edema and peripheral edema. He had no history of abdominal disorders until he suddenly developed progressive mid-abdominal pain over the prior 12 hours. He vomited once and refused his last meal. He had no bowel movement during the previous night and complained of severe, noncrampy pain around the umbilicus.

His history is significant for a prior duodenal ulcer, chronic obstructive pulmonary disease, and prior appendectomy and cholecystectomy. His medications include digoxin, furosemide, ranitidine, and subcutaneous heparin.

Physical examination reveals an elderly white man in obvious abdominal distress. The pulse rate is 110/min, respiration rate is 24/min, and blood pressure is 160/90 mm Hg. Examination of the head, eyes, ears, nose, and throat is unrevealing. Neck veins are mildly distended. He has bibasilar rales. Cardiac examination reveals atrial fibrillation, left ventricular enlargement, and a soft S_3 gallop. He has bilateral cervical bruits and femoral bruits but no abdominal bruit. His abdomen is diffusely tender with hypoactive bowel sounds. There is no rebound tenderness or hepatosplenomegaly. Rectal examination reveals a firm, enlarged prostate with some asymmetry but no distinct mass. Stool in the ampulla is positive for occult blood.

Laboratory tests from the previous day show normal electrolytes and liver enzymes, but persistent mild chronic renal insufficiency. A stat blood count reveals a leukocyte count of 11,000/μL (with 59% polymorphonuclear leukocytes, 20% lymphocytes, 7% monocytes, and 14% band forms). Pancreatic amylase is five times normal. Measurement of arterial blood gases with the patient breathing room air reveals a P_{O_2} of 86 mm Hg, P_{CO_2} of 40 mm Hg, and pH of 7.29. A chest radiograph shows cardiomegaly, vascular redistribution, and resolving pulmonary edema. An abdominal radiograph shows nonspecific gas and no evidence of subdiaphragmatic air.

What study would you order next?

(A) Pancreatic ultrasonography
(B) Abdominal computed tomography
(C) Upper gastrointestinal endoscopy
(D) Colonoscopy
(E) Abdominal angiography

Abdominal Pain Question 3

A 22-year-old legal secretary presents with lower abdominal pain. She recalls having symptoms since childhood with a tendency toward diarrhea whenever she is "stressed out." Rectal bleeding or fevers do not accompany her symptoms, which keep her up at night and are often progressive through the day. She avoids eating until dinner, after which she notes abdominal distention and gaseousness. She has always been thin but describes a large abdomen "as if she were pregnant." The symptoms are worse around her menstrual period, which has been regular and also painful for several years, such that she is often confined to bed for the first day of menstruation. She has been to several physicians over the past years and has had an upper gastrointestinal barium study and two barium enemas; she was told the tests were normal. She was told that she had a spastic colon and tried bran but stopped eating bran because of increased distention. Her only medication is ibuprofen taken for chronic headaches and dysmenorrhea.

She has no other significant medical history and is presenting because she is engaged and her fiancé is concerned about the symptoms she has each night when they are together. She lives alone. Her parents were divorced when she was 13. She has one older sister who was diagnosed with ulcer disease, although she never underwent diagnostic studies. She smokes one pack of cigarettes daily but does not drink alcohol (her father was an alcoholic).

The physical examination shows only diffuse, lower abdominal tenderness without a palpable mass. The rectal examination is described as painful but is otherwise normal. There is formed stool in the ampulla; the stool is negative for occult blood.

What would be the most important diagnostic procedure to define the cause of her symptoms?

(A) More detailed social history
(B) Colonoscopy
(C) Pelvic ultrasonography
(D) Abdominal/pelvic computed tomography
(E) Laparoscopy

Abdominal Pain Question 4

An 80-year-old woman, who lives in a nursing home, fell 3 days ago and has been receiving narcotics for severe back pain associated with at least one compression fracture of her lumbar spine. She presents with severe constipation and a grossly distended abdomen. She is afebrile; her abdomen is not tender but is distended and tympanitic to percussion, with diminished bowel sounds. Abdominal radiographs show a dilated colon to the sigmoid

colon. The cecum measures 10 cm in diameter. Flexible sigmoidoscopy reveals normal bowel.

The appropriate management of this patient is:

(A) Admission to the hospital for emergency cecostomy
(B) Admission to the hospital for emergency colectomy
(C) Outpatient emergency colonoscopy
(D) Outpatient rectal corticosteroids or mesalamine
(E) Admission to the hospital, insertion of a naso-gastric tube, and frequent turning of the patient in bed

Abdominal Pain Question 5

A 53-year-old woman presents with a long history of dyspepsia, fullness, and belching. An endoscopy at another hospital shows severe antral erythema and a small hiatal hernia, but no ulcer. Because of her long history of dyspepsia, a serum gastrin test and serum IgG test for *Helicobacter pylori* are done. The serum gastrin test result is 1800 pg/mL (normal, up to 150 pg/mL), and the test for *H. pylori* is negative.

The next test that should be done in this patient is:

(A) Push enteroscopy
(B) Secretin stimulation test
(C) Test for gastric acid secretion
(D) Angiography of the pancreas
(E) Endoscopic ultrasonography

Abdominal Pain Question 6

A 36-year-old man with a long history of Crohn's disease is hospitalized with a recurrent attack of abdominal pain. He has a long history of alcohol abuse, which he claims relieves his abdominal pain. He has been taking low-dose prednisone (5 mg/d) and 6-mercaptopurine (100 mg/d) for 2 years and calcium supplements to prevent calcium oxalate urinary crystals. Abdominal radiograph shows pancreatic calcification.

The most likely cause of his pancreatic calcification is chronic pancreatitis due to:

(A) 6-Mercaptopurine
(B) Alcohol
(C) Corticosteroids
(D) Hypercalcemia
(E) Oxalosis

Abdominal Pain Question 7

A 70-year-old woman is hospitalized with severe abdominal pain but without rebound tenderness or a palpable mass. Her temperature is 39.8 °C (103.6 °F); pulse rate is 104/min; blood pressure is

100/60 mm Hg; and she is slightly tachypneic. Five months ago she had an attack of right upper quadrant pain lasting about 7 hours. A flat-plate radiograph of the abdomen shows distended bowel loops. Ultrasonography is inconclusive due to overlying gas shadows, and computed tomography (CT) shows an edematous pancreas. Blood cultures are taken.

Laboratory studies:

Leukocyte count	18,000/μL
Serum calcium	7 mg/dL
Serum bilirubin	8.2 mg/dL
Serum alkaline phosphatase	300 U/L
Serum alanine aminotransferase	350 U/L
Serum aspartate aminotransferase	300 U/L
Serum amylase	3010 U/L

The most appropriate treatment for this patient is:

(A) Oral antibiotics and observation
(B) Intravenous antibiotics and consultation for endoscopic retrograde cholangiopancreatography (ERCP)
(C) Intravenous vancomycin
(D) Intravenous hydration and octreotide therapy
(E) Rehydration only

Abdominal Pain Question 8

A 17-year-old sexually active female adolescent presents to the office with a 4-day history of a dull bilateral abdominal pain, intermittent vomiting, and fever with temperature to 38 °C (100.4 °F). On questioning, she admits to anorexia, fatigue, and a vaginal discharge, but denies colicky pain, diarrhea, dysuria, urgency, and frequency. On physical examination, she appears uncomfortable and dehydrated. Resting pulse rate changes from 92/min in the supine position to 120/min in the sitting position. Abdominal examination is normal except for bilateral lower quadrant tenderness to deep palpation. Pelvic examination reveals a purulent cervical discharge, pain on motion of the cervix, bilateral adnexal tenderness, and a fullness in the right adnexa that cannot be fully characterized because of the patient's obesity. Urine pregnancy test is negative.

The most appropriate course of action is:

(A) Admit the patient to the hospital and begin intravenous cefoxitin and doxycycline.
(B) Administer ceftriaxone, 125 mg intramuscularly, and prescribe doxycycline, 100 mg orally twice a day for 7 days. Arrange for outpatient follow-up in 2 weeks.
(C) Administer ceftriaxone, 250 mg intramuscularly, and prescribe doxycycline, 100 mg orally twice a day for 14 days. Arrange for outpatient follow-up in 2 weeks.
(D) Prescribe ofloxacin, 400 mg orally twice a day for 14 days. Arrange for outpatient follow-up in 2 weeks.
(E) Provide azithromycin, 1 g orally, as a single, witnessed dose. Arrange for outpatient follow-up in 2 weeks.

Abdominal Pain Question 9

A 48-year-old man is admitted to the hospital for evaluation of suddenly worsening abdominal pain. He had been well until 1 year ago when he developed Raynaud's phenomenon. Nine months ago, he began having episodes of palpable purpura over his feet and pretibial area, and 4 months ago he developed a left footdrop, followed 2 weeks later by numbness over the dorsum of the right foot. One month ago he began noticing periumbilical pain about a half hour after meals. The patient's medical history is remarkable for a surgical procedure done on the left ankle, requiring transfusion, after a motorcycle accident 20 years ago.

Physical examination is notable for blood pressure of 170/100 mm Hg, palpable purpura over the lower extremities, motor and sensory deficits of the left peroneal nerve, and a sensory deficit in the distribution of the right anterior tibial nerve. Examination of the stool for occult blood is positive.

Laboratory studies:

Hematocrit	33%
Serum creatinine	1.6 mg/dL
Erythrocyte sedimentation rate	76 mm/h
Serum rheumatoid factor	512 IU/mL
Fluorescent test for antinuclear antibody	Negative

Which one of the following tests is most likely to be positive in this patient?

(A) Antibodies to double-stranded DNA
(B) Antibodies to hepatitis C virus
(C) Antibodies to parvovirus B19
(D) Antineutrophil cytoplasmic antibodies
(E) Antibodies to HIV

Abdominal Pain Questions 10-11

A 33-year-old white man presents to the emergency department 4 hours ago with acute epigastric pain and nausea and vomiting of 24 hours' duration. You see an obviously uncomfortable young man twisting on the gurney trying to get comfortable. Vital signs include a temperature of 37.2 °C (98.9 °F), pulse rate of 130/min, respiration rate of 22/min, blood pressure of 124/72 mm Hg, and an oxygen saturation of 90% on room air. The patient has epigastric tenderness on physical examination but no peritoneal signs. The cardiac examination is normal, but the patient has mild bibasilar rales. Right upper quadrant ultrasonography shows no biliary tract obstruction. He has had no recent infections. The patient received 4 liters of fluid before your arrival. His urine output has been 120 mL since his arrival in the emergency department.

Laboratory studies:

Hematocrit	36%
Leukocyte count	18,000/μL
Platelet count	114,000/μL
Lactate dehydrogenase	453 U/L
Alkaline phosphatase	97 U/L
Total bilirubin	0.6 mg/dL
Blood glucose	204 mg/dL
Blood urea nitrogen	26 mg/dL
Pao_2	59 mm Hg
Amylase	600 U/L
Calcium	9.2 mg/dL

Question 10

The most likely cause of this patient's problem is:

(A) Gallstone pancreatitis
(B) Alcoholic pancreatitis
(C) Infectious pancreatitis
(D) Autoimmune pancreatitis

Question 11

The most appropriate therapy for this patient would be:

(A) Aggressive fluid resuscitation, bowel rest, monitoring in the intensive care unit, and analgesics
(B) Aggressive fluid resuscitation, nasogastric suction, bowel rest, and ward hospitalization
(C) Analgesic medication and outpatient follow-up the next day
(D) Immediate gastroenterology consultation for endoscopic retrograde cholangiopancreatography (ERCP)

ACID–BASE

Acid–Base Question 1

An 83-year-old woman is brought to the hospital from a nursing home because of stupor developing 3 days after starting antibiotics for a fever and urinary tract infection. Physical examination shows a temperature of 38.6 °C (101.5 °F), a pulse rate of 100/min, a respiration rate of 12/min, and a blood pressure of 115/80 mm Hg. She is stuporous and disoriented to time and place. The rest of the physical examination is normal.

Laboratory studies:

Hemoglobin	12.1 g/dL
Hematocrit	43%
Leukocyte count	15,000/µL
Plasma glucose	95 mg/dL
Serum electrolytes	
Sodium	167 meq/L
Potassium	4.3 meq/L
Chloride	120 meq/L
Bicarbonate	29 meq/L
Blood urea nitrogen	26 mg/dL
Serum creatinine	1.0 mg/dL
Urinalysis	
Specific gravity	1.020
Glucose	Negative

The most likely explanation for the hypernatremia is:

(A) Osmotic diuresis
(B) Diuretic agents
(C) Lack of access to electrolyte-free water
(D) Hypertonic sodium administration
(E) Nephrogenic diabetes insipidus

Acid–Base Question 2

A 28-year-old woman with cystic fibrosis is admitted to the hospital because of rapidly increasing respiratory distress, increased cough, and increased production of purulent sputum. One month earlier, she had operative reduction of colonic intussusception; postoperatively, her respiratory status was felt to be stable clinically.

Physical examination shows a cachectic, dyspneic young woman with clubbing. She has a pulse rate of 130/min and regular, a respiration rate of 28 to 30/min, and a blood pressure of 110/70 mm Hg. The neck veins are distended; there is a right ventricular heave, and crackles are present. She has 2+ pitting edema to the knees. Chest radiograph shows a new right lower lobe infiltrate. Treatment with antibiotics and diuretics is intensified.

Laboratory studies:

Serum electrolytes	
Sodium	130 meq/L
Potassium	5.2 meq/L
Chloride	86 meq/L
Bicarbonate	38 meq/L
Blood urea nitrogen	17 mg/dL
Serum creatinine	0.6 mg/dL
Arterial blood gases on room air	
Po_2	35 mm Hg
Pco_2	69 mm Hg
pH	7.40
Urinalysis	
Specific gravity	1.020

The most likely acid-base diagnosis on admission is:

(A) Mixed metabolic acidosis and metabolic alkalosis
(B) Mixed metabolic alkalosis and respiratory acidosis
(C) Mixed metabolic alkalosis and respiratory alkalosis
(D) Mixed metabolic acidosis and respiratory acidosis
(E) Acute respiratory acidosis

Acid–Base Questions 3-5

For each patient described below, select the most likely associated set of chemical values (A-C) (each answer may be used more than once or not at all):

	Serum					Urine			
	Na$^+$ (meq/L)	K$^+$ (meq/l)	Cl$^-$ (meq/L)	HCO$_3^-$ (meq/L)	Creatinine (mg/dL)	Na$^+$ (meq/L)	K$^+$ (meq/L)	Cl$^-$ (meq/L)	pH
(A)	136	2.5	110	16	1.0	35	25	30	6.5
(B)	135	2.2	88	35	0.8	15	30	<10	6.0
(C)	140	2.9	95	32	1.3	40	40	60	5.5

3. A 46-year-old man presenting with new-onset hypertension has a blood pressure of 150/105 mm Hg and takes no medication.

4. A 28-year-old female dancer has weakness and fatigue. She has had no other medical illness. She has a blood pressure of 90/60 mm Hg. She is emaciated on physical examination, and deep tendon reflexes are weak but present.

5. A 35-year-old woman presents to the emergency room with renal colic. She had passed several renal stones before but had never been evaluated to find a reason for the nephrolithiasis.

Acid–Base Question 6

A 24-year-old woman is admitted to the hospital after having had a seizure in a shopping mall. She had bitten her tongue and has a new contusion over the left zygomatic arch. She is postictal. Her blood pressure is 100/60 mm Hg, serum sodium is 124 meq/L, serum potassium is 4.8 meq/L, and there is a mild metabolic acidosis. Acute adrenal insufficiency is suspected.

The best initial test for this disorder is:

(A) Insulin tolerance
(B) Metyrapone stimulation
(C) Urine free cortisol
(D) Cosyntropin stimulation

Acid–Base Question 7

An 80-year-old demented man who lives in a nursing home is brought to the emergency room because he gradually became comatose over a 24-hour period. On physical examination his pulse rate is 112/min and his blood pressure is 90/50 mm Hg.

Laboratory studies:

Blood urea nitrogen	79 mg/dL
Plasma glucose	1900 mg/dL
Serum sodium	140 meq/L
Serum potassium	5.0 meq/L
Serum chloride	108 meq/L
Serum bicarbonate	22 meq/L
Serum creatinine	3.0 mg/dL

Which one of the following therapeutic principles should be followed?

(A) Initial fluid replacement should be 0.45% sodium chloride because his coma is caused by hyperosmolarity.
(B) All fluid replacement should be 0.45% sodium chloride because the calculated serum osmolality is so high.
(C) All fluid replacement should be 0.9% sodium chloride because the normal serum sodium concentration indicates a state of isotonic dehydration.
(D) Initial fluid replacement should be 0.9% sodium chloride because his intravascular volume is low.
(E) Initial treatment should be an intravenous bolus of 50 units of regular insulin because his plasma glucose concentration is so high.

Acid–Base Question 8

A 64-year-old male smoker presents to the Emergency Department because of cough, anorexia, vomiting, fatigue, and weight loss, all progressive over the past 3 months. Physical examination shows a cachectic man in mild respiratory distress with a temperature of 38.1 °C (100.6 °F), and rhonchi in the right upper lobe.

Laboratory studies:

Hematocrit	48%
Leukocyte count	14,600/μL, with a left-shift
Blood urea nitrogen	56 mg/dL
Serum calcium	12.8 mg/dL
Serum phosphorus	2.7 mg/dL
Serum creatinine	1.8 mg/dL
Serum albumin	2.9 g/dL

Chest radiograph shows a 6-cm right hilar mass and a right upper lobe infiltrate. He is admitted to the hospital for intravenous antibiotics and further evaluation.

The most appropriate immediate therapeutic step for his hypercalcemia is to administer:

(A) Pamidronate, intravenously
(B) Calcitonin, subcutaneously
(C) Furosemide, intravenously
(D) Solute diuresis with sodium chloride, intravenously
(E) Plicamycin, orally

Acid–Base Question 9

You are asked to see a 17-year-old boy in the hospital Medical Intensive Care Unit who had closed-head trauma 3 days ago. The surgeons have been treating the patient with normal saline, 4 L/d for 2 days, to correct a serum sodium of 126 meq/L, but the hyponatremia continues to worsen with this regimen.

Laboratory studies:

Blood urea nitrogen	8 mg/dL
Serum electrolytes	
Sodium	122 meq/L
Potassium	4.5 meq/L
Chloride	100 meq/L
Bicarbonate	25 meq/L
Serum creatinine	1 mg/dL

The test most likely to confirm the diagnosis is:

(A) Thyroid-stimulating hormone and free thyroxine
(B) Urine sodium
(C) Simultaneous serum and urine osmolality
(D) Plasma renin activity

Acid–Base Question 10

A 49-year-old woman had a radical hysterectomy and radiation therapy for advanced cervical carcinoma 2 years ago. Her serum calcium concentration is now 11.0 mg/dL, whereas it had been normal 1 year ago.

The laboratory measurement most likely to yield a result below the normal range is:

(A) Serum parathyroid hormone-related protein
(B) Serum parathyroid hormone
(C) 24-hour urine calcium excretion
(D) Serum 25-hydroxyvitamin D
(E) Urine pyridinoline and deoxypyridinoline (collagen cross-links)

ACUTE RENAL FAILURE

Acute Renal Failure Question 1
A 75-year-old woman is admitted to the hospital for dysuria and confusion. The patient is oriented to person but not time or place. She has a history of cervical cancer, treated with total hysterectomy and radiation 18 months ago. Previous evaluation in her private physician's office 3 months ago showed her serum creatinine concentration was 1.0 mg/dL.

Physical examination shows a temperature of 36.2 °C (97.2 °F), a regular pulse rate of 98/min, a regular respiration rate of 20/min, and a blood pressure of 110/60 mm Hg. There is no orthostasis. There is no neck vein distention at 45 degrees, and the chest is clear. S_1 and S_2 are normal, without gallop or murmur. Liver span is 18 cm, and the edge is three finger breadths below the right costal margin. The spleen tip is palpable below the left costal margin. There is shifting dullness and bowel sounds are present. There is no abdominal rigidity or rebound. Distal pulses are present. There is 2+ pedal edema. Cranial nerves and reflexes are normal, and the neurologic examination did not elicit focal findings.

Laboratory studies:

Hematocrit	30.7%
Leukocyte count	7300/μL
Platelet count	142,000/μL
Serum electrolytes	
Sodium	131 meq/L
Potassium	5.7 meq/L
Chloride	98 meq/L
Bicarbonate	15 meq/L
Serum calcium	7.2 mg/dL
Serum phosphorus	6.8 mg/dL
Blood urea nitrogen	65 mg/dL
Serum creatinine	7.3 mg/dL
Urinalysis	
Specific gravity	1.011
Glucose	Negative
Protein	Trace
Blood	Negative
Ketones	Negative
Microscopic	0 to 1 erythrocytes per high-power field (hpf), 0 to 1 leukocytes/hpf, no cellular casts
Sodium	28 meq/L
FE_{Na}	4.1%
Osmolality	168 mosm/kg
4-hour urine volume	40 mL

The most appropriate initial step in the clinical management of this patient is:

(A) Renal ultrasound
(B) Renal biopsy
(C) A trial of normal saline at 300 mL/h for 2 hours
(D) Continuous arteriovenous hemofiltration
(E) Renal scintigraphy

Acute Renal Failure Question 2
A 65-year-old woman with chronic hypertension and a baseline blood urea nitrogen of 14 mg/dL and serum creatinine of 1.4 mg/dL has a sigmoid resection for diverticular disease. Three days postoperatively, the blood urea nitrogen is 26 mg/dL and the serum creatinine is 1.8 mg/dL. The postoperative course has been smooth without any hypotension, heart failure, or unusual fever.

What is the most likely reason for the change in the serum creatinine measurement?

(A) The change is within the range of error of the measurement method for creatinine.
(B) The change is due to increased release of creatinine from muscle after surgery.
(C) The change represents a significant decline in renal function.
(D) The change is the result of asymptomatic bacteriuria secondary to a Foley catheter used during and after surgery.

Acute Renal Failure Question 3
A 62-year-old man is found to have a blood urea nitrogen of 35 mg/dL and a serum creatinine of 2.0 mg/dL on his annual check-up.

Laboratory studies:

Hematocrit	24%
Leukocyte count	8200/μL
Platelet count	332,000/μL
Plasma glucose	88 mg/dL
Serum electrolytes	
Sodium	138 meq/L
Potassium	3.5 meq/L
Chloride	113 meq/L
Bicarbonate	22 meq/L
Urinalysis	
Protein	1+

Microscopic	3 to 4 leukocytes per high-power field
24-hour urine protein excretion	3.4 g
Creatinine clearance	48 mL/min

The most likely diagnosis is:

(A) Membranous nephropathy
(B) Amyloidosis
(C) Multiple myeloma
(D) Lead nephropathy

Acute Renal Failure Question 4

A 36-year-old man with a history of hypertension, injection drug use, and noncompliance calls your office for an urgent visit because of 3 days of shortness of breath, nausea, and weakness. You have followed him for progressive renal failure due to HIV nephropathy. Two months ago, his blood urea nitrogen was 65 mg/dL and serum creatinine was 7.8 mg/dL. Plans were being made to initiate dialysis soon. You suspect the patient may have become uremic, prepare to see him, and order a set of tests. In the emergency room, he has no response to 320 mg of furosemide given intravenously.

Physical examination shows a temperature of 36.6 °C (98.0 °F) and a blood pressure of 170/105 mm Hg. The patient is alert and somewhat dyspneic. There are crackles in both mid-lung fields. Cardiac examination shows an S_4 without a rub or murmur. The abdomen is without palpable organomegaly or tenderness. Extremities show 3+ pedal edema.

Laboratory studies:

Serum electrolytes	
Sodium	130 meq/L
Potassium	5.8 meq/L
Chloride	95 meq/L
Bicarbonate	15 meq/L
Blood urea nitrogen	80 mg/dL
Serum creatinine	9.0 mg/dL
Arterial blood gases on room air	
P_{O_2}	55 mm Hg
P_{CO_2}	28 mm Hg
pH	7.34

Chest radiograph shows cardiomegaly. There is cephalization of vessels with bilateral pleural effusions. Electrocardiogram shows left ventricular hypertrophy and nonspecific ST-T changes.

Which one of the following findings in this patient would dictate a need to initiate dialysis immediately?

(A) Blood urea nitrogen and serum creatinine concentrations
(B) P_{O_2} measurement
(C) Serum potassium concentration
(D) Serum bicarbonate concentration

Acute Renal Failure Questions 5-6

A 71-year-old woman who has had nocturia for several years is admitted to the hospital because of increasing weakness and frequency of urination. She had been well until 2 days ago, when she felt weak and could not climb the stairs in her apartment house. She has a duodenal ulcer diagnosed 30 years ago, which remitted after intensive antacid therapy. She has been taking Tums® for osteoporosis after reading about it in a popular magazine, and she takes bicarbonate of soda for heartburn. She has a 60–pack-year smoking history.

Physical examination shows an elderly, frail woman who is oriented to person but not to place or time. She has a regular pulse rate of 106/min, changing to 122/min on standing, and a blood pressure of 100/80 mm Hg, changing to 80/50 mm Hg on standing. There is no neck vein distention or hepatojugular reflux. The chest is clear, and S_1 and S_2 are normal. The abdomen is normal. There is no edema or focal neurologic signs. A chest radiograph is normal except for osteopenia.

Laboratory studies:

Hematocrit	41.4%
Mean corpuscular volume	Normal
Serum electrolytes	
Sodium	152 meq/L
Potassium	3.0 meq/L
Chloride	100 meq/L
Bicarbonate	39 meq/L
Blood urea nitrogen	98 mg/dL
Serum creatinine	7.1 mg/dL
Serum calcium	14.4 mg/dL
Serum phosphorus	6.3 mg/dL
Serum 1,25-dihydroxyvitamin D	30 pg/mL
Serum parathyroid hormone	16 pg/mL
Urinalysis	
Specific gravity	1.007
Glucose	Absent
Protein	Trace
Ketones	Trace
Sodium	49 meq/L
Creatinine	70 mg/dL
Osmolality	260 mosm/kg
6-hour urine volume	640 mL

Renal ultrasonogram shows normal-sized kidneys without evidence of hydronephrosis.

Question 5

The clinical and laboratory findings are most consistent with:

(A) Vitamin D intoxication
(B) Chronic renal insufficiency
(C) Multiple myeloma
(D) Milk-alkali syndrome
(E) Primary hyperparathyroidism

Question 6

Which one of the following therapies is most likely to worsen the hypercalcemia in this patient?

(A) Thiazide diuretic agents
(B) Infusion of normal saline
(C) Hypotonic fluids
(D) Calcitonin

Acute Renal Failure Question 7
A 50-year-old woman is admitted to the hospital because of vomiting. She has a 3-year history of peptic ulcer disease treated with cimetidine. Six months ago, outpatient laboratory studies showed a serum creatinine concentration of 1.1 mg/dL. Physical examination shows a well-developed, well-nourished woman with temperature of 37.2 °C (99.0 °F), regular pulse rate of 96/min, changing to 132/min on standing, regular respiration rate of 16/min, and blood pressure of 130/80 mm Hg, changing to 80/70 mm Hg on standing. Chest and cardiac examinations are normal. Examination of the abdomen shows periumbilical and epigastric tenderness without rebound or rigidity. Bowel sounds are hyperactive. There is no edema. Distal pulses and skin are normal.

Laboratory studies:

Hematocrit	34.3%
Leukocyte count	12,300/µL, with 6% eosinophils
Platelet count	210,000/µL
Serum electrolytes	
Sodium	137 meq/L
Potassium	3.3 meq/L
Chloride	100 meq/L
Bicarbonate	29 meq/L
Blood urea nitrogen	38 mg/dL
Serum creatinine	2.4 mg/dL
Urinalysis	
Specific gravity	1.022
Protein	1+
Blood	1+
Microscopic	5 to 10 erythrocytes per high-power field (hpf), 8 to 10 leukocytes/hpf, with occasional clumps, and a few leukocyte casts

Sodium	12 meq/L
Culture	No growth
Examination of the stool for occult blood	Weakly positive

Upper gastrointestinal series shows obstruction of the pyloric outlet.

In addition to volume repletion with normal saline, which of the following initial courses of action is best?

(A) Treat the patient with corticosteroids.
(B) Order diagnostic renal biopsy.
(C) Discontinue cimetidine and observe the patient.
(D) Treat the patient with intravenous antibiotics.
(E) Order emergency ultrasonography.

Acute Renal Failure Question 8
A 46-year-old man is admitted to the hospital because of syncope. He also has cardiomyopathy, mild cirrhosis, and chronic renal insufficiency due to polycystic kidney disease. He has chronic headaches for which he takes various over-the-counter medications. On admission, his left ventricular ejection fraction is 20%. Medications include captopril, warfarin, bumetanide, and metolazone.

He has a temperature of 36.6 °C (98.0 °F), a pulse rate of 76/min, and a blood pressure of 110/70 mm Hg supine and 90/60 mm Hg standing. The patient is alert; his chest is clear. Cardiac examination is normal. The abdomen is nontender to palpation; extremities show 1+ edema.

Laboratory studies:

	2 Months Ago	Admission
Serum electrolytes		
Sodium	135 meq/L	136 meq/L
Potassium	4.1 meq/L	4.3 meq/L
Chloride	98 meq/L	95 meq/L
Bicarbonate	22 meq/L	21 meq/L
Blood urea nitrogen	60 mg/dL	96 mg/dL
Serum creatinine	4.2 mg/dL	5.7 mg/dL
Urinalysis		
Protein	1+	
Microscopic	2 to 5 erythrocytes per high-power field (hpf), 2 to 5 leukocytes/hpf	

The most likely cause of the worsening azotemia is:

(A) Renal artery stenosis
(B) Prerenal azotemia
(C) Natural progression of polycystic kidney disease
(D) Acute pyelonephritis
(E) Allergic interstitial nephritis

Acute Renal Failure Questions 9-13

For each clinical diagnosis below, select the most likely findings on urinalysis (A-E) (each answer may be used more than once or not at all):

	Specific Gravity	Protein	Blood	Microscopic
(A)	1.010	Trace	Negative	1 to 3 leukocytes/hpf, many pigmented granular casts, 5 to 10 renal tubular cells/hpf, occasional renal tubular cell casts
(B)	1.025	4+	3+	10 to 15 erythrocytes/hpf, 3 to 8 leukocytes/hpf, 2 to 3 erythrocyte casts/hpf
(C)	1.012	1+	2+	20 to 30 erythrocytes/hpf, 15 to 25 leukocytes/hpf, Hansel's stain positive for eosinophils (5% of leukocytes)
(D)	1.020	1+	1+	10 to 15 erythrocytes/hpf, 20 to 25 leukocytes/hpf, and leukocyte casts
(E)	1.007	Negative	Negative	0 to 3 erythrocytes/hpf, 1 to 3 leukocytes/hpf

9. Acute tubular necrosis

10. Acute interstitial nephritis

11. Obstructive uropathy

12. Acute glomerulonephritis

13. Acute pyelonephritis

ALTERED MENTAL STATUS

Altered Mental Status Question 1

The nurse on duty at night in a 120-bed nursing home calls you about an 86-year-old woman with Alzheimer's disease, congestive heart failure, degenerative joint disease, and the recent onset of depression. The nurse says that the patient had become agitated that afternoon and her behavior has worsened to the point that she is intermittently screaming and acting physically aggressive toward other residents. The patient's medications include digoxin, 0.25 mg/d; furosemide, 40 mg/d; naproxen potassium, 250 mg three times daily; and nortriptyline, 10 mg twice daily.

What is the most appropriate management of the patient at this point?

(A) Increase the dose of nortriptyline to 25 mg twice daily, and order a nortriptyline level in 5 to 7 days.
(B) Prescribe haloperidol, 0.5 mg twice daily and every 6 hours as needed.
(C) Prescribe oxazepam, 1 mg twice daily and 1 mg every 6 hours as needed.
(D) Send the patient to the emergency room for a medical evaluation.
(E) Contact the consultant psychiatrist who prescribed the nortriptyline for advice.

Altered Mental Status Question 2

A daughter brings her 86-year-old mother to your office and states that over the last 6 months her mother has become increasingly forgetful. Symptoms include frequently repeating conversations just completed and difficulty managing financial affairs. The patient is taking no medications. History, physical examination, and neurologic testing of motor, sensory, and cerebellar function show no abnormalities. The patient is alert and oriented times 3.

The next most appropriate step is to:

(A) Order an imaging study of the brain.
(B) Reassure the daughter that mild memory disorders are normal for persons of advanced age.
(C) Do a structured mental status examination.
(D) Refer the patient to a neurologist.
(E) Refer the patient to a psychiatrist.

Altered Mental Status Question 3

An 89-year-old woman is brought to your office by her relatives, who noticed that recently the patient's house had become very messy, that she seemed distracted and irritable, and that she was having memory problems. The patient has lived alone and been self-sufficient since the death of her husband 10 years ago. There is no history of the patient having fallen or having suffered any other trauma. She has hypertension and osteoarthritis, for which she has been taking chlorthalidone, 25 mg/d; atenolol, 25 mg/d; and ibuprofen, 800 mg/d.

Physical examination shows a thin woman with temporal muscle wasting. She has decreased short-term memory and appears to lack insight; there are no focal neurologic findings. Laboratory studies show elevated serum alanine aminotransferase and mean corpuscular volume and low-normal serum albumin. You discontinue the patient's medications and ask her relatives to bring her to your office in 1 week.

In the follow-up visit 1 week later, her relatives report that there is no change in her mental status.

What is the most likely cause of the patient's mental deterioration?

(A) Subdural hematoma
(B) Alzheimer's disease
(C) Alcohol abuse
(D) Multi-infarct dementia

Altered Mental Status Question 4

You are asked by an orthopedic surgeon to evaluate the acute onset of altered mental status in his patient, a 70-year-old retired physician who underwent a successful total knee replacement for osteoarthritis 4 days earlier. Except for mild anxiety attributed to his hospital stay, the patient has been doing very well, participating in daily physical therapy. Last night he became confused and agitated, with visual hallucinosis, and his symptoms continue to worsen during the day. He has a history of diabetes, borderline hypertension, and smoking. His medication at home includes insulin; current medications include insulin, subcutaneous heparin, morphine as needed, acetaminophen, and stool softener. He is wearing pneumatic compression stockings.

On examination, he is tremulous, agitated, and confused, and appears to have visual hallucinosis. Temperature is 37.2 °C (99 °F); pulse rate is 104/min; respiratory rate is 16/min; and blood pressure is 170/94 mm Hg. The knee incision is clean. Except for his mental status, he has a normal physical examination, including neurologic examination. Blood count and electrolytes are normal, except for a glucose level of 170 mg/dL. Oxygen saturation on room air is 97%; electrocardiography reveals sinus tachycardia of 100 with nonspecific ST-T–wave changes.

What is the next best step in the management of this patient?

(A) Order computed tomography of the head.
(B) Measure serial creatine kinase isoenzymes.
(C) Perform lumbar puncture.
(D) Discontinue morphine.

Altered Mental Status Question 5
A 56-year-old male accountant presents with a 2- to 3-month history of difficulty at work. His colleagues note that he has become "less productive" and several tax returns that he recently prepared were incorrect. At home, his wife has noted that he has been misplacing objects, and on one occasion, he was unable to understand how to operate the automatic garage door opener. Recently, he drove to the wrong field to watch his daughter play soccer and was unable to find his way home.

He has a history of poorly controlled hypertension. His only medication is amlodipine. He scored a 26/30 on the Mini-Mental State Examination (MMSE), losing points in orientation and memory, but the remainder of his neurologic examination is normal.

Which of the following diagnostic tests should be obtained next?

(A) Single-photon emission computed tomography of the brain
(B) Magnetic resonance imaging of the brain
(C) Cerebrospinal fluid analysis
(D) Electroencephalography

Altered Mental Status Question 6
A previously healthy 35-year-old auto mechanic presents to your office on a Wednesday because he lost consciousness while at work 2 days ago. He recalls working on a carburetor and then awakening in an ambulance with headache, muscle aches, and a sore tongue. His coworkers saw him lying on the floor of the garage shaking. This episode lasted 2 to 3 min-

utes, followed by moaning, thrashing, and poor responsiveness. He was then evaluated at a local hospital: blood chemistries, electrolytes, and a complete blood count were normal, as was computed tomography of the head.

Currently, on physical examination, his temperature is 37.5 °C (99.5 °F), pulse rate is 72/min, respiration rate is 18/min, and blood pressure is 130/86 mm Hg. Neurologic examination is normal. Magnetic resonance imaging of the brain is normal.

Which one of the following factors would necessitate antiepileptic drug therapy in this patient?

(A) Significant alcohol use over the weekend
(B) A history of a single febrile seizure
(C) Toxicity screen positive for cocaine
(D) Left temporal slowing on electroencephalography
(E) Family history of epilepsy

Altered Mental Status Question 7
A healthy 20-year-old woman presents to your office because she lost consciousness while donating blood. She says that she began to feel queasy and lightheaded while donating blood and then fainted. The phlebotomist reports that the patient had several jerking movements and a brief episode of whole body stiffening. The patient recovered after being placed in a head-down position but had a slight headache. She has no previous history of such episodes, but she tends to become ill at the sight or smell of blood. On physical examination, her temperature is 38 °C (100.4 °F), pulse rate is 92/min, respiration rate is 22/min, and blood pressure is 110/70 mm Hg. General physical and neurologic examinations are normal.

Which of the following is the next most appropriate step?

(A) Order an electroencephalogram.
(B) Begin sodium valproate.
(C) Order magnetic resonance imaging of the brain.
(D) Begin phenytoin.
(E) Reassure the patient that she simply fainted.

Altered Mental Status Questions 8-11
For each patient with confusion described below, select the most likely diagnosis (A-E) (each answer may be used more than once or not at all):

(A) Parkinson's disease
(B) Alzheimer's disease
(C) Creutzfeldt-Jakob disease
(D) Normal-pressure hydrocephalus
(E) Vascular dementia

8. A 62-year-old previously healthy electrician is brought to your office by his wife for evaluation of confusion and gait difficulties. Shortly after the patient retired 3 years ago, his wife noticed that he was frequently repeating himself during casual conversation and that he was forgetting where he left his tools. He is continent, and in most of his activities of daily living, he is independent; however, his wife reports that his muscles seem stiff and that he seems to be gradually slowing down.

On neurologic examination, he is alert but oriented only to person. His speech is fluent with frequent paraphasic errors. Naming, comprehension, judgment and short-term recall are impaired. He is unable to demonstrate how to open a lock or light a candle. His cranial nerve and sensory examinations are normal. Motor examination reveals bradykinesia, increased tone and normal strength. Reflexes and plantar responses are normal. His gait is characterized by stooped posture, short steps, and decreased arm swing.

9. A 76-year-old-man with hypertension and coronary artery disease presents to your office after falling several times at home. The patient was well until 2 years ago when his son noted mild confusion and occasional non-sense words while on an annual fishing trip. He did well for the next 18 months, at which time he became more forgetful and began having difficulty with his gait and coordination, particularly with his right arm and leg. His examination is notable for a blood pressure of 155/95 mm Hg and an irregular pulse. He has marked difficulty in naming objects and repeating phrases, and he is able to recall only 2 of 3 objects beyond 5 minutes. He scored 25 out of 30 points on the Mini-Mental State Examination (MMSE). He has a right pronator drift and right extensor plantar response.

10. An 82-year-old woman presents to your office for her annual evaluation. She has a history of progressive memory loss and confusion beginning 2 years ago, and another physician diagnosed her with senile dementia. She is currently no longer able to maintain her residence at an assisted-living apartment because she has forgotten to shut off her stove on several occasions, and she has recently developed urinary incontinence. Over the last month, her gait has become unsteady and she has had several falls.

Her examination reveals evidence of a moderate dementia with decreased spontaneous speech, poor memory, particularly in retrieval, and marked impairment in judgment, insight, and sequencing tasks. Her cranial nerve examination is normal. Motor examination reveals diffuse paratonia without weakness. She has no tremor. She has marked difficulty in initiating gait, but once started, she is able to walk at a brisk pace with normal arm swing.

11. A 64-year-old woman with hypertension and osteoarthritis is brought to your office by her husband because of increased confusion and falls. Three years ago she developed a tremor in her left hand but never sought medical attention. Her husband is now concerned about her increasing forgetfulness and that routine tasks take her twice as long as before. She has fallen on several occasions at home, usually when changing positions or making sharp turns.

Her examination reveals a blood pressure of 150/90 mm Hg. Her neurologic examination reveals normal orientation but decreased fluency, slowed response times, hypophonia, and poor verbal recall. She scores 23 out of 30 points on the Mini-Mental State Examination (MMSE). Findings on the cranial nerve examination are normal. The motor examination shows mild bradykinesia, full power, and a slight, rhythmic tremor of both hands, more prominent on the left, which does not change with movement. Reflexes and plantar responses are normal. She has a narrow-based gait with stooped posture, short steps, and has marked difficulty in turning.

Altered Mental Status Questions 12-15
For each patient with the sudden onset of mental status changes, select the most likely location of cerebral infarction (A-D) (each answer may be used more than once or not at all):

(A) Dominant frontal lobe
(B) Thalamus
(C) Head of the caudate nucleus
(D) Nondominant parietal lobe

12. A 76-year-old man with atrial fibrillation is brought to your office by his wife following the sudden onset of agitation and confusion. He believes his wife is plotting to have him committed. He is talkative but unable to provide a coherent history. On examination, his pulse rate is 78/min and irregular, and his

blood pressure is 135/80 mm Hg. He is disoriented and mildly agitated. His concentration is poor, and he is easily distracted. The remainder of his neurologic examination is normal.

13. A 75-year-old man is brought to your office by his wife because of a change in his behavior. He is typically active in his retirement, but 5 days ago, he became withdrawn and uninterested in his usual activities. He even declined to speak to his grandchild on the telephone last night. His history is significant for hypertension, osteoarthritis, and angina pectoris. On physical examination, his blood pressure is 170/90 mm Hg. He is quiet and answers in short phrases when spoken to; cognitive function is grossly intact.

14. A 74-year-old woman is brought to your office by her husband after she suddenly stopped talking during breakfast. Her husband reports that she seemed to understand his question but would not respond verbally. He also notes that her right arm seems limp. On examination, her pulse is 72/min and regular, and blood pressure is 150/92 mm Hg. She is mute but able to follow simple commands. She could not write or copy words and had mild weakness in her right arm. Her plantar responses are flexor bilaterally.

15. A 66-year-old hypertensive woman who is recovering from a laparoscopic cholecystectomy suddenly became unresponsive on the third postoperative day. On examination, her pulse is 80/min and regular, and her blood pressure is 145/85 mm Hg. She is unresponsive to voice but briefly opens her eyes and attempts to vocalize following vigorous tactile stimulation. Her pupils are 3 mm in diameter and reactive, and her ocular movements are full except for markedly decreased up-gaze. The remainder of the findings on the cranial nerve examination are normal. Her muscle power and tone appear normal and symmetric.

Altered Mental Status Questions 16-19
For the presenting cognitive deficits described below, select the most likely associated condition (A-E) (each answer may be used more than once or not at all):

(A) Delirium
(B) Alzheimer's dementia
(C) Vascular dementia
(D) Parkinson's disease–associated dementia
(E) Major depression

16. A 70-year-old man presenting with driving accidents and getting lost over the past year.

17. A 75-year-old man presenting with memory loss, aphasia, and personality changes over the past year.

18. A 75-year-old woman presenting with problems with memory and falls after treatment with lorazepam for grief reaction.

19. A 70-year-old woman presenting with problems with memory, slow speech, planning and executing tasks, and falls.

Altered Mental Status Question 20
A 73-year-old man presents to the emergency room because of a mild speech disturbance and right facial weakness that began 2 hours ago. He has a history of coronary angioplasty and is taking aspirin, 325 mg daily. On physical examination, the patient is afebrile, pulse rate is 68/min, and blood pressure is 130/85 mm Hg. A left carotid bruit is present. He has mild anomic aphasia and a right pronator drift. By the end of the examination, his neurologic deficits resolve, and his examination is normal. Findings on computed tomography of the brain are normal. An angiogram shows an 80% stenosis of the origin of the left internal carotid artery. The patient is treated with intravenous heparin.

What is the next most appropriate treatment for this patient?

(A) Increased aspirin dose
(B) Ticlopidine
(C) Warfarin
(D) Tissue plasminogen activator
(E) Carotid endarterectomy

Altered Mental Status Question 21
A 68-year-old woman is brought to the emergency room because of the sudden onset of altered speech and impaired gait. She has a history of poorly controlled hypertension and diabetes mellitus. On physical examination, her blood pressure is 190/100 mm Hg. Her speech is difficult to understand, but she follows commands well. There is mild left-sided weakness and considerable ataxia. The sensory examination is unremarkable.

What is the most likely diagnosis?

(A) Left posterior inferior cerebellar artery occlusion
(B) Right middle cerebral artery occlusion
(C) Left cerebellar hemorrhage
(D) Right pontine lacunar infarction
(E) Right thalamic lacunar infarction

ANEMIA

Anemia Question 1

A 66-year-old woman comes to your office because her vitamin B_{12} level was recently found to be low (110 ng/L). She has had no symptoms except for some forgetfulness, which she thinks is no worse than her husband's. Her dietary intake is adequate. She was found to have hyperglycemia 6 years ago, and she therefore cut down on sweets and starches and stopped eating red meats, which she replaces with fish or chicken. She has no history of other illnesses or hospitalizations.

Findings on the physical examination are normal, except for diminution in vibratory sense in her toes. She scores well on the Mini-Mental State Examination (29 points out of a possible 30).

Laboratory studies:

Hemoglobin	12.9 g/dL
Mean corpuscular hemoglobin concentration	33.8 g/dL
Mean corpuscular volume	92 fL
Leukocyte count	7200/µL, with a normal differential and no evidence of hyper-segmented neutrophils on the blood smear
Platelet count	215,000/µL
Blood urea nitrogen	15 mg/dL
Plasma glucose (fasting)	108 mg/dL
Serum bilirubin (total)	0.6 mg/dL
Serum folate	9.8 µg/L
Serum lactate dehydrogenase	175 U/L
Serum vitamin B_{12}	125 ng/L
Serum methylmalonic acid	395 nmol/L (normal, 80 to 370 nmol/L)

The most appropriate response to this patient's findings is:

(A) Reassure her that the low vitamin B_{12} level is clinically insignificant.
(B) Ask her to include red meat in her diet and return in 6 months to re-evaluate her vitamin B_{12} level.
(C) Prescribe vitamin B_{12}, 10 µg/d orally.
(D) Do a Schilling test and start treatment with vitamin B_{12}, 1000 µg intramuscularly.
(E) Arrange for endoscopy and gastric analysis for acid output.

Anemia Question 2

A 64-year-old woman is hospitalized because of progressive shortness of breath and palpitations over the past few weeks. She has also noted a yellow tinge to her eyes during this time.

She occasionally drinks wine excessively but says that she has abstained since the onset of her symptoms. For the last 6 months she has not eaten meat or fish, and her diet has consisted mostly of toast with margarine, tea, and an occasional banana. She says her Social Security checks do not stretch as far as they used to.

Findings on the physical examination show mild scleral icterus in a pale, blue-eyed, gray-haired, disheveled woman. The pulse rate is 110/min, and the respiration rate is 22/min. Crackles that do not clear with coughing are heard at both lung bases, and there is mild pitting edema at both ankles. The rest of the examination, including a neurologic evaluation, is normal.

Laboratory studies:

Hemoglobin	5.1 g/dL
Packed cell volume	15%
Mean corpuscular hemoglobin concentration	34.0 g/dL
Mean corpuscular volume	112 fL
Erythrocyte distribution width	21.0%
Platelet count	109,000/µL
Leukocyte count	4600/µL with a normal differential

Which of the following blood levels are most likely in this patient?

	Vitamin B_{12}	Folate	Methylmalonic acid	Homocysteine
(A)	Low	Normal	High	High
(B)	Low	Normal	Normal	High
(C)	Normal	Low	High	Normal
(D)	Normal	Low	Normal	High
(E)	Normal	Normal	Normal	Normal

Anemia Question 3

A 34-year-old woman presents to your office with a 1-week history of generalized weakness, easy fatigability, and shortness of breath. One hour ago, she developed a headache and a left hemiparesis. Two days ago, she noted easily bruisability and bleeding gums. Three days ago, she developed a fever with a temperature to 38.8 °C (102 °F), not associated with shaking chills. A history reveals that she had no previous serious illnesses, and the review of systems is normal.

On physical examination, the patient's temperature is 40 °C (104 °F), the pulse rate is 70/min, and the blood pressure is 120/70 mm Hg. There are scattered purpuric and petechial lesions over both lower extremities. In addition, there are scattered purpuric lesions over the soft palate and fresh blood along the gingiva. Cardiopulmonary examination is normal except for a grade 2/6 high-pitched ejection-type systolic murmur at the base and left sternal border. There is a mild left hemiparesis and hemihypesthesia with hyperactive reflexes and pathologic toe signs on the left.

Laboratory studies:

Hemoglobin	6 g/dL
Mean corpuscular volume	80 fL
Erythrocyte distribution width	20%
Leukocyte count	15,000/μL, with 88% neutrophils, 2% lymphocytes, and 10% monocytes
Reticulocyte count	200,000/μL
Platelet count	9000/μL
Serum creatinine	1.0 mg/dL
Total serum bilirubin	3.0 mg/dL
Direct bilirubin	0.2 mg/dL
Lactate dehydrogenase	3500 U/L
Urinalysis	Protein, 2+; erythrocytes, 30 to 40 per high-power field; leukocytes, 5 per high-power field

The most likely diagnosis of this patient's disorder is:

(A) Acute leukemia
(B) Bacterial endocarditis
(C) Thrombotic thrombocytopenic purpura
(D) Hemolytic-uremic syndrome
(E) Systemic lupus erythematosus

Anemia Question 4

A 72-year-old man has had increasing fatigue over the past few weeks. He has a hemoglobin level of 5.1 g/dL and is hospitalized. He was healthy until 1 to 2 months ago, when he began to feel tired. He takes no medications and does not abuse alcohol. He denies melena, hematochezia, or any other blood loss, and he has had no recent chest pain or dizziness. His diet is somewhat limited because he lives alone and cooks for himself, which he has not been able to do as well recently because of his fatigue. His history is normal except for knee surgery 15 years ago. The family history is unremarkable.

In the recumbent position the patient has a pulse rate of 90/min and a blood pressure of 110/72 mm Hg. In the upright position the patient has a pulse rate of 98/min and blood pressure of 104/68 mm Hg. His respiration rate is 18/min. The remainder of the findings on physical examination are normal, except for pallor and a smooth tongue.

Laboratory studies:

Hemoglobin	5.3 g/dL
Mean corpuscular volume	122 fL
Leukocyte count	4100/μL
Reticulocyte count	58,000/μL (1.2% corrected)
Platelet count	125,000/μL
Total bilirubin	1.9 mg/dL
Direct bilirubin	0.3 mg/dL
Serum lactate dehydrogenase	2750 U/L
Examination of stool for occult blood	Negative

Electrocardiogram is normal, and chest radiography shows borderline cardiomegaly. Blood is drawn for serum vitamin B_{12} and folate determinations.

The most appropriate immediate management for this patient's anemia is:

(A) Transfuse 1 unit of packed erythrocytes and re-evaluate to decide if further transfusions are needed.
(B) Transfuse 3 units of packed erythrocytes to bring the hemoglobin above 8 g/dL.
(C) Transfuse 5 units of packed erythrocytes to bring the hemoglobin above 10 g/dL.
(D) Do not transfuse, but treat immediately with subcutaneous erythropoietin.
(E) Do not transfuse, but monitor the patient's vital signs, and begin vitamin treatment.

Anemia Question 5

A 47-year-old woman, who is new to the area, comes to your office to have her ferrous sulfate prescription refilled and to have her blood tested. She has taken iron irregularly ever since she was diagnosed with anemia after her first pregnancy more than 20 years ago. She usually took one pill a day, but she ran out shortly after her move 1 month ago. She says that she has been anxious about her new job and has been eating poorly for the past few months because of job stress. She is otherwise healthy and has had no blood counts done in 15 years.

Her menstrual cycles have been regular, with periods lasting 3 days with "moderate flow"; she uses two to three pads daily. She has 3 children, aged 18 to 24 years, and believes she may be entering menopause. She is a vegetarian, but she eats eggs and dairy products. The patient does not know of any anemia in her family but believes her mother also took iron pills.

Findings on physical examination are normal.

Laboratory studies:

Hemoglobin	11.4 g/dL
Packed cell volume	33%
Mean corpuscular hemoglobin concentration	34.6 g/dL
Mean corpuscular volume	72 fL
Erythrocyte distribution width	13.0%
Leukocyte count	6900/µL
Platelet count	288,000/µL
Serum ferritin	166 µg/L
Serum iron	84 µg/dL
Iron-binding capacity	260 µg/dL
Percent iron saturation	32%

As a result of the findings, the following additional tests are done: thyroid-stimulating hormone level is 1.55 IU/L, and hemoglobin electrophoresis shows hemoglobin A, with 1.8% hemoglobin A_2, and 1.5% hemoglobin F.

The most likely diagnosis is:

(A) No hematologic disorder
(B) Recurrent iron deficiency
(C) Anemia of chronic disease
(D) α-Thalassemia
(E) β-Thalassemia

Anemia Question 6

A 54-year-old woman presents to your office with fever and persistent bleeding from a dental extraction done 3 weeks ago. The patient has felt well for the past month with no fevers or weight loss, but she has had some fatigue that she attributes to long hours at work. Seven years ago she was noted to be pancytopenic and was diagnosed with aplastic anemia. She was treated with antithymocyte globulin, cyclosporine, and prednisone and had a complete hematologic recovery.

Physical examination shows a pale, middle-aged woman. There is no lymphadenopathy or hepatosplenomegaly.

Laboratory studies:

Hemoglobin	8.2 g/dL
Mean corpuscular volume	117 fL
Leukocyte count	3100/µL, with 21% segmented neutrophils, 10% band forms, 68% lymphocytes, and 1% monocytes
Platelet count	36,000/µL

Peripheral blood morphology shows hypogranular and hyposegmented neutrophils. The erythrocyte morphology shows both anisocytosis and poikilocytosis with some teardrop cells.

The most likely diagnosis is:

(A) Recurrent aplastic anemia
(B) Chronic lymphocytic leukemia
(C) Myelodysplasia
(D) Vitamin B_{12} deficiency
(E) Miliary tuberculosis

Anemia Question 7

A 42-year-old black woman is referred to your office because of increasing fatigue. Fourteen months ago, she was found to be anemic after presenting to her doctor's office because of a 2-month history of fatigue. At that time, the referring physician noted a past history of iron deficiency. The patient also reported heavy menses as a teenager and the fact that she took iron for several years. Her menstrual blood loss had not been excessive recently. Laboratory tests are shown below. Because of the low vitamin B_{12} level, an anti-intrinsic factor antibody was assayed and found to be present, and a serum gastrin level was found to be 761 ng/L. A Schilling test was not done.

The patient was treated with vitamin B_{12} (six 1000-µg injections for 3 weeks), and she was taught to give herself monthly vitamin B_{12} injections of 1000 µg each.

Eight months ago, she returned for a follow-up visit. The results of the diagnostic tests are shown below.

Today, she says that her menstrual periods have recently become heavier. She has had no weight loss, abdominal pain, or change in appetite, although there may have been some increased constipation. She insists that she has faithfully given herself monthly vitamin B_{12} injections, although she only uses 0.5 mL instead of 1 mL to save money. The physical examination is normal.

Laboratory studies:

	14 Months Ago	8 Months Ago	Today
Hemoglobin	6.8 g/dL	13.6 g/dL	11.1 g/dL
Mean corpuscular hemoglobin concentration	34.0 g/dL	33.2 g/dL	33.6 g/dL
Mean corpuscular volume	123 fL	87 fL	94 fL
Erythrocyte distribution width	17.6%	13.0%	13.3%
Platelet count	149,000/μL	258,000/μL	266,000/μL
Leukocyte count	5100/μL	6600/μL	6200/μL, with a normal differential
Serum vitamin B_{12}	111 ng/L	—	—
Folate level	19.2 μg/L	—	—
Stool for occult blood	—	—	Negative

At this point you should:

(A) Measure serum vitamin B_{12} and give the patient a 1000-μg vitamin B_{12} injection.
(B) Give the patient oral folic acid, 1 mg daily.
(C) Request endoscopy to rule out gastric cancer.
(D) Order thyroid function tests.
(E) Schedule a Schilling test.

Anemia Questions 8-11

For each statement below select the associated transfusion-transmitted infectious agent (A-E) (each answer may be used more than once or not at all):

(A) Hepatitis C virus
(B) Human T-cell lymphotropic virus, types I and II
(C) Cytomegalovirus
(D) Bacterial contamination
(E) HIV

8. Present in 1/202,000 to 1/2,778,000 donated units

9. Cause(s) severe morbidity and even mortality in immunosuppressed patients

10. Produce(s) asymptomatic disease or mild illness but may cause cirrhosis with liver failure

11. Usually cause(s) no detectable adverse effect, but about three acutely fatal transfusion-transmitted cases occur annually in the United States

Anemia Questions 12-16

For each type of acute transfusion reaction listed below, select the associated mechanism of action (A-E) (each answer may be used more than once or not at all):

(A) Erythrocyte incompatibility
(B) Immune reaction to plasma proteins
(C) Antibody to donor leukocyte antigens
(D) Occasionally antibody to IgA, but often mechanism is unknown
(E) Volume overload

12. Febrile, nonhemolytic reaction

13. Hemolytic reaction

14. Urticaria

15. Pulmonary congestion

16. Anaphylaxis

Anemia Questions 17-20

For each of the disorders described below, select the most likely complete blood count and chemistry results (A-E) (each answer may be used more than once or not at all):

	Hgb (g/dL)	MCV (fL)	WBC (/μL)	Platelets (/μL)	Retic (cells/μL)	Bili (total) (mg/dL)	Bili (direct) (mg/dL)	LDH (U/L)
(A)	14.5	105	6500	100,000	50,000	0.8	0.2	200
(B)	4.5	105	2500	50,000	15,000	0.5	0.2	200
(C)	4.5	105	2500	50,000	15,000	2.5	0.2	800
(D)	4.5	105	6500	450,000	250,000	2.5	0.2	800
(E)	4.5	75	6500	100,000	250,000	1.5	0.2	500

17. Aplastic anemia

18. Autoimmune hemolytic anemia

19. Direct acute effect of alcohol abuse

20. Bacterial overgrowth in the small intestine

Anemia Question 21

A 43-year-old man comes to your office for the first time with leg swelling and fatigue. He had been followed previously by a nephrologist, because he had nephrotic syndrome due to membranous glomerulopathy proved by biopsy. He is able to continue working but has diminished energy and poor exercise tolerance. He has increasing leg swelling, especially at the end of the day. He had taken a blood pressure medication in the past but has not taken any medication for the last 3 years. On physical examination, the patient is pale with a pulse rate of 80/min and a blood pressure of 170/110 mm Hg. The lungs are clear, and the heart is normal. The abdomen is obese, and there is 4+ pitting edema of the extremities.

Laboratory studies:

Hemoglobin	10.5 g/dL
Hematocrit	30%
Mean corpuscular volume	88 fL
Leukocyte count	6500/μL
Platelet count	260,000/μL
Plasma glucose	120 mg/dL
Serum electrolytes	
Sodium	135 meq/L
Potassium	5.5 meq/L
Chloride	105 meq/L
Bicarbonate	21 meq/L
Blood urea nitrogen	45 mg/dL
Serum creatinine	3.5 mg/dL
Urinalysis	
Protein	4+
Microscopic	2 to 5 erythrocytes per high-power field (hpf), 2 to 5 leukocytes/hpf

The best explanation for this patient's anemia is:

(A) Iron deficiency
(B) Hemodilution from volume expansion
(C) Erythropoietin deficiency
(D) Decreased erythrocyte survival

Anemia Questions 22-26

For the patients with chronic renal failure described below, select the type of anemia most likely to be present (A-E) (each answer may be used more than once or not at all):

(A) Normocytic normochromic anemia
(B) Microcytic hypochromic anemia with iron deficiency
(C) Microcytic hypochromic anemia with positive hemosiderin-laden macrophages in pulmonary secretions
(D) Microangiopathic hemolytic anemia
(E) No anemia

22. A 45-year-old man with rapidly progressive glomerulonephritis with linear deposit of IgG antibody along glomerular basement membrane

23. A 52-year-old woman with chronic renal failure

24. A 64-year-old man with chronic renal failure with "saturnine" gout

25. A 38-year-old man with polycystic kidney disease

26. A 40-year-old woman with malignant hypertension

Back Pain

Back Pain Question 1

A 42-year-old male auto mechanic developed acute, severe low back pain while at work 3 days ago. The pain began suddenly while he was straining to remove a bolt from a car engine. The pain was most severe in his right low back and radiated through his right buttock and down the posterior aspect of his right leg to his knee. He has received partial relief from lying down and has been taking acetaminophen with codeine left over from a previous prescription for pain associated with a broken toe. He has had previous episodes of low back pain but none this severe and none associated with pain down his leg. He has no history of bowel and bladder dysfunction. He has come to your office now because he is anxious to return to work.

Physical examination reveals a muscular man in moderate distress leaning over the examination table. He has significant difficulty moving around secondary to his pain. His temperature is 37 °C (98.6 °F), pulse rate is 84/min, and blood pressure is 142/92 mm Hg. His back examination shows muscle spasm and tenderness in the lower lumbar region to the right of the spine. He is most comfortable lying on the examination table with knees partially flexed. The straight-leg maneuver with the right leg increases his back pain at elevation to 45 degrees. Back pain is also increased with the straight-leg maneuver on the left leg. Sensation is intact to pin prick, and deep tendon reflexes are 2+ at both knees and ankles. He is able to walk on his heels and toes but does so with apprehension.

In addition to analgesics, what is the best management approach for this patient?

(A) Surgical consultation
(B) Magnetic resonance imaging of lumbosacral spine
(C) Radiography of the lumbosacral spine
(D) Physical activity as tolerated
(E) Bed rest

Back Pain Question 2

A 60-year-old man with severe neck and back pain and a 30-year history of ankylosing spondylitis is helped into your office by his wife. His pain began after a coughing spell, which caused him to fall in his bathroom at home, but he did not strike his head. He also has noted very fleeting tingling in his arms and legs. The back pain is most pronounced in the interscapular region. His medical history is notable for hypertension and chronic bronchitis secondary to cigarette smoking. He is taking indomethacin and enalapril.

Physical examination reveals a pallid man in obvious pain. His temperature is 37 °C (98.6 °F), pulse rate is 100/min, respiration rate is 20/min, and blood pressure is 170/100 mm Hg. He has a rigid spine with dorsal kyphosis and very limited chest expansion on inspiration. His lung examination reveals bibasilar crackles and distant breath sounds. Cardiac examination reveals a grade 2/6 diastolic decrescendo murmur at the base. Neck examination reveals severely limited rotation, flexion, and extension. Back examination reveals paraspinal muscle spasm in the interscapular region. Pulses are intact at the groin, and deep tendon reflexes are intact at the biceps, triceps, knee, and ankle.

The most likely diagnosis is:

(A) Acute aortic insufficiency
(B) Muscle strain
(C) Thoracic aortic dissection
(D) Traumatic spinal fracture
(E) Spontaneous pneumothorax

Back Pain Question 3

A 75-year-old jeweler with long-standing back symptoms comes to you for help. The patient started having back symptoms about 30 years ago when he would periodically "throw out his back" and would require bed rest for 2 or 3 days before the symptoms would go away. Between episodes he was completely healthy except for occasional low-grade back aches after prolonged automobile rides. About 20 years ago he started having back symptoms every day, which were worse after prolonged activity and relieved by lying down. He started taking acetaminophen as needed and was functional despite the pain. About 3 months ago, his low back pain began to occasionally awaken him from sleep and was unrelieved by lying down. Medical, familial, and social histories are unremarkable.

Physical examination shows an overweight man with normal vital signs and normal findings. Lumbar spine flexion is normal for his age. Rectal examination is normal. Laboratory studies show normal hematocrit, hemoglobin, complete blood count, serum calcium, serum phosphorus, liver function tests, and kidney function.

The most likely diagnosis is:

(A) Lumbar spinal stenosis
(B) Malignancy involving the spine
(C) Osteoporosis
(D) Herniated disc

Back Pain Question 4
A 79-year-old retired surgeon presents with chronic and recent exacerbation of low back pain. He has had chronic back symptoms that are usually worse with use, on prolonged airplane rides, and after shoveling snow. The symptoms are completely relieved by bed rest and time. In the last 2 years, however, the quality of his pain has changed. He has back pain radiating to both buttocks, which comes on with walking a half block and is relieved by sitting down for more than several minutes. He is otherwise healthy.

On physical examination, his vital signs are normal. His pulses are normal. Examination of his back shows flattened lumbar lordosis; straight–leg-raising tests are negative bilaterally; and there are no neuro-motor deficits of the lower extremities. A rectal examination shows a smooth, slightly enlarged prostate without nodules. The remainder of the physical examination is normal.

Laboratory studies show normal complete blood count and Westergren erythrocyte sedimentation rate of 25 mm/h; urinalysis is normal.

Radiographs show grade 1 spondylolisthesis at L4–L5, multilevel disc-space narrowing, facet osteoarthritis, and normal soft tissue and bone density.

The most likely diagnosis is:

(A) Abdominal aneurysm
(B) Lumbar spinal stenosis
(C) Metastatic cancer to spine
(D) Peripheral vascular disease
(E) Multiple myeloma

CANCER

Cancer Question 1
Which one of the following statements about melanoma is correct?

(A) The incidence of melanoma is increasing by 20% per year.
(B) Measuring suspicious lesions every 6 to 12 months is recommended.
(C) Melanomas greater than 0.75 mm in depth are seldom cured by surgery.
(D) Slow enlargement of a lesion excludes melanoma.
(E) Melanoma risk factors include light skin and hair color.

Cancer Question 2
What is the most important prognostic indicator of survival for a patient with malignant melanoma?

(A) Sex of the patient
(B) Tumor thickness
(C) Age of the patient
(D) Location of the lesion
(E) Diameter of the lesion

Cancer Question 3
A 47-year-old woman with a history of breast cancer presents for routine evaluation. Three years ago she underwent a left lumpectomy with axillary node dissection followed by adjuvant chemotherapy with doxorubicin and cyclophosphamide and breast irradiation for management of a 2.5-cm infiltrating duct cancer, which involved one of eleven axillary lymph nodes and did not express estrogen and progesterone receptors. A review of systems is negative.

Physical examination shows a well-appearing woman with a well-healed left lumpectomy scar and an absence of axillary or supraclavicular adenopathy. Chest and abdominal examinations are normal.

What one of the following diagnostic tests would you recommend for this patient?

(A) Bone scan
(B) Bilateral mammography
(C) Chest radiograph
(D) Measurement of serum tumor markers

Cancer Question 4
A 30-year-old man who is in excellent health comes to your office for a routine examination. His mother died of colon cancer at age 41 years; his 38-year-old brother was recently diagnosed with colon cancer; and his maternal aunt had ovarian cancer. Physical examination is normal, and examination of the stool is negative for occult blood. A complete blood count is normal.

Which one of the following statements is true about this patient?

(A) His sister is at increased risk for breast cancer.
(B) Colon cancer in his family is more likely to arise in the proximal bowel.
(C) He should undergo a prophylactic colectomy.
(D) He likely has a condition associated with a mutation in BRCA2.
(E) He should have an annual colonoscopy beginning at age 35 years.

Cancer Question 5
Which one of the following statements is true about prostate cancer?

(A) Community screening through prostate-specific antigen (PSA) assay has been proven to improve survival in randomized clinical trials.
(B) Age-specific normal ranges for PSA increase with the age of the patient.
(C) Transrectal ultrasonography is a highly sensitive and specific screening tool.
(D) Digital rectal examination is a reliable screening test for prostate cancer.
(E) Randomized clinical trials have proved radical prostatectomy to yield a 15% survival benefit at 5 years compared with radical radiotherapy for matched patients.

Cancer Question 6
A 59-year-old man presents with cough, dyspnea, and facial edema of 2 weeks' duration. He has a 40–pack-year smoking history. Except for an anteroseptal myocardial infarction 4 years ago, he has been healthy.

Physical examination reveals a blood pressure of 130/85 mm Hg and normal heart sounds with a pulse rate of 72/minute, but there is reduced air entry in the right middle chest, dilated veins in the upper chest, and a slightly tender liver palpable 3 cm below the costal margin. The results of hematology and chemistry screens (including liver function tests) are normal, but a chest CT scan shows a central right upper lobe mass, with collapse and extensive mediastinal adenopathy. Blood gases are within normal limits, but spirometry shows an obstructive pattern.

The next step in the management of this patient would be:

(A) Immediate radiotherapy
(B) Immediate chemotherapy
(C) Bronchoscopy
(D) Mediastinoscopy
(E) Intravenous furosemide

Cancer Questions 7-8
Question 7

A 70-year-old man with advanced hormone-refractory prostate cancer presents with multifocal pain, which he grades as 5/10. He has been treated by bilateral orchiectomy and radiotherapy to the right hemipelvis. His prostate-specific antigen (PSA) concentration is 100 ng/mL, and a bone scan shows multiple "hot spots," with a distribution that includes thoracolumbar spine, pelvis, ribs, and long bones. Apart from a serum alkaline phosphatase of 400 U/mL, the results of hematology and chemistry tests are normal.

The patient has been using occasional extra-strength acetaminophen with some improvement of pain, but recently this medication has been ineffective and his pain has increased dramatically.

The next step in the management of this patient should be:

(A) Luteinizing hormone-releasing hormone agonist
(B) Palliative radiotherapy
(C) Parenteral morphine infusion
(D) Nonsteroidal anti-inflammatory drugs (NSAIDs) with opioids for breakthrough pain
(E) Diazepam

Question 8

After an initial improvement in his symptoms with treatment, the condition of the patient deteriorates, and he has further back pain accompanied by increasing weakness of the lower limbs and severe constipation despite the use of stool softeners.

The next step in management should be:

(A) Cytotoxic chemotherapy
(B) Referral for physical therapy
(C) MRI of the spine
(D) Increased laxatives
(E) Referral for radioactive strontium

Cancer Question 9

A 42-year-old mother of three young children presents with a hoarse voice, a dry cough, and hemoptysis. She has not lost weight recently and has no constitutional symptoms. There is no relevant medical history, but her father died of cancer of the larynx and an aunt had breast cancer. She has smoked 25 cigarettes per day since the age of 16 years.

Physical examination reveals a clinically normal cardiovascular system, but a fixed left-sided upper lobe inspiratory wheeze, with scattered left upper lobe crepitations. There is no evidence of peripheral lymph node enlargement and no clinical evidence of metastases. However, indirect laryngoscopy shows a paralyzed left vocal cord. The results of hematology and chemistry screens are normal. A CT scan shows a 4-cm left upper lobe spiculated mass, with left-sided mediastinal lymph node enlargement.

The next step in the management of this patient should be:

(A) Mammography
(B) Bronchoscopy and mediastinoscopy
(C) Fine-needle biopsy of the mass
(D) Two-week therapeutic trial of antibiotics
(E) Thoracotomy with resection of the mass and mediastinal lymph node

Cancer Question 10

A 65-year-old woman presents with malignant ascites. For which one of the following possible causes of her condition is potentially curative therapy available?

(A) Colon carcinoma
(B) Ovarian carcinoma
(C) Breast cancer
(D) Gastric carcinoma

Cancer Question 11

A 48-year-old woman who had occult blood discovered in her stool was diagnosed with cancer of the sigmoid colon. The tumor was excised, and an end-to-end anastomosis of her remaining bowel was performed. The pathology review demonstrated the cancer to be a 5-cm polyploid lesion with invasion of the bowel wall but not beyond the muscularis.

Twenty lymph nodes were identified, and none contained cancer.

Laboratory tests, including measurement of carcino-embryonic antigen, ultrasonography of the liver, and chest radiography are normal.

What is the best therapeutic option for this patient at this time?

(A) Radiation therapy to the colon in the region of the previous cancer
(B) Adjuvant chemotherapy with 5-fluorouracil (5-FU) and levamisole
(C) Adjuvant chemotherapy with 5-FU and leucovorin
(D) Annual evaluation and colonoscopy
(E) Daily nonsteroidal anti-inflammatory drug therapy to suppress further polyp formation

Cancer Question 12

A 58-year-old woman has had cough and increased shortness of breath for 6 weeks. She also reports a 6-lb weight loss. Physical examination is unremarkable. Complete blood count and liver function tests are normal. Blood gases show a Po_2 of 88 mm Hg, Pco_2 of 38 mm Hg, and pH of 7.4. Chest radiograph shows a 3-cm right mid-lung mass. CT scan of the chest shows a right middle lobe mass measuring 3.3 cm in diameter. Three mediastinal lymph nodes are seen and measure 1, 1.5, and 1.5 cm in diameter, respectively. Bronchoscopy shows a mass in the right mid-lobe bronchus. Biopsy specimen shows squamous cell carcinoma.

What is the most appropriate action now?

(A) CT scan of the brain and abdomen
(B) Pulmonary function tests
(C) Thoracotomy
(D) Mediastinoscopy
(E) Neoadjuvant (preoperative) chemotherapy

Cancer Question 13

A 36-year-old woman with no previous medical history presents with an eczematoid scaly eruption on her left nipple. She says that she has recently taken up jogging and this has irritated her breast.

On physical examination, she has a 1-cm reddened and slightly crusted lesion on the left nipple. There is no discharge or masses or other abnormalities on either breast. Topical skin treatment with emollients and corticosteroids is prescribed, and she is told to return for re-examination in 2 weeks. At representation 2 weeks later, the crust is somewhat decreased, but the scaly eruption on the nipple is still present, although somewhat diminished. She has continued to jog.

Which of the following is the best course of management?

(A) Continue topical therapy.
(B) Continue topical therapy, and recommend she wear a running bra or consider stopping her jogging program.
(C) Continue topical therapy, but add an antifungal agent.
(D) Order a mammogram, and refer her to a surgeon for biopsy.
(E) Order a mammogram, and if negative, continue topical therapy.

Cancer Question 14

A 40-year-old man with ulcerative colitis involving the entire colon diagnosed 20 years ago has had intermittent flares that have been easily controlled as an outpatient by increasing doses of 5-ASA and occasional corticosteroids. He has been undergoing colonoscopic surveillance every other year. At his most recent surveillance, performed during an acute flare, some biopsy specimens reveal definite inflammation and low-grade dysplasia.

The appropriate next step in the patient's management is:

(A) Refer to a surgeon for immediate colectomy.
(B) Ask for a second opinion from a pathologist expert in inflammatory bowel disease.
(C) Repeat the colonoscopy with segmental biopsies.
(D) Treat the active colitis, and repeat surveillance as soon as the colitis is quiescent or within 3 months.

Cancer Questions 15-18

For each patient with breast cancer described below, select the recommended local therapy (A-D) (each answer may be used more than once or not at all):

(A) Regular breast examination and annual mammography
(B) Breast radiotherapy
(C) Modified radical mastectomy with or without reconstruction
(E) Lumpectomy with axillary dissection and breast radiotherapy

15. A 39-year-old woman presents with a 1.5-cm infiltrating ductal carcinoma. She had mantle radiotherapy at the age of 16 years for stage IIA Hodgkin's disease.

16. A 42-year-old woman undergoes biopsy for a palpable mass. Pathologic examination shows a fibroadenoma and lobular carcinoma in situ.

17. A 65-year-old woman is found to have a 1.5-cm infiltrating ductal carcinoma by needle-localization biopsy of a mammographically detected lesion.

18. A 47-year-old woman is found to have a cluster of microcalcifications on screening mammography. Biopsy specimen shows a 2.0-cm ductal carcinoma in situ without invasion and with negative margins of excision.

Cancer Questions 19-22

For each gastrointestinal malignant condition shown below, select the associated etiologic factor (A-E) (each answer may be used more than once or not at all):

(A) Schistosomiasis
(B) Tobacco use
(C) *Helicobacter pylori* infection
(D) Human papillomavirus infection
(E) Hepatitis C infection

19. Gastric lymphoma

20. Squamous cell carcinoma of the anus

21. Hepatocellular carcinoma

22. Pancreatic adenocarcinoma

CHEST PAIN

Chest Pain Question 1

A 59-year-old man with hypertension, hyperlipidemia, and a positive family history is seen in your office 2 weeks after an uncomplicated non–Q-wave myocardial infarction of uncertain location. A low-level exercise stress test before discharge was negative for ischemia to a peak pulse rate of 92/min. Seven months previously, he was able to accomplish 11 minutes of exercise, according to the standard Bruce protocol, but stopped because of knee pain at a peak pulse rate of 145/min and a systolic blood pressure of 210 mm Hg without chest discomfort, diagnostic electrocardiographic changes, or important arrhythmias. He has remained stable on a medical regimen of aspirin, β-blockers, an angiotensin-converting enzyme inhibitor, and an hydroxymethylglutaryl coenzyme A (HMG-CoA) reductase inhibitor. Arrangements are made for his enrollment in a program of cardiac rehabilitation, but he telephones 1 week later to report three episodes of mild central chest discomfort during the early morning hours. These symptoms are similar to, but less intense than, those associated with his myocardial infarction.

The most appropriate strategy would be:

(A) Repeat low-level exercise stress testing
(B) Repeat symptom-limited exercise stress testing using the standard Bruce protocol
(C) Coronary angiography
(D) Ambulatory electrocardiographic monitoring

Chest Pain Question 2

A 54-year-old man presents with exertional chest pain of 3 weeks' duration. His risk factors include a 30–pack-year history of smoking and type 2 diabetes mellitus for 2 years that has been controlled with glyburide. Physical examination is unremarkable and includes good peripheral pulses. An exercise electrocardiogram shows 2 mm of horizontal ST-segment depression at 5 METs. You place the patient on aspirin, metoprolol, and nitroglycerin as needed, with advice to quit smoking before angiography.

The patient's symptoms persist in spite of treatment. You suggest he will probably need revascularization and refer him to a cardiologist. Coronary angiography shows proximal two-vessel disease (left anterior descending and right coronary arteries) with normal left ventricular function.

Based on published literature, which of the following is recommended?

(A) Percutaneous transluminal coronary angioplasty (PTCA)
(B) PTCA and rotablation
(C) Coronary artery bypass graft
(D) Directional atherectomy

Chest Pain Question 3

A 62-year-old man presents for a general health examination. He reports three episodes of left precordial chest discomfort over the past month while using the treadmill at his health club. He has noticed no other problems. He has not seen a physician in 22 years.

On physical examination, his height is 172.7 cm (68 in), and his weight is 75.8 kg (167 lb). His pulse rate is 74/min and regular, and blood pressure is 150/100 mm Hg in both arms. The retinal arterioles appear mildly narrowed. The left ventricular impulse is slightly sustained. There is an S_4. The remainder of the examination is normal. A resting electrocardiogram shows a sinus rhythm with left atrial enlargement, prominent left ventricular voltage, and minor, nonspecific T-wave flattening in leads 1, aVL, V_5, and V_6.

The next step in the treatment of this patient should be:

(A) Admission to a chest pain observation unit
(B) Exercise stress testing
(C) Dobutamine echocardiography
(D) Initiation of medical treatment and exercise stress testing
(E) Coronary angiography

Chest Pain Question 4

A 45-year-old man is seen in consultation for severe chest pain and exertional dyspnea. When he was 8 years old, hypertrophic cardiomyopathy was diagnosed echocardiographically, and his activities have been limited since childhood. He had previously been treated with atenolol, 100 mg three times daily, but he was unable to tolerate this because of severe fatigue, depression, and sexual dysfunction. Currently he is taking verapamil, 120 mg three times daily.

He reports substernal chest pain and shortness of breath while climbing one flight of stairs or walking less than one block and is now considering medical disability.

Physical examination shows a trim man. His pulse rate is 56/min, and blood pressure is 120/80 mm Hg. His carotid pulse is 3+ with rapid upstroke and a bisferiens character. Jugular venous pressure is seen at 8 cm H_2O with prominent a waves. His lungs are clear. His cardiac examination shows a point of maximal intensity that is laterally displaced beyond the mid-clavicular line. There is a 2+ left ventricular heave. S_1 is normal, and S_2 is paradoxically split. There is a palpable and audible S_4. A grade 3/6 systolic ejection murmur is heard at the left sternal border and radiates to the carotid arteries; this murmur increases with Valsalva's maneuver. A grade 2/6 apical holosystolic murmur is also present. His abdomen is free of organomegaly or ascites. There is no peripheral edema.

Chest radiograph shows mild cardiomegaly (cardiac/thoracic ratio is 14/24 cm). There is left ventricular prominence, and both lung fields are clear. Electrocardiography shows sinus bradycardia, left atrial enlargement, marked left ventricular hypertrophy with a strain pattern, and frequent premature ventricular contractions. There are 2-mm Q waves seen in leads II, III, and aVF. Echocardiography, which had been done the preceding year, shows marked concentric left ventricular hypertrophy (septal wall thickness of 18 mm, posterior wall thickness of 14 mm). There is marked systolic anterior motion of the mitral valve; 2+ mitral regurgitation is also present. Mild right ventricular hypertrophy and biatrial enlargement are evident. There is a resting left ventricular aortic outflow gradient of 40 mm Hg by Doppler ultrasonography; this gradient increases to 95 mm Hg during a Valsalva's maneuver.

The most appropriate next treatment option is:

(A) Addition of amiodarone
(B) Addition of metoprolol
(C) Insertion of a ventricular pacemaker (ventricular demand inhibited [VVI] pacing)
(D) Insertion of an atrioventricular sequential pacing system (dual-chamber [DDD] pacing)
(E) Septal myotomy-myectomy

Chest Pain Question 5

A 36-year-old woman presents to the emergency department for the second time in a week with pleuritic chest and left shoulder discomfort and a low-grade fever. She had been involved in an argument with her boyfriend 6 days previously during which he grabbed her by both upper arms and shook her

violently for about 30 seconds. She did not experience any appreciable external trauma. On physical examination, her pulse rate is 100/min and regular, and blood pressure is 94/70 mm Hg. Her left iris is green, and her right iris is blue. She is slender with a straight back and a slight pectus excavatum. The palate is high-arched, and the fingers are longer than yours despite the fact that she is 3 inches shorter. She is in no acute distress. There is a pericardial friction rub. A chest radiograph shows an increase in the transverse dimension of the cardiac silhouette and a small left pleural effusion. An electrocardiogram shows a sinus rhythm with diffuse J-point elevation and PR-segment depression in lead 2.

Which one of the following tests should you order?

(A) Erythrocyte sedimentation rate
(B) Creatine kinase determination
(C) Echocardiogram
(D) Antinuclear antibody titer
(E) D-dimer test

Chest Pain Question 6

A 75-year-old woman presents with a history of mild stable angina pectoris for 5 years and an inferior myocardial infarction 2 years ago. In the fall of the year 3 months ago, she noted precordial heaviness climbing the stairs with packages. Now in the cold weather, she is taking sublingual nitroglycerin every day. She denies dyspnea, palpitations, or peripheral edema. Her medications include metoprolol, 50 mg twice daily; aspirin, 325 mg/d; and nitroglycerin as needed.

On physical examination, her pulse rate is 56/min and regular, and blood pressure is 130/76 mm Hg. Carotid arteries are firm without bruits, jugular venous pulses are normal, and lungs are clear. The apical impulse is palpable, with a presystolic wave. S_1 and S_2 are normal. An S_4 is easily audible. There is no hepatic enlargement or peripheral edema. Pulses below the femur are palpable but decreased.

Laboratory studies:

Hemoglobin	13.0 g/dL
Hematocrit	38%
Cholesterol (fasting)	198 mg/dL
Triglycerides	130 mg/dL
HDL cholesterol	44 mg/dL
Calculated LDL cholesterol	128 mg/dL
Thyroid-stimulating hormone	2.6 μU/mL

The electrocardiogram shows the old inferior infarct. After discussion of treatment options, the patient strongly opposes an invasive strategy.

Which of the following would be most appropriate additional therapy?

(A) Nifedipine
(B) Long-acting nitrate
(C) Verapamil
(D) Amlodipine
(E) Increase in metoprolol

Chest Pain Question 7

A 53-year-old woman presents with a history of intermittent chest pain for 3 years. The pain is described as a nonradiating, pressing ache in the left parasternal and upper left chest. There is no relationship with eating, and the pattern is not predictable. It occurs when she is carrying packages, during stress, and at rest. The ache lasts 10 to 30 minutes and is followed by a sense of fatigue. She is frightened by the pain and has presented to the emergency room three times; each time she was sent home without advice. She is convinced something is wrong. Her last menstrual period was 4 years ago. There is no family history of coronary heart disease, diabetes, hypertension, or stroke.

On physical examination, she appears well. She is 163 cm (64 in) tall and weighs 57 kg (125 lb). Her pulse rate is 76/min, and blood pressure is 128/76 mm Hg. The carotid and jugular pulses are normal. The breasts are normal. There is a slight amount of tenderness in the left costochondral junction, but this is not exactly the same symptom as her chief complaint. Heart sounds are normal, and there is no murmur, S_3, or S_4. The abdomen and extremities are normal.

Laboratory studies include a normal complete blood count; cholesterol, 180 mg/dL; and high-density lipoprotein (HDL) cholesterol, 49 mg/dL. Electrocardiogram is normal. An exercise thallium-201 study using single-photon emission computed tomography (SPECT) shows a 1-mm horizontal ST-segment depression at 6 METs and an equivocal fixed anterior defect thought possibly to be due to breast attenuation.

You refer the patient to a cardiologist, who does a catheterization. The cardiologist reports the coronary arteries are clean; left ventricular ejection fraction is 55% with good wall motion; and left ventricular end-diastolic pressure is 17 mm Hg.

What is the most effective treatment for this patient?

(A) Estrogen
(B) Nitroglycerin
(C) Anxiolytic agent
(D) β-blocker
(E) Nonsteroidal anti-inflammatory drug

Chest Pain Question 8

A 74-year-old man presents to the emergency room because he suddenly developed severe substernal chest pain associated with diaphoresis about 1 hour ago after finishing his breakfast. Four years ago he was diagnosed with temporal (giant cell) arteritis. At that time, he was successfully treated with prednisone, which was discontinued after 18 months. He takes no medications and stays active by playing golf twice a week.

On physical examination the patient is writhing in pain. His temperature is 36.6 °C (98.0 °F), pulse rate is 120/min, respiration rate is 28/min, and blood pressure is 150/90 mm Hg. The jugular veins are normal. The lungs are clear. Cardiac examination is normal, except for tachycardia. Pulses are intact. The remainder of the examination is normal.

Portable chest radiograph is normal. The electrocardiogram shows tachycardia and minimal ST-T–wave changes.

The most likely diagnosis is:

(A) Acute myocardial infarction
(B) Acute pericarditis
(C) Acute esophagitis
(D) Aortic dissection
(E) Esophageal rupture

Congestive Heart Failure

Congestive Heart Failure Question 1

A 38-year-old man is seen in the emergency department for sudden onset of rapid heart beat and lightheadedness. He has been HIV positive for 5 years and has been taking zidovudine for the past 18 months. His most recent CD4 cell count was 375/μL.

Physical examination reveals a well-appearing man with mild dyspnea. His pulse rate is 110/min, irregularly irregular, and his blood pressure is 130/80 mm Hg. Jugular venous pressure is 10 cm H_2O. Fine crackles are audible at both lung bases. On cardiac examination, there is a diffuse point of maximal intensity and a grade 2/6 holosystolic apical murmur. The patient's abdomen and extremities are normal. Laboratory studies include positive serologies for toxoplasma and varicella and cytomegalovirus. Serum creatine kinase is 600 U/L, with the MB fraction less than 1%. The patient's electrocardiogram shows atrial fibrillation with a rapid ventricular response rate and a pronounced interventricular conduction defect. Echocardiogram shows a mildly dilated, globally hypokinetic left ventricle; mild right ventricular dilatation and hypokinesis are also present. Left ventricular ejection fraction is 35%.

What is the most likely diagnosis?

(A) HIV cardiomyopathy
(B) Cytomegalovirus myocarditis
(C) Cardiac toxoplasmosis
(D) Zidovudine-induced cardiotoxicity
(E) Tachycardia-induced cardiomyopathy

Congestive Heart Failure Question 2

A 61-year-old man requires intubation in the Emergency Department for respiratory distress. He has had a known heart murmur for 20 years and receives endocarditis prophylaxis. His wife reports two weeks of progressive dyspnea and weight gain, culminating in severe rest dyspnea.

On physical examination his pulse rate is 104/min and regular; blood pressure is 80/50 mm Hg. Jugular venous pressure is 5 cm H_2O, and the carotid arteries show a small volume. Crackles are audible two thirds up from the lung bases bilaterally. There is a 1+ left ventricular heave, normal S_1, and single S_2. A 1/6 systolic ejection murmur is audible at the base and apex. An S_3 is also present. The extremities show no edema but are cool and mottled.

Chest radiograph shows mild cardiomegaly, interstitial edema, and moderate-sized bilateral effusions. The patient's electrocardiogram is shown on the next page.

What is the most likely diagnosis?

(A) Acute mitral regurgitation
(B) Recent anterior myocardial infarction
(C) Aortic stenosis
(D) Infarct-related ventricular septal defect

Congestive Heart Failure Question 3

A 69-year-old man with no history of cardiac disease is admitted to the hospital with acute pulmonary edema. Over the previous month, he had noted progressive dyspnea with exertion and had received treatment for a presumed pulmonary infection. On admission, his pulse rate is 126/min and regular, respiration rate is 44/min, and blood pressure 138/80 mm Hg. He is diaphoretic and slightly dusky. His neck veins are not visible while he is sitting upright. There are crackles bilaterally to the apices. The cardiac impulse cannot be felt, and the heart tones are inaudible. He has no palpable abdominal aortic aneurysm. There is no peripheral edema. Electrocardiogram shows a sinus tachycardia with a minor intraventricular conduction defect, small nondiagnostic Q waves in the inferior leads, and nonspecific ST-T-wave abnormalities.

Treatment for pulmonary edema with oxygen, morphine sulfate, and furosemide is begun, and intubation is avoided. A myocardial infarction is excluded by serial enzyme measurements and electrocardiography. Echocardiogram shows mild left ventricular cavity dilatation with multiple regional wall motion abnormalities, an estimated ejection fraction of 25% to 30%, and mild mitral regurgitation. Further history obtained after stabilization includes an elevated serum cholesterol concentration and a positive family history of coronary artery disease. He quit smoking cigarettes approximately 10 years ago. Ethanol intake had been minimal.

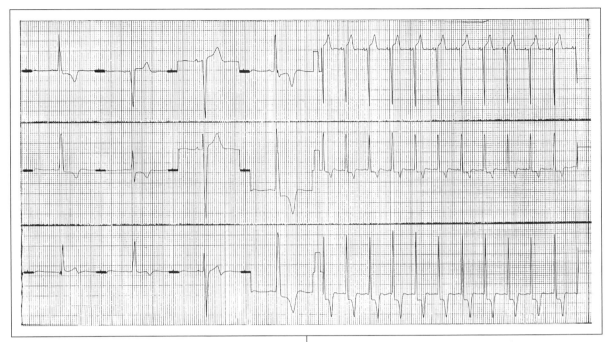

Question 2

The following day, he has transient dyspnea at rest.

What is the most appropriate diagnostic strategy at this point?

(A) Repeat echocardiography to assess left ventricular function and mitral regurgitation
(B) Dobutamine echocardiography to screen for the presence of myocardial ischemia
(C) Radionuclide perfusion imaging to assess viability and reversible ischemia
(D) Cardiac catheterization with hemodynamic assessment and coronary angiography

Congestive Heart Failure Question 4
A 42-year-old man presents because of increasing abdominal girth and lower-extremity edema. A decade ago he underwent treatment for Hodgkin's disease that included mantle field radiation therapy and MOPP chemotherapy.

Physical examination shows a pulse rate of 84/min and blood pressure of 100/70 mm Hg. There is dullness to percussion and absent tactile fremitus at the right base; bronchial breathing is detected 2 cm below the right scapular angle. The external jugular veins are not observed with the patient at 45 degrees. The cardiac impulse is not detected; the left border of cardiac dullness is in the fifth left interspace 7 cm from the midsternal line. The heart sounds are distant. There are no murmurs; a dis-

crete sound is noted in early-middiastole in the fifth left interspace about 7 cm from the midsternal line. There is 3+ pitting edema bilaterally to the thighs.

What is the most likely diagnosis?

(A) Effusive pericarditis
(B) Occult constrictive pericarditis
(C) Constrictive pericarditis
(D) Idiopathic dilated cardiomyopathy
(E) Restrictive cardiomyopathy

Congestive Heart Failure Question 5
An 87-year-old woman is seen in consultation for increasing exertional dyspnea. She has a 10 year history of mild hypertension and has had non–insulin-dependent diabetes mellitus for the past 8 years. She has no chest pain but has had worsening shortness of breath while climbing stairs or walking two to three blocks. Her medications include conjugated estrogen and metformin.

Physical examination shows an obese woman. The pulse rate is 60/min and regular, and blood pressure is 140/60 mm Hg. Her chest shows fine bibasilar rales. A 1+ left ventricular heave is palpable, and a prominent S_4 is audible. There is no murmur. No hepatomegaly, ascites, or peripheral edema is noted.

Electrocardiogram shows sinus rhythm, borderline left ventricular hypertrophy, and nonspecific repolarization abnormalities. Chest radiograph reveals normal heart size and mild interstitial edema.

33

Laboratory studies show blood urea nitrogen, 18 mg/dL, and serum creatinine, 1.1 mg/dL. Echocardiogram shows mild concentric left ventricular hypertrophy; posterior and septal wall thickness is 12 mm. The left atrium is mildly dilated (42 mm). Left ventricular function is hyperdynamic. There is minimal sclerosis of the aortic valve leaflets, with normal motion.

An exercise test is done and is terminated at 4 minutes for marked dyspnea and fatigue. At peak exercise, the pulse rate is 90/min and blood pressure is 165/80 mm Hg. Technetium 99m sestamibi imaging discloses normal myocardial perfusion. Treatment is initiated with furosemide, 40 mg daily. During a follow-up visit at 1 month, the patient reports modest improvement in her dyspnea but is still unable to climb one flight of stairs. Blood pressure is 130/84 mm Hg. Laboratory studies now show blood urea nitrogen, 36 mg/dL, and serum creatinine, 1.2 mg/dL.

The most effective treatment option at this point would be:

(A) Increase in furosemide dosage
(B) Addition of an angiotensin-converting enzyme (ACE) inhibitor
(C) Addition of a β-blocker
(D) Addition of a calcium channel antagonist
(E) Addition of an oral or transdermal nitrate preparation

Congestive Heart Failure Question 6
A 70-year-old man presents with 6 months of worsening dyspnea on exertion and fatigue. He has a longstanding history of congestive heart failure and three previous myocardial infarctions. Despite treatment with digoxin, escalating doses of furosemide, and enalapril (20 mg) twice daily, his symptoms continue to progress. There is no history of angina. An exercise test with thallium imaging done within the last year showed extensive anterior, septal, and inferior scars but no evidence for reversible myocardial ischemia.

Physical examination shows a frail, cachectic, mildly dyspneic man. His pulse rate is 105/min and regular, and blood pressure is 82/50 mm Hg. His head, eyes, ears, nose, and throat examination shows mild facial wasting. There is no central cyanosis. His neck veins are elevated at 12 cm H_2O with prominent V waves. His chest is clear. Cardiac examination shows a diffuse point of maximal intensity. There is a palpably dyskinetic apex. S_1 is soft, S_2 is narrowly split, and a modest increase in intensity of the pulmonic component is noted. There is a grade 2/6 holosystolic murmur at the left sternal border apex and loud

S_3 and S_4. A mildly tender liver edge descends 3 cm below the right costal margin, with a total span of 13 cm. There is no ascites, but 2+ peripheral edema is present to midcalf.

Laboratory studies show blood urea nitrogen of 56 mg/dL, and a serum creatinine of 1.5 mg/dL. Chest radiograph shows marked cardiomegaly, small bilateral pleural effusions, and 2+ pulmonary vascular redistribution. There are no pulmonary infiltrates. Electrocardiogram shows sinus tachycardia, left atrial enlargement, and intraventricular conduction defect. QS waves are evident in leads V_1 to V_4, and II, III, and aVF.

His physician prescribes metoprolol, 6.25 mg twice daily. The dosage is slowly increased over the next month to 25 mg orally twice daily. The patient questions the purpose of this new medication.

What is the most accurate statement about the proven effects of metoprolol therapy in this patient?

(A) His heart failure symptoms are likely to improve.
(B) There is a 25% chance that he will not tolerate the medication.
(C) His left ventricular ejection fraction is likely to fall during long-term therapy.
(D) His exercise tolerance is unlikely to change.
(E) His 1-year survival will be improved.

Congestive Heart Failure Question 7
A 52-year-old man is referred for evaluation of 3 months of worsening shortness of breath. He denies any associated chest pain. He had a normal stress test 1 year ago. Two months ago when he noted palpitations his pulse rate was 138/min and irregular. Treatment was begun with digoxin once daily, and he was advised to return for follow-up. Five years ago he discontinued his pattern of one or two beers over the weekend. There is a 10-year history of hypertension (highest reading, 150/90 mm Hg) that has been controlled with medication.

On physical examination, the patient's pulse rate is 165/min and irregularly irregular; blood pressure is 130/85 mm Hg. Bibasilar crackles are present. On cardiac examination, the point of maximal intensity is diffuse; an S_3 and a grade 1/6 holosystolic murmur are audible at the apex.

The serum digoxin level is 0.2 ng/dL. Chest radiograph shows modest cardiomegaly, interstitial edema, and small bilateral pleural effusions. Electrocardiogram shows atrial fibrillation with a ventricular response rate of 165/min, poor R-wave progression, conduction delay, and nonspecific repolarization abnormalities. Echocardiography shows four-chamber enlargement, global left and right ventricular hypokinesis, and left ventricular ejection fraction of 30%.

What is the most likely diagnosis?

(A) Hypertensive heart disease
(B) Alcoholic cardiomyopathy
(C) Ischemic heart disease
(D) Idiopathic dilated cardiomyopathy
(E) Tachycardia-induced cardiomyopathy

Congestive Heart Failure Question 8

A 58-year-old man who has recently been hospitalized for decompensated heart failure asks to see you before discharge to discuss an exercise program. His history includes three myocardial infarctions. He denies any symptoms of angina pectoris during the past year but has limited his activities on a friend's advice. Other medical problems include diet-controlled diabetes mellitus and mild obstructive lung disease. Following a 5-pound diuresis, he can ambulate in the hospital hallway for 15 minutes with only mild dyspnea and a fall in oxygen saturation from 97% to 92%. Discharge medications will include digoxin, furosemide, lisinopril, transdermal nitrate, glyburide, and theophylline.

The patient is a mildly cachectic man who appears older than his stated age. His pulse rate is 98/min and regular, and blood pressure is 85/50 mm Hg. Head, eyes, ears, nose, throat examination reveals mild facial wasting. There is no circumoral cyanosis. His chest shows an increase in anteroposterior diameter and has scattered end-expiratory wheezes. On cardiac examination, his point of maximal intensity is moderately displaced, and there is a loud summation gallop. A grade 2/6 holosystolic murmur is noted at the apex and radiates to the axilla. His liver is nontender and descends 2 cm below the right costal margin, with a span of 14 cm. There is 1+ peripheral edema.

Laboratory studies show blood urea nitrogen, 55 mg/dL, and serum creatinine, 1.9 mg/dL. Chest radiograph shows moderate cardiomegaly, small bilateral pleural effusions, hyperexpansion consistent with obstructive lung disease, and mild pulmonary vascular redistribution. Electrocardiogram shows sinus rhythm, left atrial enlargement, intraventricular conduction defects (QRS = 0.11), evidence for old inferior and anterolateral myocardial infarctions, and diffuse ST- and T-wave abnormalities consistent with digoxin effect. Echocardiography shows markedly impaired left ventricular contractility with segmental variation. The inferior wall is akinetic; the apex is dyskinetic; the anterior wall is markedly hypokinetic. Overall, left ventricular ejection fraction is 18%. There is moderate mitral regurgitation and mild tricuspid regurgitation. Right ventricular function appears normal.

Which exercise regimen is most beneficial for this patient?

(A) Aerobic exercise training should be avoided because it will increase his risk of sudden cardiac death.
(B) Aerobic exercise training may be safely undertaken but is unlikely to improve his functional capacity.
(C) Aerobic exercise training should be avoided because it will lead to more rapid disease progression.
(D) Aerobic exercise training may be safely undertaken and may improve exercise capacity and decrease heart failure symptoms.
(E) Physical activity should be limited and frequent bed rest encouraged.

Congestive Heart Failure Question 9

A 45-year-old male cattle farmer is admitted to your service on a Saturday afternoon with fever and mild confusion of 3 days' duration. He had been in his usual state of good health until 4 days ago when he felt ill at dinner. His wife states that he went to bed early but awakened at 3 am with a shaking chill. Over the next 2 days, he had occasional shaking chills without other symptoms. On the evening of admission his wife noted that he was confused and brought him to the Emergency Department.

On physical examination, his temperature is 38.9 °C (102 °F), pulse rate is 115/min, respiration rate is 24/min, and blood pressure is 120/60 mm Hg. He appears flushed and his sclerae are mildly injected. There is a petechia in the right conjunctival sac and two splinter hemorrhages in the nail beds of the right hand. No crackles are noted in the lung fields. The mean venous pressure is approximately 9 cm H_2O. S_1 and S_2 are normal in intensity, and a short soft diastolic decrescendo murmur is noted. The abdominal examination is normal, and there is no edema.

Laboratory studies show a leukocyte count of 15,000/μL with a left shift; the blood chemistries are normal. Urinalysis shows 6 to 10 erythrocytes and 5 to 8 leukocytes per high-power field. The chest radiograph shows a normal heart size and no pulmonary infiltrates. The electrocardiogram shows sinus tachycardia, normal axis and intervals, and normal QRS complexes. The T waves are flattened in the lateral leads; there is no left ventricular hypertrophy.

You make a tentative diagnosis of infective endocarditis, order three sets of blood cultures, and start the patient on ampicillin(sulbactam sodium, 3.0 g every 6 h. An echocardiogram is requested for Monday. On Sunday afternoon you are notified that all blood cultures are growing gram-positive cocci and that final identification and sensitivities will be available in the morning. Six hours after this news, you are informed that the patient is tachypneic (32/min, with labored respirations) and "doesn't look too well." Physical examination shows pulse rate of 120/min and regular; blood pressure of 120/80 mm Hg; and pulse oximetry of 88%. S_1 and S_2 are muffled, the decrescendo murmur is perhaps somewhat shorter, and an extra heart sound is present. The electrocardiogram is unchanged.

The most important next step in the management of this patient is:

(A) Change antibiotics
(B) Call a cardiothoracic surgeon
(C) Obtain further blood cultures
(D) Administer furosemide

CHRONIC OBSTRUCTIVE PULMONARY DISEASE

Chronic Obstructive Pulmonary Disease
Question 1

A 72-year-old man presents because of extreme exertional dyspnea and fatigue that have progressed over the past 3 years. Chronic obstructive pulmonary disease had been diagnosed 3 years earlier based upon spirometry, and oxygen (1 L/min) was prescribed for mild arterial hypoxemia (Pao_2 = 52 mm Hg). Fifteen years earlier he had an episode of severe chest pain that was diagnosed to be a myocardial infarction. He has smoked 2 packs of cigarettes daily for 20 years.

On physical examination he appears chronically ill. His neck veins are distended to the angle of the mandible while sitting up. Chest examination reveals a mild decrease in the intensity of the breath sounds over both lung fields. Cardiac examination shows a palpable left parasternal heave and a grade 3/6 holosystolic murmur, which is best heard along the left sternal border. Ascites and peripheral edema are also present.

Pulmonary function and arterial blood gas studies:

Forced vital capacity (FVC)	4.2 L (98% of predicted)
Forced expiratory volume in 1 second (FEV$_1$)	2.6 L (78% of predicted)
Pao_2	56 mm Hg
$Paco_2$	32 mm Hg
pH	7.41

A chest radiograph shows large pulmonary arteries. An electrocardiogram shows Q waves in II, III, and aVF. Echocardiography with contrast shows enlargement of the right atrium and right ventricle as well as severe pulmonary arterial hypertension with an estimated systolic pulmonary artery pressure of 78 mm Hg. There is no evidence of mitral stenosis or an atrial septal defect. The left ventricle appears normal. Ventilation/perfusion lung scans show six segmental perfusion defects, with three matched and three mismatched abnormalities on the ventilation scan.

The most appropriate diagnostic recommendation at this time is:

(A) Transesophageal echocardiography
(B) Cardiac catheterization
(C) Methacholine challenge test
(D) Pulmonary angiography
(E) Helical CT scan of the chest

Chronic Obstructive Pulmonary Disease
Question 2

A 63-year-old woman presents because of recurrent episodes of right upper quadrant pain for 3 weeks. She also has cough productive of two tablespoons of sputum daily as well as exertional dyspnea when she hurries on level ground. She has been smoking two packs of cigarettes daily for 43 years.

On physical examination the intensity of breath sounds is diminished over all lung fields. She has tenderness to palpation in the right upper quadrant. Three years ago her forced expiratory volume in 1 second (FEV$_1$) of 1.12 L was 33% of predicted. The patient's oxygen saturation while she is breathing room air now is 92%. Ultrasonography of the abdomen shows two large gallstones.

The most appropriate management plan for this patient is:

(A) Laparoscopic cholecystectomy
(B) Preoperative spirometry and arterial blood studies
(C) Preoperative spirometry and total lung capacity measurement
(D) No surgery
(E) Preoperative spirometry, arterial blood studies, and measurement of single-breath carbon monoxide diffusing capacity (DLco)

Chronic Obstructive Pulmonary Disease
Questions 3-6
For each patient described below, select the most appropriate management option (A-E) (each answer may be used more than once or not at all):

(A) Room air arterial blood gas study
(B) Screening overnight pulse oximetry
(C) Room air arterial blood gas study and exercise pulse oximetry in 1 to 3 months
(D) Exercise pulse oximetry
(E) Indefinite continuous long-term oxygen therapy

3. A 62-year-old man with known severe chronic obstructive pulmonary disease presents to your office 2 days after discharge from the hospital where he was treated successfully with inhaled bronchodilators and oral corticosteroids for an acute exacerbation of chronic airflow obstruction. At hospital discharge, his exercise tolerance had returned to baseline (he could walk 50 yards in the hallway with mild dyspnea). Room air arterial blood gas studies on discharge showed PaO_2 of 44 mm Hg, $PaCO_2$ of 39 mm Hg, and pH of 7.43. Current medications include ipratropium, four puffs four times a day; albuterol, one to four puffs as needed; prednisone, 40 mg each day for 3 more days; and nasal oxygen, 2 L/min, to be increased by 1 L/min for exercise and sleep.

4. A 66-year-old man presents to your office for follow-up of chronic obstructive pulmonary disease. At a routine office visit 1 year ago he was noted to have a chronic productive cough, decreased intensity breath sounds in all lung fields, and a 100–pack-year smoking history. Spirometry confirmed severe airflow obstruction. Room air arterial blood gas studies showed PaO_2 of 47 mm Hg, $PaCO_2$ of 40 mm Hg, and pH of 7.42. The patient stopped smoking, intensive bronchodilator therapy was initiated, and long-term oxygen therapy with nasal oxygen, 2 L/min, was started. Room air arterial blood gas studies 3 months later showed PaO_2 of 50 mm Hg, $PaCO_2$ of 38 mm Hg, and pH of 7.40. Two weeks ago, preoperative room air blood gas studies showed PaO_2 of 58 mm Hg, $PaCO_2$ of 36 mm Hg, and pH of 7.44. The surgeon returns him to your office for re-evaluation of long-term oxygen therapy.

5. A 67-year-old woman who previously lived in another state presents to your office requesting a prescription for long-term oxygen therapy. She has a 5-year history of symptomatic chronic obstructive pulmonary disease. Despite smoking cessation and intensive therapy with inhaled ipratropium and albuterol and oral theophylline, she now experiences marked dyspnea and fatigue with household chores. Two weeks ago her previous physician did spirometry that confirmed severe airflow obstruction. Her hematocrit was 47%. Her room air arterial blood gas studies then showed PaO_2 of 58 mm Hg, $PaCO_2$ of 39 mm Hg, and pH of 7.41. She was started on oxygen therapy, 2 L/min 24 hours per day. She believes that her dyspnea and energy level are markedly improved after 2 weeks of oxygen therapy. Her physical examination is remarkable only for diffusely diminished breath sounds.

6. A 68-year-old woman presents to your office with a 6-year history of progressive exertional dyspnea associated with chronic cough productive of 15 mL of mucoid sputum each day. She has smoked three packs of cigarettes per day for 50 years. Her only current medication is albuterol, two puffs four times a day and as needed. Physical examination reveals a thin, cachectic woman with diffusely diminished breath sounds and expiratory wheezing in all lung fields but no other abnormalities. Hematocrit is 44%. Spirometry shows forced vital capacity (FVC) of 80% of predicted, forced expiratory volume in 1 sec (FEV_1) of 31% of predicted with no improvement after bronchodilators, and FEV_1/FVC ratio of 33%. Office pulse oximetry reveals oxygen saturation of 91%.

**Chronic Obstructive Pulmonary Disease
Questions 7-10**
For each patient described below, select the most likely flow-volume loop (A-D) (each answer can be used more than once or not at all):

(A)

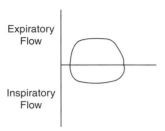

(B)

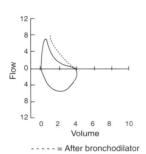

----- = After bronchodilator

(C)

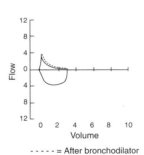

----- = After bronchodilator

(D)

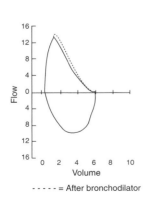

----- = After bronchodilator

7. A 34-year-old woman who has dyspnea at rest and hoarseness after being intubated for 20 days for aspiration pneumonia

8. A 70-year-old woman who smoked two packs of cigarettes daily for 50 years and who has severe exertional dyspnea and diminished intensity of breath sounds on chest auscultation

9. A 40-year-old male nonsmoker who has wheezing and a persistent cough accompanied by episodic dyspnea

10. A previously healthy 65-year-old man who has exertional dyspnea

**Chronic Obstructive Pulmonary Disease
Question 11**
A 59-year-old woman presents with obstructive lung disease. She has had progressive dyspnea with exercise to the point where she now becomes short of breath walking short distances. She has an FEV_1 of 0.82 L, which is 65% of predicted. She has no history of occupational exposures but does tell you that she had hay fever as a child and her father died of emphysema. She smoked one pack of cigarettes per day beginning at age 16 but she quit approximately 13 years ago.

Which one of the following test results is likely to differentiate emphysema from asthma in this patient?

(A) The presence of reversible component (>13% improvement of FEV_1) on pulmonary function testing after administration of albuterol by nebulizer
(B) Increased residual volume
(C) Decreased carbon dioxide diffusing capacity (DLco)
(D) Positive methacholine bronchial challenge
(E) Allergy skin testing

**Chronic Obstructive Pulmonary Disease
Questions 12-15**
A 75-year-old retired woman with chronic bronchitis presents to your office because of an acute exacerbation of her bronchitis. The patient has increased sputum volume of dark color and thick consistency. The patient also has diabetes mellitus, hypertension, peptic ulcer disease, and gastroparesis. Her medications include furosemide, cimetidine, and cisapride. You elect to treat the bronchitis with an antibiotic. Given her other medications, you must consider drug–drug interactions.

For each of the following potential adverse events select the most likely causal agent (A-D) (each answer may be used more than once or not at all):

(A) Ciprofloxacin
(B) Cephalexin
(C) Clarithromycin
(D) Norfloxacin

12. Ventricular arrhythmia

13. Theophylline toxicity

14. Clinical failure secondary to inadequate spectrum of activity

15. Clinical failure secondary to poor antibiotic concentration

Chronic Obstructive Pulmonary Disease
Question 16

A 69-year-old man with end-stage emphysema has severe persistent dyspnea at rest. He has no cough, chest pain, orthopnea, or edema. He has more than a 90–pack-year smoking history but quit smoking 3 years ago. He has a 9-year history of emphysema that is slowly progressing, and for the past 15 months has required 2 L of continuous oxygen. His medications include theophylline extended-release capsules, 300 mg twice daily; albuterol by metered-dose inhaler with a spacer device, two puffs four times daily; ipratropium bromide by metered-dose inhaler, four puffs four times daily; and furosemide, 20 mg/d. He uses the proper technique with the metered-dose inhalers. He was given an empirical trial of prednisone, 40 mg/d, for 2 weeks without significant improvement in his symptoms or results on spirometry.

The physical examination shows a barreled-chested thin man with a respiration rate of 22/min with pursed-lip and diaphragmatic breathing. His breath sounds are diffusely diminished without wheeze or rhonchi. The cardiac examination reveals a prominent P_2 without jugular venous distention. Arterial blood gases (with the patient receiving 2 L of oxygen) are pH, 7.36; Po_2, 62 mm Hg; and Pco_2, 52 mm Hg; Hco_3 is 29 meq/L, and oxygen saturation is 90%.

Chest roentgenogram show hyperinflated lungs with bullae but is otherwise normal. Spirometry shows forced expiratory volume in 1 second (FEV_1) of 500 mL, forced vital capacity (FVC) of 2.6 L, and FEV_1/FVC of 20%, with no significant response to bronchodilators.

The best therapy to manage this patient's symptoms is:

(A) Add beclomethasone by inhaler
(B) Substitute a hand-held nebulizer for the metered-dose inhaler to deliver his inhaled medications
(C) Begin a short-term trial of codeine, 30 to 60 mg every 6 hours as needed
(D) Increase the flow of oxygen to 3 L/min
(E) Give lorazepam, 1 mg three times daily as needed

COUGH

Cough Question 1

A 20-year-old woman with a history of atopic dermatitis has perennial symptoms of nasal congestion with nocturnal coughing. Her cat sleeps in her carpeted bedroom that contains several live plants. Nasal examination reveals bilateral boggy pale-blue mucosa; FEV_1 is 75% of predicted and FVC is 90% predicted. Examination of the chest is normal.

Which one of the following procedures would you do next to evaluate the patient's nasal congestion and cough?

(A) Total eosinophil count
(B) Total IgE level
(C) Skin testing to mite, mold, and animal dander
(D) Provocation–neutralization therapy

Cough Questions 2-5

For each patient with cough described below, select the most appropriate management option (A-E) (each answer may be used more than once or not at all):

(A) Obtain a chest roentgenogram
(B) Prescribe an antihistamine–decongestant
(C) Order a methacholine challenge test
(D) Prescribe trimethoprim–sulfamethoxazole
(E) Prescribe guaifenesin–dextromethorphan elixir

2. A 24-year-old man with no chronic medical problems presents with a nagging cough. One week ago, he developed rhinorrhea, sore throat, myalgias, and a dry cough. Some of the symptoms have resolved, but his cough is keeping him awake at night. He has been taking acetaminophen, cough lozenges, and oxymetazoline nasal spray. On examination, his temperature is 36.7 °C (98.2 °F), throat and tympanic membranes are normal, and there is no cervical adenopathy. Auscultation of his lungs is unremarkable.

3. A 32-year-old woman presents with a persistent cough for the past 3 months. She is a non-smoker, takes no chronic medications, and is otherwise healthy. She has noticed some rhinorrhea alternating with nasal congestion, and she takes occasional antacids for episodic dyspepsia. She denies dyspnea or wheezing. On examination, she is afebrile, and the nose, ears, throat, and lungs are normal.

4. A 64-year-old man with chronic bronchitis presents with 1 week of rhinorrhea, ear fullness, and worsening cough. Initially dry, his cough now is productive of a modest amount of yellowish-white sputum. His medications include inhaled ipratropium bromide four times daily, a β-adrenergic agonist inhaler as needed, and enalapril for chronic hypertension. On examination, his temperature is 36.5 °C (97.8 °F), his ears, throat, and nose are normal, and he has no sinus tenderness. He is barrel-chested with distant breath sounds diffusely and a few scattered rhonchi. There are no crackles or areas of dullness.

5. A 42-year-old man presents with an episodic but nagging cough for the past year. The cough is typically dry. He reports no nasal symptoms, dyspnea, wheezing, dyspepsia, or heartburn. He has seen several physicians previously, and trials of chlorpheniramine, pseudoephedrine, erythromycin, and terpin hydrate have failed. His physical examination is normal.

Cough Question 6

A 65-year-old man presents to your office with a 1-month history of cough. He has otherwise felt well and denies weight loss, chest or abdominal pain, headache, neurologic symptoms, and bone pain. He has a 55–pack-year history of smoking but stopped smoking approximately 4 years ago. Physical examination, including stool examination for occult blood, is normal.

Chest roentgenogram shows a 2.5-cm peripheral nodule in the right upper lobe; a comparison film from 8 years ago was normal. Spirometry shows an FEV_1 of 1.7 L (65% predicted) with an FVC of 3.0 L (75% predicted). Arterial blood gas results on FIO_2 of 0.21 are PO_2, 75 mm Hg; PCO_2, 42 mm Hg; and pH, 7.39. Chest CT scan shows a 2.5-cm peripheral lung mass and a 1.8-cm mediastinal lymph node in the pretracheal, retrocaval region. Laboratory data include hematocrit 41%, alkaline phosphatase 75 U/L, aspartate aminotransferase 34 U/L, alanine aminotransferase 26 U/L, and calcium 9.5 mg/dL.

The most appropriate plan at this time is:

(A) Quantitative perfusion lung scan
(B) Mediastinoscopy by a traditional suprasternal approach
(C) Wedge resection of the mass
(D) Right upper lobectomy
(E) Radiation therapy

Cough Question 7
As a part-time college health physician for a small community college, you are asked to consult with the nurse practitioner about a 19-year-old man with a chronic cough of 10 months' duration that is unresponsive to antihistamines, bronchodilators, and antibiotics. The young man reports no production with the cough and states that the cough is not exacerbated by exercise.

On examination, the patient is 5'5" and weighs 115 lb. Although thin, he appears healthy. He is afebrile, and lungs are clear. Examination of head, eyes, ears, nose, and throat is normal.

The patient should be investigated further for which one of the following?

(A) Postnasal drip
(B) Sarcoidosis
(C) Stress
(D) Cystic fibrosis
(E) Gastrointestinal reflux

DEPRESSION

Depression Question 1

A 72-year-old woman is brought to your office by her family because they are concerned that she has become "a hermit" and refuses to go out of her house. She formerly was mobile and active, worked in her yard, visited neighbors, and drove her car to go shopping. Three months ago, the patient had a minor automobile accident on the way to the grocery. Two months ago, while walking on an uneven drive-way, she fell and reports that she may have tripped. She says she no longer enjoys playing with her bridge club because she has trouble understanding her partner's bids. She reports diminished appetite and early morning awakening.

Physical examination shows moderately decreased visual acuity, presence of bilateral lens opacities, and impacted cerumen in both ears. The neurologic and the cardiovascular examinations are normal. All laboratory tests are normal, but electrocardiography shows occasional extra-systoles. You suspect this woman is depressed.

The most likely underlying cause for all of her symptoms is:

(A) Apathetic hyperthyroidism
(B) Alzheimer's disease
(C) Combined visual and hearing defects
(D) Sick sinus syndrome
(E) Labyrinthitis

Depression Question 2

A 60-year-old engineer is referred to you for evaluation of weight loss. He was well until 6 months earlier, when he noticed increasing fatigue, decreased appetite, loss of ability to concentrate, and an increasingly troublesome headache affecting the occiput and neck. The headache is relieved by lying down and sleeping, but it has been of such severity that he sleeps many hours during the day, yet rises fatigued. He is concerned about the possibility of brain tumor, and fears the onset of Alzheimer's disease; his work is suffering. He is particularly worried about becoming a burden to his wife and children, and no longer participates with them in former favored activities, such as going to the movies or dining out. He reports no delusions or hallucinations.

The patient takes no medications, and states that he does not use illicit or over-the-counter drugs. Physical examination, including complete blood count, is normal.

What is the next best step in the management of this patient?

(A) Measure antinuclear antibodies.
(B) Measure vitamin B_{12} and thyroid function.
(C) Obtain computed tomography of the brain.
(D) Begin therapeutic trial with a psychostimulant.
(E) Begin therapeutic trial with an antidepressant.

Depression Questions 3-5

For each patient described below, select the best therapy (A-D) (each answer can be used more than once or not at all):

(A) Immediate referral to a psychiatrist
(B) Antidepressant medication
(C) Short-acting benzodiazapine sleep medication
(D) Regular counseling by a primary care physician

3. A 26-year-old married woman who has been in good health has not slept for the past 5 nights and has been crying regularly. Her mother died 2 weeks ago and the patient has two young children at home. Physical examination is entirely normal. She is sad and cries easily. Her husband, who is with her, is very concerned.

4. A 45-year-old single man who has been in good health has had trouble sleeping at night and has been drinking heavily. His mother died 2 months ago. He says he has had thoughts of hurting himself. He is unshaven and disheveled, but physical examination is otherwise entirely normal.

5. A 30-year-old single woman comes to your office because of new onset of chest pain, which began shortly after she lost her job 2 weeks ago. The pain is nonexertional and seems to occur more often when she is home alone. She has also had trouble sleeping and has little energy. Her physical examination is normal.

Depression Question 6

A 36-year-old woman presents with chronic tiredness and difficulty sleeping. She denies any new stresses in her life, but worries about her two children, her house payments and other bills, her elderly mother's health, and her husband's recent job change. She is irritable and bothered by frequent headaches. Although she knows some of her worries are unreasonable, she cannot get her mind off them.

The most likely diagnosis in this patient is:

(A) Obsessive–compulsive disorder
(B) Major depression
(C) Adjustment disorder with anxious mood
(D) Hypochondriasis
(E) Generalized anxiety disorder

Depression Question 7

You are seeing a 74-year-old woman whose husband died of myocardial infarction 4 weeks ago. She does not feel like going out socially but has been receiving family and close friends. She stays in bed, in her room, or around the house most of the day. She feels somewhat depressed and has occasional difficulty falling asleep. She can describe the events leading up to her husband's death in detail, as well as the funeral and other events that occurred afterward. While crying somewhat, she expresses some guilt for not having had sufficient time to talk with her husband and for not realizing that he was so sick. She has no wish or plan to commit suicide.

The woman has been in good health and has not previously suffered from major depression or other psychological difficulties requiring treatment. She was married to her husband for 43 years, and they had two children: one, a daughter, lives in another state and visited for a week after the death; the other, a son, lives locally and has been in constant contact with his mother. The woman does not work but has been a volunteer at her church and several other activities. She currently does not feel like volunteering but thinks that she will probably resume doing so in several months.

Which one of the following statements best characterizes this patient's current condition?

(A) She is experiencing an acute grief reaction.
(B) Depression requiring treatment has likely become superimposed on her grief reaction.
(C) She has entered a period of fairly normal grieving, which may continue for 6 to 12 months.
(D) Her crying and inactivity suggest that she will likely have a complicated grief reaction.
(E) Her feelings of guilt suggest that grieving will be more prolonged and severe than is usual with normal bereavement.

Depression Question 8

A 63-year-old man comes to the office 3 months after having a large anterior wall myocardial infarction. His medications include a β-blocker and aspirin. The patient complains of overwhelming fatigue, loss of appetite, and difficulty sleeping for the past 2 months. Since his myocardial infarction, he has had trouble concentrating and has been quite anxious. He has no dyspnea on exertion, chest discomfort, palpitations, or edema.

On physical examination, the blood pressure is 160/72 mm Hg, pulse rate is 56/min and regular, and the respiration rate is 12/min. On auscultation of the chest, there are no crackles; the heart beat is regular and there are no murmurs or gallops. No edema is present.

At this time, you would:

(A) Stop the β-blocker
(B) Begin nortriptyline
(C) Begin methylphenidate
(D) Begin paroxetine
(E) Begin lorazepam

Depression Question 9

A 28-year-old man presents with persistent fatigue for the past 9 months. The clinical finding or test result most helpful in distinguishing major depression from chronic fatigue syndrome would be:

(A) Normal complete blood count
(B) Sleep disturbance
(C) Normal Epstein-Barr virus and other viral serologic titers
(D) Previous history of major depression
(E) Therapeutic response to antidepressant medication

Depression Questions 10-14
For each patient described below, select the most likely diagnosis (A-E) (each answer may be used more than once or not at all):

(A) Major depression
(B) Atypical major depression
(C) Seasonal affective disorder
(D) Depression not otherwise specified (NOS)
(E) Dysthymia

10. A 42-year-old woman admits to feeling depressed today. She describes episodes lasting for a few days several times each month on average, going back for many years. During these episodes she feels depressed but continues to function in her work as an accountant and does not suffer psychomotor retardation, suicidal ideation, worthlessness, guilt, or inability to concentrate. She has mild insomnia at times, and her weight and appetite are stable. When feeling depressed, she also feels mildly to moderately fatigued.

11. A 42-year-old woman felt well until about 6 weeks ago, when her brother with whom she is close was diagnosed with leukemia. Since then, she has been tired and has lost interest in her work and in reading and gardening. She has lost 5 to 10 pounds and is not interested in food. She tends to awaken about 4 or 5 AM and has difficulty falling back asleep. She denies being suicidal, though she admits to "normally" thinking of death at times.

12. A 42-year-old woman presents with her third episode of fatigue, loss of interest, and feeling depressed. The symptoms come each year around November. The patient is losing interest in her work, notes that her appetite is poor, and admits to awakening early in the morning and having difficulty falling asleep.

13. A 42-year-old woman presents with fatigue and a 6.8-kg (15-lb) weight gain. She says she tends to oversleep in the mornings, and on returning home from her work as an accountant, she finds herself constantly snacking and overeating. Her mood is labile, and she has burst into tears several times due to conflicts with fellow workers. She has trouble making decisions. She has also lost interest in gardening and reading and finds that nothing seems to give her pleasure.

14. A 42-year-old woman admits to being depressed off and on for a number of years. She has some intense episodes, similar to this one, lasting weeks to months at a time, but she is virtually always somewhat "down." She has mild insomnia, but in the past month has been awakening more often in the early morning and has difficulty returning to sleep. There has been no change in her weight or appetite. For a long time she has lacked much pleasure or exhilaration in life, but she denies having difficulty in concentrating more than occasionally, and denies any excessive guilt or thoughts of suicide.

DIABETES MELLITUS

Diabetes Mellitus Question 1

A 45-year-old man has had type 1 diabetes mellitus for 27 years. Three years ago, he was found to have background diabetic retinopathy, microalbuminuria, and hypertension. He was therefore changed from a conventional to an intensive treatment regimen with four injections of insulin daily. In the past year, he has noted complete loss of warning signs of hypoglycemia and has had two episodes of nocturnal hypoglycemia, requiring help from the emergency medical service. He has been treated with enalapril and metoprolol for his hypertension and because of a myocardial infarction 6 months ago.

On physical examination his blood pressure is 160/96 mm Hg. Hemoglobin A_{1c} is 6.1% (normal, 4.0% to 6.0%), and morning plasma cortisol is 20 µg/dL.

Which of the following is the best course of action?

(A) Continue an intensive insulin regimen; however, emphasize meticulously avoiding hypoglycemia for several months and allow hemoglobin A_{1c} to increase to 7.1%.
(B) Stop the intensive regimen and maintain hemoglobin A_{1c} around 9.0% by switching to a conventional program of two injections of NPH and regular insulin daily.
(C) Add an α-adrenergic antagonist to offset the blunting effect of the β-blocker on sensing and responding to hypoglycemia.
(D) Treat with a sympathomimetic drug such as ephedrine to restore autonomic catecholamine warning signs of hypoglycemia.

Diabetes Mellitus Question 2

A 32-year-old woman is admitted to the hospital in a semi-comatose, volume-depleted state, exhibiting marked air hunger. She has had type 1 diabetes mellitus for 12 years and ran out of insulin 3 days ago. Her plasma glucose is 1075 mg/dL, serum bicarbonate is 4.5 meq/L, and arterial blood gases include a Pco_2 of 23 mm Hg and a pH of 6.90. Serum potassium is 3.8 meq/L.

After 4 hours of treatment that includes standard doses of insulin (10 units/h), fluids, intravenous potassium chloride (10 meq/L), plus 150 meq/L of sodium bicarbonate, the patient's pH increases to 7.10. However, she suddenly develops respiratory failure followed by cardiac arrest.

What is the most likely therapeutic misjudgment?

(A) She was given too much potassium chloride and had suppression of all cardiac pacemaker activity.
(B) She was given too little potassium chloride and developed respiratory muscle paralysis followed by ventricular fibrillation.
(C) She was given too little insulin in the face of an unusually high plasma glucose concentration and developed cerebral edema.
(D) She was given too much bicarbonate, which led to cerebrospinal fluid acidosis and suppression of the brain stem respiratory center.
(E) She should have been given her potassium as potassium phosphate in order to prevent respiratory muscle paralysis from hypophosphatemia caused by insulin administration.

Diabetes Mellitus Question 3

A 56-year-old man presents with a 7-year history of type 2 diabetes mellitus. He has been taking glyburide since the onset of his diabetes, 10 mg in the morning and 5 mg in the evening. His height is 170 cm (67 in), and his weight is 106.8 kg (235 lb). His hemoglobin A_{1c} is 9.8 %, and fasting plasma glucose is 252 mg/dL.

Which of the following is most likely to improve his glycemia?

(A) Increase glyburide to 10 mg twice daily.
(B) Substitute metformin, 500 mg three times daily, for the glyburide.
(C) Substitute NPH insulin, 30 units every morning, for the glyburide.
(D) Decrease glyburide to just 10 mg every morning, and add NPH insulin, 20 units at bedtime.
(E) Add acarbose, 100 mg before each meal, to his glyburide.

Diabetes Mellitus Question 4

A previously well 26-year-old man presents with 4 weeks of polyuria and polydipsia that were followed by 36 hours of nausea and vomiting, culminating in 8 hours of stupor. On physical examination he is hypotensive and volume-depleted and has Kussmaul's respiration. His plasma glucose is 640 mg/dL, Pco_2 is 16 mm Hg, and arterial pH is 6.95. Serum electrolytes show potassium of 3.9 meq/L, bicarbonate of 6 meq/L, anion gap of 26, and phosphorus of 3.0 mg/dL. After 8 hours of insulin infusion at 10 U/h, potassium chloride administration at 10 meq/h, and fluid resuscitation, his blood pressure has normalized, and his plasma glucose has decreased to 82 mg/dL, potassium has decreased to 3.1 meq/L, bicarbonate has increased to 16 meq/L, and phosphorus has decreased to 0.9 mg/dL. The patient now has muscle pain and a creatine kinase level of 2000 U/mL.

What is the most appropriate treatment now?

(A) Discontinue insulin and give 50 mL of 50% glucose and 10 meq/h potassium phosphate as a bolus.
(B) Decrease insulin to 5 U/h, change fluids to 5% glucose in 0.45% saline, and increase potassium chloride to 15 meq/h.
(C) Continue insulin at 10 U/h, change intravenous fluids to 10% glucose in water, and continue potassium chloride at 10 meq/h.
(D) Decrease insulin to 1 U/h, change fluid to 10% glucose, and increase potassium chloride to 15 meq/h.
(E) Decrease insulin to 1 U/h, change fluid to 5% glucose in 0.45% saline, and give 80 mmol of phosphate as potassium phosphate over the next 6 hours.

Diabetes Mellitus Question 5
A 48-year-old man presents with a 6-week history of polyuria, polydipsia, fatigue, and muscle weakness. He has lost 22.7 kg (50 lb) in the preceding 6 months without dieting. He denies symptoms of infection. He has no family history of diabetes. On physical examination, he is 172.7 cm (68 in) tall and weighs 93 kg (205 lb). His body mass index is 32. He has no signs of Cushing's syndrome or acromegaly. Hemoglobin A_{1c} is 13%, fasting plasma glucose is 352 mg/dL, and thyroid function test results are normal. Urinalysis shows 5% glucose and moderate ketones. After stimulation with glucagon, his C-peptide level is 0.3 nM.

Which one of the following statements regarding his diabetes is correct?

(A) He has type 1 diabetes mellitus and will require permanent insulin treatment.
(B) He has type 2 diabetes mellitus and should be treated initially with a weight reduction diet to ameliorate his obesity.
(C) He has type 2 diabetes mellitus, and metformin is the drug of choice because it will facilitate weight loss.
(D) He has type 2 diabetes mellitus and will almost certainly respond to a conventional starting dose of a sulfonylurea drug.
(E) It is unclear whether he has type 1 or type 2 diabetes mellitus, but his history and current metabolic state indicate an initial need for insulin treatment.

Diabetes Mellitus Question 6
A 29-year-old woman, gravida III para II, is referred to you because she was found to have gestational diabetes on routine screening 26 weeks into her third pregnancy. She has no family history of diabetes. Her previous pregnancies were uncomplicated, and the infant birth weights were normal.

Which of the following should you tell her?

(A) If she requires insulin treatment, she will likely be switched to an oral hypoglycemic drug after delivery.
(B) She is at no increased risk of developing diabetes later in life because her family and obstetrical histories are negative.
(C) Her child may be born small for gestational age if she does not control her plasma glucose.
(D) Her child will need monitoring for diabetes starting at birth.
(E) A glucose tolerance test done at 6 to 8 weeks post partum will likely show her to be nondiabetic.

Diabetes Mellitus Question 7
A 54-year-old man with alcoholism and type 2 diabetes mellitus treated with glyburide, 20 mg/d, is brought to the emergency room in a coma after a 24-hour drinking binge, during which he reportedly ate nothing. His plasma glucose is 18 mg/dL.

The preferred management of this patient is:

(A) Administer 25 to 50 g of glucose intravenously, followed by a high-carbohydrate meal, observation for 4 hours, and discharge.
(B) Administer 25 g of glucose intravenously, followed by 5% glucose in water at 80 mL/h for 4 hours, and discharge.
(C) Administer 1 mg of glucagon intravenously or subcutaneously every hour for 4 hours, followed by a high-carbohydrate meal, and discharge.
(D) Administer 25 g of glucose and 100 mg of hydrocortisone intravenously, followed by a high-carbohydrate meal, and discharge.
(E) Administer 25 g of glucose intravenously, followed by hospital admission and a maintenance infusion of 10% glucose in water.

Diabetes Mellitus Question 8

A 43-year-old woman who has had type 1 diabetes mellitus for 26 years has early satiety, nausea, frequent vomiting after meals, and constipation. Her weight has decreased 2.7 kg (6.0 lb) in the past 3 months. She has noted increasing episodes of hypoglycemia, some of them symptomatic. Physical examination shows pulse rate of 90/min, supine, and 92/min, standing, and blood pressure of 144/88 mm Hg, supine, and 106/62 mm Hg, standing. Medications include long-acting verapamil, 240 mg daily, and enalapril, 15 mg daily.

Laboratory studies:

Hemoglobin A_{1c}	8.1%
Blood urea nitrogen	52 mg/dL
Serum potassium	5.6 meq/L
Serum creatinine	3.4 mg/dL

Which of the following is most likely to relieve her symptoms?

(A) Dialysis
(B) Changing the verapamil to labetalol
(C) Doxycycline
(D) Metoclopramide
(E) Ranitidine

Diabetes Mellitus Question 9

A 26-year-old traveling salesman who has had type 1 diabetes mellitus for 12 years has been taking 14 units of NPH insulin at breakfast and 6 units before supper. He takes regular insulin in doses ranging from 2 to 12 units before breakfast, lunch, and supper, depending on premeal blood glucose. Recent average self-monitored blood glucose levels are 112 mg/dL before breakfast, 52 mg/dL before lunch, 205 mg/dL before supper, and 68 mg/dL at bedtime. He has hypoglycemic symptoms before lunch and the need to eat a large snack at 1600 h and at bedtime. You ask him to determine blood glucose levels 1.5 hours after breakfast and after supper and find averages of 281 mg/dL and 310 mg/dL, respectively. His hemoglobin A_{1c} is 8.2%.

Which of the following is most likely to improve his blood glucose profile?

(A) Decrease his morning NPH dose.
(B) Move his evening NPH dose to bedtime.
(C) Change his regular insulin to lisproinsulin.
(D) Increase his regular insulin dose at breakfast, lunch, and supper.

Diabetes Mellitus Question 10

Which of the following statements is true about the use of angiotensin-converting enzyme (ACE) inhibitors on angiotensin II receptor antagonists in diabetic patients?

(A) ACE inhibitors, when compared with other antihypertensive agents, have been shown to reduce proteinuria and delay the progression of renal disease in type I insulin-dependent diabetic patients.
(B) ACE inhibitors have not been shown to prevent the development of proteinuria in type II adult-onset diabetic patients who are normotensive and who have microalbuminuria.
(C) Common side effects of ACE inhibitors include cough and hypokalemia.
(D) Common side effects of angiotensin II receptor antagonists include cough and hyperkalemia.

Diabetes Mellitus Question 11

Which one of the following statements about microalbuminuria in the clinical care of diabetic patients is correct?

(A) Microalbuminuria is considered abnormal when the urine excretion of albumin exceeds 30 mg/d (> 15 µg/min) on two consecutive measurements.

(B) Microalbuminuria is a unique small–molecular-weight prealbumin found in the urine of diabetic patients.

(C) Abnormal microalbumin concentrations in a juvenile-onset diabetic patient have not yet been shown to be a marker for future diabetic nephropathy.

(D) Microalbuminuria is not present if the routine urinalysis is negative for protein.

Diabetes Mellitus Question 12

In the United States, the major cause of renal failure in patients who start dialysis is:

(A) Chronic glomerulonephritis
(B) Hypertension
(C) Chronic interstitial nephritis
(D) Diabetes mellitus
(E) Polycystic kidney disease

Deep Venous Thrombosis

Deep Venous Thrombosis Question 1

A 33-year-old woman in the thirtieth week of an otherwise normal pregnancy presents with a painful right leg. There is no history of either trauma or insect bites, although she and her husband were camping in a state park 2 weeks ago. Physical examination reveals normal pulse and blood pressure. The lungs are clear to percussion and auscultation. The mean jugular venous pressure is 9 cm H_2O. S_1 is single and normal in intensity; S_2 splits normally, with the aortic valve component louder than the pulmonic valve component. A grade 2/6 systolic crescendo-decrescendo murmur is heard at the second left interspace. No diastolic murmurs or gallops are heard. The abdomen is gravid. The right leg is swollen and tender at the level of the calf, where there is mild to moderate tenderness. Homans' sign is positive in the right leg. There is 2+ pitting edema of the right leg and 1+ pitting edema of the left leg.

An electrocardiogram is normal. The patient is sent for emergent venous ultrasonography of her lower extremities, and 2 hours later the radiologist reports that she has deep venous thrombosis of the veins in the right leg.

What is the most appropriate next step for this patient?

(A) Intravenous heparin for 7 days followed by warfarin
(B) Intravenous heparin until the conclusion of pregnancy
(C) An inferior vena cava filter
(D) A venogram

Deep Venous Thrombosis Question 2

You are asked to see a 47-year-old man who was hospitalized because he developed a proximal deep venous thrombosis following a 1-hour airplane flight. He has no risk factors for venous thromboembolism besides the 1-hour flight. The patient has been otherwise healthy and has had no weight loss, fevers, or excessive fatigue, and he does not smoke or drink.

A review of his family history indicates that a maternal uncle had a venous thrombosis following hip replacement surgery at age 72 years, and his paternal grandfather had a major stroke at age 68 years.

Physical examination shows a trim, healthy-appearing man, 187 cm (74 in) tall and weighing 79.5 kg (175 lb). Findings on the chest and abdominal examinations are normal. His leg is mildly swollen, and the calf is tender to deep palpation.

Laboratory studies:

Protein C activity	69%
Protein S activity	85%
Antithrombin III activity	81%
Activated protein C resistance assay	2.4
Fibrinogen concentration	434 mg/dL
Homocysteine	8.6 µmol/L
Prothrombin time	12.1 sec
Activated partial thromboplastin time	30.6 sec

Hexagonal phospholipid neutralization test (for a lupus anticoagulant) is negative. In addition, findings on a complete blood count are normal, stool guaiac test for occult blood is negative, and findings on chest radiography are normal.

For how long and at what intensity should this patient be treated with oral anticoagulant therapy?

(A) Six months, international normalized ratio (INR) of 2 to 3
(B) Six weeks, INR of 2 to 3
(C) Three months, INR of 2 to 3
(D) Six months, INR of 2.5 to 3.5
(E) Lifelong treatment, INR of 1.5 to 2, plus 325 mg of aspirin daily

Deep Venous Thrombosis Question 3

A 56-year-old previously healthy man presents to your office because of the development of painful swelling in his left calf after a vigorous game of racquetball. He has no history of venous thromboembolism, and he has no chest pain or shortness of breath. He smokes a pack of cigarettes per day and drinks two highballs before dinner each night.

Findings on physical examination are normal, except for edema, calf tenderness, and a dusky discoloration of his left lower leg. Pulses are intact bilaterally. The results of a complete blood count and a prothrombin time and activated partial thromboplastin time are normal.

Ultrasonography shows a deep venous thrombosis involving the calf and popliteal veins on the left. The patient adamantly refuses hospitalization for treatment of his deep venous thrombosis because he is too busy at the office.

An appropriate regimen of home treatment for deep venous thrombosis would include:

(A) Heparin, 5000 units every 12 h subcutaneously, plus warfarin, 15 mg started immediately
(B) Aspirin, 325 mg, and warfarin, 15 mg, both administered immediately
(C) Low–molecular-weight heparin administered in prophylactic doses (for example, enoxaparin, 30 mg subcutaneously every 12 h) and warfarin, 15 mg started immediately
(D) Low–molecular-weight heparin in subcutaneous therapeutic doses, monitored with daily heparin assays (anti-Xa) for the first 3 days, plus warfarin, 15 mg started that evening
(E) Low–molecular-weight heparin given in subcutaneous therapeutic doses with no laboratory heparin monitoring, plus warfarin, 5 to 10 mg started that evening

Deep Venous Thrombosis Question 4

A 62-year-old man presents with sudden arterial oxygen desaturation, shortness of breath, and pain in his posterior chest 3 days after he underwent four-vessel coronary artery bypass graft surgery for extensive coronary artery disease. He has been maintained postoperatively with subcutaneous heparin for deep venous thrombosis prophylaxis.

Physical examination shows him to be comfortable and in no acute distress. His pulse is 86/min and regular, and his blood pressure is normal at 120/80 mm Hg. Examination of his right posterior chest shows an intermittent friction rub. Cardiac examination is normal. There is no evidence of splenomegaly.

Laboratory studies show a hematocrit of 31%, a leukocyte count of 16,500/μL, and a platelet count of 56,000/μL. A heparin-induced thrombocytopenia test is strongly positive. Pulmonary angiography shows a right-sided, moderate-sized pulmonary embolus. Duplex ultrasonography of the right lower extremity reveals a proximal deep venous thrombosis.

What therapy should be started after the subcutaneous heparin is stopped?

(A) Administer therapeutic doses of intravenous heparin along with platelet transfusions to increase the platelet count to greater than 100,000/μL.
(B) Insert an inferior vena cava filter below the renal veins, administer danaparoid (a heparinoid), and start oral anticoagulant agents.
(C) Give a bolus of intravenous streptokinase to lyse pulmonary emboli, followed by antiplatelet therapy with ticlopidine to block platelet aggregation.
(D) Administer therapeutic doses of subcutaneous low–molecular-weight heparin.
(E) Stop all antithrombotic therapy, remove heparin-coated catheters, and begin low-dose aspirin plus standard-dose ticlopidine.

Deep Venous Thrombosis Question 5

You are asked to evaluate a 27-year-old woman with a 10-year history of systemic lupus erythematosus (SLE) who was admitted to the hospital for her third episode of deep venous thrombosis. She has no history of excessive bleeding. She has been treated in the past with plaquenil and low doses of prednisone, and her previous episodes of venous thrombosis were treated with heparin followed by warfarin for 3 to 6 months.

Physical examination shows evidence of a left deep venous thrombosis. In addition, her left knee is slightly swollen and warm. Laboratory studies are obtained before antithrombotic treatment is started.

Laboratory studies:

Hematocrit	32%
Mean corpuscular volume	79 fL
Leukocyte count	7600/μL
Platelet count	135,000/μL
Prothrombin time	13.6 sec
Activated partial thromboplastin time	43 sec
Serum creatinine	1.5 mg/dL
Urinalysis	Protein 1+

Confirmatory studies show that the prolonged activated partial thromboplastin time (aPTT) is due to the presence of a lupus anticoagulant.

Standard heparin is started with a 5000-unit bolus along with 1200 U/h intravenously by continuous infusion. An aPTT 6 hours later is more than 120 seconds.

What is the best way to administer and monitor heparin therapy in this patient?

(A) Stop heparin therapy for 1 hour, then decrease the heparin infusion to 1000 U/h, and repeat the aPTT in 6 hours.
(B) Do a heparin (anti-Xa) assay on the plasma sample with the aPTT more than 120 seconds. If the heparin level is within therapeutic range, continue heparin at that dose regardless of the aPTT.
(C) Progressively decrease the dose of heparin and aim for an aPTT range of 80 to 100 seconds.
(D) Stop heparin, insert an inferior vena cava filter, and start warfarin, 15 mg orally.
(E) Stop heparin and administer low–molecular-weight heparin in therapeutic doses with monitoring to achieve an aPTT of 1.5 to 2.0 times the control.

Deep Venous Thrombosis Question 6
A 37-year-old woman who is 6 months pregnant develops superficial phlebitis of the greater saphenous vein approximately 2 cm above the knee. The vein is firm, red, warm, and tender to palpation.

The optimal management of this patient's condition would be:

(A) Surgical consultation to ligate the greater saphenous vein
(B) Constant-infusion heparin therapy
(C) Ultrasonography of the greater saphenous vein and local therapy
(D) Thrombolytic therapy
(E) Aspirin therapy

Deep Venous Thrombosis Question 7
A 65-year-old man with a history of myocardial infarction complicated by left ventricular failure presents to the emergency room with shortness of breath that began today. He underwent resection of an adenocarcinoma of the colon 12 days ago.

On physical examination he appears to be in moderate distress; his pulse rate is 112/min, respiration rate is 30/min, and blood pressure is 112/70 mm Hg. Chest examination reveals diminished breath sounds over the right posterolateral chest and a few late inspiratory crackles at the base of the right and left lungs. The point of maximal impulse is in the anterior axillary line, and a grade 2/6 holosystolic murmur can be heard best at the apex with radiation to the axilla. There is 1+ bilateral pitting edema of the lower extremities and no calf tenderness.

Arterial blood gas studies:

Pa_{O_2}	51 mm Hg
Pa_{CO_2}	28 mm Hg
pH	7.47
$P(A-a)_{O_2}$	64 mm Hg

A chest radiograph shows a small right pleural effusion, volume loss in the right lower lobe, and mild bilateral perihilar lung edema. An electrocardiogram shows sinus tachycardia with no acute changes. Lung ventilation-perfusion scan results indicate a low probability for acute pulmonary embolism.

What is the most appropriate diagnostic test for this patient?

(A) Serial impedance plethysmography
(B) Compression duplex ultrasonography of both lower extremities
(C) Surface echocardiography
(D) Pulmonary angiography
(E) Diuretics, oxygen, and a repeat chest radiograph in 24 hours

Deep Venous Thrombosis Questions 8-11
For each patient described below, select the most appropriate management strategy (A-E) (each answer may be used more than once or not at all):

(A) Treat as an outpatient with enoxaparin, 1 mg/kg subcutaneously every 12 h for at least 5 days, overlapped with warfarin (titrated to international normalized ratio [INR] of 2.0 to 3.0) for at least 4 days. Continue warfarin for 6 months. Then discontinue warfarin after re-evaluation.
(B) Treat as an inpatient with therapeutic intravenous heparin for at least 5 days, overlapped with warfarin (titrated to INR of 2.0 to 3.0) for at least 4 days. Continue warfarin for 6 months. Then discontinue warfarin after re-evaluation.
(C) Treat as an inpatient with therapeutic intravenous heparin for at least 5 days, overlapped with warfarin (titrated to INR of 2.0 to 3.0) for at least 4 days. Continue warfarin for 3 months. Then re-evaluate before discontinuing warfarin.
(D) Test for factor V Leiden (activated protein C resistance) after at least 3 months of warfarin and after warfarin has been discontinued. Give inpatient therapeutic intravenous heparin for at least 5 days and titrate warfarin to INR of 2.0 to 3.0. Maintain therapeutic warfarin indefinitely.
(E) Treat as an inpatient with therapeutic intravenous heparin for at least 5 days, overlapped with warfarin (titrated to INR of 2.0 to 3.0) for at least 4 days. Maintain therapeutic warfarin indefinitely.

8. A 15-year-old boy, an adopted child, presents with a swollen, painful left leg. Routine laboratory studies, including complete blood count and urinalysis, and chest radiograph are normal. Acute proximal deep venous thrombosis (DVT) involving the popliteal vein is confirmed by compression ultrasonography.

9. A 35-year-old woman who takes oral contraceptives develops a swollen right leg 3 days after right knee arthroscopy. She took nonsteroidal anti-inflammatory drugs for a month before her arthroscopy. Physical examination discloses a large hematoma at the arthroscopy site. Edema extends from the right ankle to the mid tibia. Routine laboratory studies, including complete blood count and urinalysis, and chest radiograph are normal. Compression ultrasonography confirms acute proximal DVT.

10. A 74-year-old woman who lives alone in a small mountain community had symptomatic acute proximal DVT of the left leg confirmed by compression ultrasonography 1 year ago. Nine months ago her anticoagulant medication (warfarin) was discontinued. Her routine mammogram and Papanicolaou smear 6 months ago were normal. Now she has swelling of the right calf. Routine laboratory studies, including complete blood count, chemistry profile, and urinalysis, are normal. Compression ultrasonography confirms extensive proximal DVT.

11. A previously healthy 80-year-old man presents with a swollen left leg 2 days after flying across the United States to visit his grandchildren. On physical examination he appears pale, and his left leg is swollen. Routine laboratory studies show anemia (hemoglobin of 9.7 g/dL) and thrombocytopenia (platelet count of 110,000/µL), with a normal urinalysis and chest radiograph. Compression ultrasonography confirms acute proximal DVT.

DYSPNEA

Dyspnea Question 1

A 56-year-old man with a 25-year history of severe rheumatoid arthritis presents to your office for routine follow-up. He has noted decreased exercise capacity and progressive edema for the past 6 weeks. He has no nocturnal dyspnea, but he has progressive fatigue and some dyspnea while walking.

Physical examination shows a thin man with evidence of muscle wasting. His pulse rate is 120/min, respiration rate is 18/min, and blood pressure is 110/60 mm Hg. There is no paradoxical pulse. The jugular venous pressure is 14 cm of water, with a slight increase upon inspiration. The lungs are clear. Cardiac examination is normal except for tachycardia. The liver is palpable 3 cm below the right costal margin. No other abdominal organs are palpable. There are changes of deforming rheumatoid arthritis in the hands and feet, with rheumatoid nodules over both olecranon processes. He has 3+ pitting edema bilaterally.

The most likely diagnosis is:

(A) Pulmonary hypertension
(B) Bronchiolitis obliterans
(C) Inflammatory cardiomyopathy
(D) Constrictive pericarditis
(E) Cryptogenic cirrhosis

Dyspnea Question 2

A 26-year-old man presents for a pre-employment physical examination. He reports persistent fatigue after a viral upper respiratory illness 4 weeks ago and notes a decline in exercise capacity. Although he previously ran 5 miles per day without difficulty, he now feels dyspneic after 2 to 3 miles of vigorous running. There is no history of dizziness, syncope, or palpitations. He denies any previous medical illness and alcohol or drug usage.

Physical examination reveals a well-appearing, muscular man. His pulse rate is 94/min and slightly irregular, and his blood pressure is 100/60 mm Hg. The chest is clear to auscultation and percussion. The point of maximal intensity is diffuse and laterally displaced. An S_4 gallop and a grade 1/6 systolic murmur are audible at the apex. The abdomen and extremities are normal.

The patient's chest radiograph shows cardiomegaly (cardiac:thoracic ratio of 0.55) and clear lung fields. An electrocardiogram shows sinus rhythm, frequent premature ventricular contractions, left atrial enlargement, intraventricular conduction defects, poor R-wave progression, and nonspecific ST- and T-wave abnormalities. An echocardiogram shows global left and right ventricular hypokinesis, left ventricular end-diastolic dimension of 60 mm, and left ventricular ejection fraction of 32%.

Initial medical treatment should consist of which of the following?

(A) Furosemide
(B) Enalapril
(C) Digoxin
(D) Amiodarone
(E) β-blocker

Dyspnea Question 3

A 28-year-old woman presents with mild exertional dyspnea and fatigue that she has noted for the past 6 months. She has recently completed law school and is now employed in a firm where her duties require an occasional 10-hour day. She has always been active physically, but 4 months ago she gave up bicycling on weekends because she was becoming winded while cycling. Initially, she blamed her symptoms on her work, but recently she has noted mild dyspnea while carrying grocery packages. Her medical history is remarkable for a heart murmur noted on occasions when she visited her pediatrician. She was advised that this murmur was "functional" in nature and was never told to restrict her activities.

Physical examination reveals a well-developed, well-nourished woman. Her pulse rate is 85/min, and blood pressure is 120/60 mm Hg. There is no cyanosis or clubbing. The lungs are clear. Jugular venous pressure is 8 cm H_2O. There is a prominent precordial impulse at the lower left sternal border. S_1 is single; S_2 is widely split. The aortic and pulmonic components are equal in intensity. A grade 2–6 systolic crescendo-decrescendo murmur is noted at the second-to-third left interspace. There are no diastolic murmurs or gallops. The liver is not enlarged, and there is no edema.

The patient's electrocardiogram and chest radiographs are shown.

What is the most likely diagnosis?

(A) Atrial septal defect
(B) Ventricular septal defect
(C) Valvular pulmonic stenosis
(D) Patent ductus arteriosus

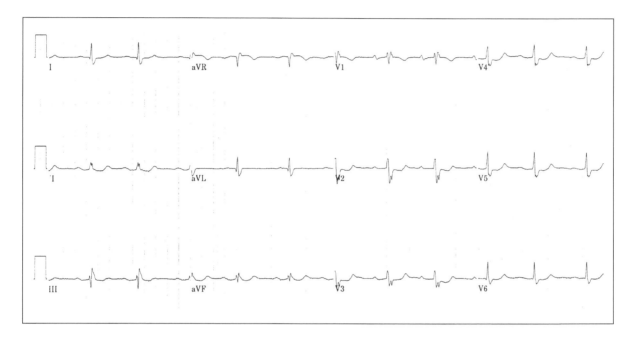

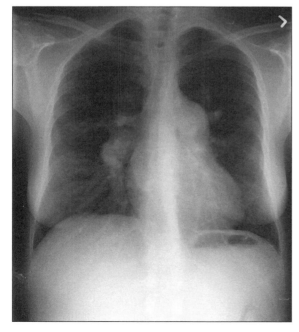

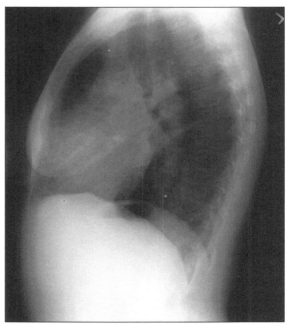

Dyspnea Questions 4-7

For the patients described below, select the pleural fluid results (A-E) that correlate with the most likely cause of pleural effusion (each answer may be used more than once or not at all):

	Appearance	Serum Protein (g/dL)	Fluid Protein (g/dL)	Serum LDH (U/L)	Fluid LDH (U/L)	Glucose (mg/dL)	pH	Amylase
(A)	Purulent	7.3	5.0	196	1000	30	7.10	Pleural fluid = serum
(B)	Hemorrhagic	6.4	3.0	160	60	80	7.38	Pleural fluid = serum
(C)	Turbid, with debris	7.1	4.0	280	1000	50	7.00	Pleural fluid = serum
(D)	Serosanguineous	6.8	1.5	272	1000	55	7.29	Pleural fluid > serum
(E)	Purulent	6.2	4.0	240	500	100	6.00	Pleural fluid > serum

4.   A patient with nephrotic syndrome develops acute dyspnea and presents with a unilateral pleural effusion.

5.   A 56-year-old woman with widely disseminated ovarian carcinoma presents with exertional dyspnea and bilateral pleural effusions that have increased over several months.

6.   A 60-year-old man presents with painful, swollen joints and an asymptomatic pleural effusion.

7.   A 56-year-old man presents with retching, severe chest pain, and a left-sided minimal pleural effusion.

Dyspnea Question 8

A 30-year-old man traveling in Colorado comes to the mountain infirmary, at which you are a consultant, with marked dyspnea and fatigue. He is from the Midwest and is vacationing with his family at a resort (peak, 9500 feet [2900 meters]). His symptoms began within a few hours of his first day snow skiing. The patient does not exercise regularly, is otherwise healthy, and has never experienced this degree of shortness of breath previously. His temperature is 36.8 °C (98 °F); pulse rate is 120/min; respiration rate is 24/min; and blood pressure is 160/94 mm Hg. Physical examination reveals diffuse lung crackles, but no heart murmur or gallop is heard. No lower extremity edema is present, and the electrocardiogram is normal.

Which one of the following is the best immediate intervention?

(A) Intravenous corticosteroids
(B) Intravenous saline
(C) Intravenous furosemide
(D) Oral acetazolamide
(E) Descent to lower altitude

Dyspnea Question 9

A 62-year-old man with severe community-acquired pneumonia requires intubation and mechanical ventilation. During the first several hours of ventilation, he develops progressive hypoxemia, hypotension (90/55 mm Hg), and oliguria, requiring placement of a pulmonary artery catheter. His most recent arterial blood gases on 60% fraction of inspired oxygen (F_{IO_2}) are as follows: Pao_2, 55 mm Hg; $Paco_2$, 35 mm Hg; pH, 7.32; and hemoglobin oxygen saturation, 85%. His blood hemoglobin concentration is 9 g/dL, lactate is 7 mg/dL, pulmonary artery occlusion pressure (PA_{OP}) is 5 mm Hg; and cardiac output is 3.0 L/min.

Which of the following interventions would produce the largest increase in his oxygen delivery (DO_2)?

(A) Institute volume infusion to increase the cardiac output to 4 L/min.
B   Add positive end-expiratory pressure (PEEP) to increase the hemoglobin oxygen saturation to 90%.
(C) Transfuse packed erythrocytes to raise the hemoglobin to 10 g/dL.
(D) Increase the F_{IO_2} to raise the hemoglobin oxygen saturation to 95%.
(E) Increase the minute ventilation to raise the pH to 7.40.

Dyspnea Question 10

A 35-year-old woman presents because of feeling light-headed while carrying her groceries up the stairs to her apartment. She also notes that she has become progressively short of breath over the last 3 months when going on walks with her husband. She has taken oral contraceptives for the past 10 years. She has no history of rheumatic fever, nor does she have orthopnea or paroxysmal nocturnal dyspnea.

On physical examination she appears healthy but overweight (body mass index = 32). Auscultatory findings include a parasternal heave just to the left of the sternum and an increase in the intensity of P_2, but the patient is clearly anxious at the time of this examination.

The chest radiograph is normal, and the electrocardiogram shows a tall R wave in lead V_1 and a deep S wave in lead V_6.

What is the most appropriate procedure for further evaluation of this patient?

(A) Spirometry
(B) Exercise electrocardiography
(C) Antinuclear antibody test
(D) Surface echocardiography
(E) Pulmonary angiography

Dyspnea Question 11

A 37-year-old woman comes to the emergency room for evaluation of sore throat, dyspnea, and a change in her voice (muffled). The dyspnea developed over the past 60 minutes. Her symptoms began 3 days ago as an isolated sore throat and have progressed over the last 24 hours. Her medications include oral contraceptive pills and cimetidine. On physical examination, the patient is anxious with an upright posture and a respiration rate of 20/min. No cervical adenopathy is present and the pharynx is mildly erythematous. Chest auscultation is normal.

The most appropriate next step in the evaluation of this patient is:

(A) Lateral neck radiographs
(B) Computed tomography of the neck
(C) Ventilation-perfusion scan
(D) Indirect laryngoscopy
(E) Lower-extremity duplex ultrasonography

Dyspnea Question 12

A 25-year-old pregnant woman with allergic rhinitis and asthma who is receiving maintenance immunotherapy and intermittent oral theophylline has been experiencing exacerbations of asthma more than three times a week. She asks about additional therapy to control the symptoms.

Which of the following would you recommend to this patient?

(A) Inhaled ipratropium bromide, two inhalations four times daily
(B) Oral low-dose corticosteroids
(C) Inhaled terbutaline or albuterol as needed with a regular schedule inhaled cromolyn sodium or beclomethasone dipropionate
(D) No form of inhaled therapy is appropriate

Dyspnea Questions 13-15

You are working in the emergency room, and the patients with asthma described below present themselves; for each patient, select the best treatment strategy (A-E) (each answer may be used more than once or not at all). (Proper arrangement for follow-up is assumed.)

(A) β_2-Agonist metered-dose inhaler (MDI)
(B) β_2-Agonist MDI and corticosteroid MDI on a regular schedule
(C) An outpatient course of systemic corticosteroids
(D) Nebulized β_2-agonist, systemic corticosteroids, and immediate hospitalization
(E) β_2-Agonist MDI and oral theophylline on a regular schedule based on blood level of the drug

13. A 35-year-old man with a 12-year history of asthma reports gradually increasing symptoms over the past 3 days, with severe dyspnea preventing sleep last night. He is sweating and sitting up on the examination table and is reluctant to lie down. His temperature is 37 °C (98.6 °F), pulse rate is 120/min, and respiration rate is 35/min. He is severely dyspneic on examination and wheezes are present. FEV_1 is 30% of predicted, P_{O_2} is 70 mm Hg, P_{CO_2} is 42 mm Hg, and pH is 7.45.

14. An 18-year-old male athlete states that he developed acute dyspnea and wheezing while he was recovering from a 10-minute conditioning run. The attack lasted about 10 minutes and terminated shortly after a mild coughing spell. Similar but milder episodes have occurred with exertion one to four times per month. He was sent to the emergency department by his coach. He appears to be comfortable; vital signs are normal; and examination of the chest is unremarkable. FEV_1 is 110% of predicted.

15. A 55-year-old male ex-smoker with a chart diagnosis of chronic obstructive pulmonary disease (COPD) has had increased exertional dyspnea and cough over the past week. He is

taking ipratropium bromide and intermittent short-acting β_2 agonist as needed. Sputum is minimal and clear. He has not smoked for 5 years. The symptoms are sufficiently bothersome to interfere with his work and seem to be progressing. He does not sleep well, but does not attribute this to breathlessness. His temperature is 37.2 °C (99 °F), pulse rate is 76/min, respiration rate is 20/min, and blood pressure is 135/80 mm Hg. He appears to be comfortable at rest. Chest examination reveals a few bilateral rhonchi and somewhat diminished breath sounds over both bases. FEV_1 is 50% of predicted, and FEV_1/FVC is 0.60. Chest radiograph is normal except for hyperlucency and a flattened diaphragm.

Dyspnea Question 16

A definitive diagnosis of asthma is established by which one of the following?

(A) Demonstrated atopic status
(B) Relief of symptoms with bronchodilator therapy
(C) Decreased FEV_1/FVC on spirometry
(D) Documented reversibility of airways obstruction
(E) Positive methacholine challenge

Dyspnea Questions 17-19

For each patient described below, select the most likely diagnosis (A-E) (each answer may be used more than once or not at all):

(A) Bronchiolitis obliterans
(B) Hypersensitivity pneumonitis
(C) Reactive airways dysfunction syndrome (RADS)
(D) Occupational asthma
(E) Organic toxic dust syndrome (OTDS)

17. One year ago, a 30-year-old janitorial worker was asked to clean an accidental spill of ammonia. After 45 minutes, he noted dyspnea and coughing. Since then, he has complained of dyspnea on exertion, chest tightness, and a dry cough triggered by tobacco smoke, cold air, and household irritants. The physical examination is normal. A chest radiograph screening spirometry test, and diffusing capacity for carbon monoxide ($DLco$) are normal. A methacholine inhalation challenge test is positive (PD_{20} of 2.5 mg/mL).

18. A 25-year-old biotechnology worker is employed in a factory that manufactures microbial enzymes from *Aspergillus* and *Bacillus subtilis*. He reports shortness of breath, fever (temperature, 37.8 °C [100.1 °F]), and myalgias beginning 4 to 6 hours after coming to work. Crackles are heard in both lung bases. A chest radiograph is normal. Spirometry shows an FVC of 66% of predicted, FEV_1 of 65% of predicted; and FEV_1/FVC of 80%; the $DLco$ is decreased to 55% of predicted. A methacholine test is deferred because of a low baseline FEV_1.

19. A 45-year-old baker reports chest tightness and dyspnea beginning 1 hour after coming to work. Respiratory symptoms improved after the work shift, but that night the patient awakens with dyspnea and wheezing. The symptoms occur only on days at work when an *Aspergillus* enzyme powder used as a leavening agent was added to dough. The physical examination is normal. A chest radiograph, screening spirometry, and $DLco$ are normal. A methacholine inhalation challenge test is positive (PD_{20} of 0.25 mg/mL).

Dyspnea Question 20

A 52-year-old man presents with persistent dyspnea and fatigue several weeks after a hospitalization for congestive heart failure. He was hospitalized with progressive orthopnea, peripheral edema, and evidence of biventricular heart failure. He has a 25–pack-year smoking history and no evidence of alcohol or drug abuse. Diffuse hypokinesis and mild to moderate mitral regurgitation were noted on echocardiogram. Cardiac catheterization showed minimal coronary artery disease, and the patient was felt to have idiopathic congestive cardiomyopathy. He was successfully treated with digoxin, 0.25 mg/d; lisinopril, 10 mg/d; furosemide, 20 mg/d; and warfarin sodium, 5 mg/d. Since discharge, he has not had chest pain, orthopnea, paroxysmal nocturnal dyspnea, or peripheral edema.

Examination during the clinic visit shows a pulse rate of 88/min, a respiration rate of 16/min, and a blood pressure of 110/74 mm Hg; his weight is unchanged from discharge. There is no jugular venous distention; the chest is clear to auscultation; and the cardiac examination reveals a grade II/VI holosystolic murmur at the apex without a ventricular gallop.

Laboratory studies:

Complete blood count	Normal
Serum electrolytes	Normal
International normalized ratio	2.6
Electrocardiography shows no change from discharge. Spirometry is normal.	
Cardiopulmonary exercise testing	
Maximum exercise capacity (VO_{2Max})	Reduced
Maximum heart rate	90% of predicted
Anaerobic threshold	Borderline low

Breathing reserve–Dyspnea   0.5
index (normal <0.6)
  (maximum ventilation/
  maximal voluntary
  ventilation)
Alveolar-arterial O$_2$ gradient   No significant
                                    desaturation

The most likely cause of dyspnea in this patient is:

(A) Chronic pulmonary emboli
(B) Deconditioning
(C) Congestive heart failure
(D) Pulmonary fibrosis
(E) Chronic obstructive pulmonary disease

Dyspnea Questions 21-23

A 72-year-old retired oil and gas producer, a lifelong nonsmoker, has a 4-month history of progressive dyspnea. He stopped playing tennis 1 year ago because fatigue limited the number of sets he could play. He was treated for depression with fluoxetine hydrochloride. At the time of his retirement 7 years ago, he underwent a complete wellness examination, and he says that he was given a "clean bill of health." However, it was reported that his cardiac stress test was limited because of breathlessness and leg fatigue, and his chest radiograph showed "mild chronic interstitial changes at the bases."

Physical examination reveals crackles at the bases of both lungs. There are no signs of deforming arthritis. Serum rheumatoid factor and antinuclear antibody determinations are negative. Urinalysis is normal. Radiographs of the sinuses and an ear, nose, and throat examination disclose no abnormalities.

A radiograph of the chest is shown.

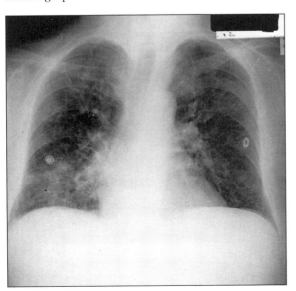

Question 21

All of the following findings would be expected in this patient EXCEPT:

(A) A diffusing capacity for carbon monoxide of less than 70% of predicted normal
(B) Abnormal compliance (static) with marked increase in elastic recoil
(C) A forced expiratory volume in 1 second (FEV$_1$) of 1.66 L (49% of predicted); forced vital capacity (FVC) of 2.62 L (64% of predicted); FEV$_1$/FVC ratio 63%
(D) Pao$_2$, 87 mm Hg; Paco$_2$, 32 mm Hg; pH, 7.48; Sao$_2$, 93% P(A-a)o$_2$, 23 mm Hg
(E) A total lung capacity of 65% or less of predicted

Question 22

The diagnosis would best be made by means of:

(A) Gallium 67 lung scanning
(B) Bronchoalveolar lavage done by fiberoptic bronchoscopy
(C) A scalene lymph node biopsy
(D) A lung biopsy
(E) Percutaneous renal biopsy with immuno-fluorescence

Question 23

After the diagnosis is confirmed, the most appropriate management is:

(A) Administration of penicillamine, orally, for at least 3 months
(B) Referral of the patient for lung transplantation
(C) Repeated chest radiographs and pulmonary function studies at 6-month intervals
(D) Advise the patient to move to a new home
(E) Administration of corticosteroids, orally, for at least 3 months

DYSURIA

Dysuria Question 1

A 68-year-old woman with psoriasis presents to your office because she has developed dysuria. She is receiving oral methotrexate, 10 mg per week, for treatment of her psoriasis. Urinalysis shows many bacteria and 40 to 60 leukocytes per high-power field.

Which of the following drugs is contraindicated for treatment of this patient's urinary tract infection?

(A) Ampicillin
(B) Trimethoprim–sulfamethoxazole
(C) Cephalexin
(D) Ciprofloxacin
(E) Amoxicillin-clavulanate

Dysuria Question 2

A 28-year-old married man had a sexual encounter with a prostitute while on a business trip in Seattle 1 week ago. After returning home, he noted a burning sensation on urination and a yellow discharge in his underwear. Microscopic examination of the discharge reveals 4+ polymorphonuclear neutrophils and many intracellular gram-negative diplococci.

Which of the following is the best course of action in the management of this patient?

(A) Give the patient a prescription for doxycycline, 100 mg orally twice a day for 7 days.
(B) Give the patient two prescriptions for ofloxacin, 300 mg orally twice a day for 7 days, one for him and one to give to his wife.
(C) Administer ceftriaxone, 125 mg intramuscularly, and azithromycin 1 g orally, draw blood for a VDRL, and arrange for his wife to be examined and treated.
(D) Administer a single oral dose of azithromycin, 2 g, draw blood for a VDRL and HIV-antibody, and arrange for his wife to be examined and treated.
(E) Administer a single oral dose of cefixime, 400 mg, draw blood for a VDRL, and arrange for his wife to be examined and treated.

Dysuria Question 3

A 22-year-old woman presents with a 2-day history of headache, fever, malaise, sore throat, dysuria, and vaginal discharge and irritation. She appears mildly toxic on physical examination. Her tonsils are enlarged bilaterally, and she has both cervical and inguinal adenopathy. Pelvic examination shows numerous shallow, painful ulcers on the labia majora and minora but is otherwise normal. Ligase chain reaction assay on freshly voided urine is negative for *Neisseria gonorrhoeae* and *Chlamydia trachomatis*.

Which of the following is the most appropriate management action?

(A) Give no treatment but counsel the patient that herpes simplex infections can recur, and that so long as she avoids having sex when ulcers are present, the risk of transmission to her sexual partner is minimal.
(B) Give no treatment but explain that not only can the infection be transmitted to sexual partners, but also there is a 10% to 20% probability of transmitting the virus to her children during future pregnancies.
(C) Give immediate treatment with acyclovir and encourage her to bring in her most recent sexual partner so that he can be treated also.
(D) Give immediate treatment with acyclovir, explain that herpes simplex infections often recur, and explain that she can transmit the virus to her sexual partner even when she has no visible ulcers.
(E) Give immediate treatment with acyclovir and explain that she will have to remain on acyclovir therapy for years or otherwise she will be able to transmit the infection to her sexual partner.

Dysuria Questions 4-8
For each patient described below, select the most appropriate management (A-E) (each answer may be used more than once or not at all):

(A) No treatment is indicated unless the patient develops fever or other signs consistent with urosepsis.
(B) Obtain a culture of the urine and then start oral treatment with trimethoprim–sulfamethoxazole, norfloxacin, or ciprofloxacin. Modify treatment as dictated by urine culture results and course. Treat for 7 days.
(C) Treat for 3 days with trimethoprim–sulfamethoxazole. Obtain urine culture only if no symptomatic response or relapse occurs.
(D) Hospitalize the patient and initiate therapy with parenteral gentamicin and ampicillin, after obtaining cultures of the urine and blood.
(E) Obtain culture of the urine and then start therapy with trimethoprim–sulfamethoxazole or a fluoroquinolone for 2 to 4 weeks.

4. An 18-year-old woman presents with urinary frequency, dysuria, and low-grade fever. Urinalysis shows pyuria and bacilli. She has never had similar symptoms or treatment for urinary tract infection.

5. An 18-year-old woman presents with her third episode of urinary frequency, dysuria, and pyuria in the past 4 months.

6. A 58-year-old man presents with his first episode of urinary frequency and dysuria. Urinalysis shows pyuria and bacilli.

7. A 24-year-old woman presents with fever, chills, nausea, vomiting, flank pain, and tenderness. Her temperature is 40 °C (104 °F), pulse rate is 120/min, and blood pressure is 100/60 mm Hg.

8. A 78-year-old woman presents with an indwelling Foley catheter and pyuria.

Dysuria Question 9
A 35-year-old man presents to your office because of a 2-week history of severe, incapacitating pain and swelling of both knees and the left ankle. Six weeks before this visit he presented with a purulent urethral discharge and dysuria. The patient was diagnosed with gonococcal urethritis and treated with an antibiotic. Following treatment, he showed significant improvement; however he noticed residual dysuria and a clear urethral discharge that lasted for 2 weeks.

Physical examination now shows bilateral conjunctivitis and signs of inflammatory synovitis of the affected joints. Joint aspiration shows a yellow turbid fluid containing 33,000 leukocytes/μL.

What is the most likely joint fluid culture result?

(A) Culture positive for *Neisseria gonorrhoeae*
(B) Culture positive for *Chlamydia trachomatis*
(C) Culture positive for *Ureaplasma urealyticum*
(D) Culture positive for *Campylobacter jejuni*
(E) Culture sterile

GASTROINTESTINAL BLEEDING

Gastrointestinal Bleeding Question 1

A 60-year-old man with cirrhosis comes to the Emergency Department 2 hours after vomiting two cups of bright red blood. Spironolactone prescribed for a history of ascites is his only medication. Physical examination shows a somnolent but arousable man with a nasogastric tube in place with bright red blood on aspiration. With the patient supine, the blood pressure is 102/68 mm Hg and the pulse rate is 92/min; with the patient sitting the blood pressure is 82/50 mm Hg and the pulse rate 115/min. The respiration rate is 14/min and temperature is 37.0 °C (98.6 °F). Further examination reveals a confused patient with asterixis, clear chest, regular heart rhythm without murmurs, and moderate abdominal distention with bulging flanks. A liver edge is detectable by ballottement 2 cm below the right costal margin.

Laboratory studies:

Serum sodium	120 meq/L
Serum potassium	5.3 meq/L
Serum bicarbonate	35 meq/L
Serum chloride	75 meq/L
Serum albumin	2.2 g/dL
Blood urea nitrogen	20 mg/dL
Serum creatinine	2.0 mg/dL

After hemodynamic stabilization with volume resuscitation, which of the following therapeutic measures would be appropriate?

(A) Intravenous octreotide infusion
(B) Empiric broad-spectrum antibiotic therapy
(C) Endoscopy for diagnosis and possible endoscopic therapy
(D) Large-volume paracentesis
(E) All of the above

Gastrointestinal Bleeding Question 2

A 66-year-old woman presents with iron deficiency anemia and stool that is positive for occult blood. She has had arthralgias for several months for which she has taken multiple NSAIDs. The physical examination is nonspecific. At colonoscopy, she is found to have multiple ulcerations in the proximal transverse colon, which on biopsy are interpreted as nonspecific inflammation. She has mild anemia; laboratory findings are otherwise unremarkable.

The most appropriate treatment would be:

(A) Sulfasalazine, 500 mg/d orally, and prednisone, 40 mg/d orally
(B) Partial colectomy
(C) Methotrexate, 25 mg intramuscularly every week
(D) Cyclosporine
(E) Discontinue NSAIDs

Gastrointestinal Bleeding Question 3

A 56-year-old man with a history of peptic ulcer disease presents to the Emergency Department with a history of three episodes of hematemesis and light-headedness in the past 24 hours. His previous ulcer was diagnosed 10 years ago by upper gastrointestinal series. He takes cimetidine intermittently for symptoms of epigastric pain. He denies previous gastrointestinal bleeding or NSAID use. He has no other medical problems and takes no medications.

His blood pressure is 100/70 mm Hg supine and 80/60 mm Hg standing; the pulse rate is 110/min supine. The hematocrit is 34%. He has no abdominal pain or tenderness. The physical examination is otherwise unremarkable.

The best initial approach to this patient is:

(A) Nasogastric aspiration to assess the level of bleeding
(B) Rapid volume replacement with normal saline
(C) Rapid blood product replacement
(D) Emergency endoscopy to identify and treat the bleeding lesion
(E) Measurement of hematocrit to estimate the volume of blood lost

Gastrointestinal Bleeding Question 4

For which one of the following conditions is therapy for *Helicobacter pylori* infection a proven benefit?

(A) NSAID-induced ulcers
(B) Peptic ulcers
(C) Nonulcer dyspepsia
(D) Gastric cancer
(E) Gastroesophageal reflux disease

Gastrointestinal Bleeding Question 5

A 55-year-old man with a mild hypertension and diabetes controlled by diet comes to the Emergency Department because he has been vomiting blood and had black tarry stools. His blood pressure and pulse are 150/90 mm Hg and 90 per minute supine and 110/70 mm Hg and 100 per minute sitting. The hematocrit is 35%; it is usually greater than 40%.

He is resuscitated with intravenous fluids, admitted to the Intensive Care Unit, and given two units of packed erythrocytes; 8 hours later he no longer has postural hypotension and is not vomiting. Naso-gastric aspirate is clear, and the hematocrit is 30%. Endoscopy shows a 1-cm duodenal ulcer with a large adherent clot.

The most appropriate treatment for the bleeding is:

(A) Surgical plication of the ulcer bed
(B) Intra-arterial vasopressin
(C) Endoscopic therapy
(D) Start therapy for ulcer disease and discharge the patient the next day
(E) Start therapy for ulcer disease and observe the patient in the hospital for further bleeding

Gastrointestinal Bleeding Question 6

A 40-year-old man has had mildly abnormal liver function tests for several years. Hepatitis C antibody was recently found to be positive. He denies intra-venous drug use. He vomited a couple of times last week after eating Mexican food and then noted melena for 2 days. He had no postural symptoms. When you see him 1 week later, his stool is brown but positive for occult blood. The liver and spleen are not enlarged, and there are no spider angio-mata or ascites. The hematocrit, which is normally 43% to 45%, is 38%. You arrange an endoscopy. The gastroenterologist detects no varices but "portal hypertensive gastropathy"; otherwise the endoscopy is normal.

Which of the following treatments is most appro-priate to prevent rebleeding?

(A) Interferon-α
(B) Sclerotherapy
(C) Propranolol
(D) Transjugular intrahepatic portasystemic stent (TIPS)
(E) Portocaval shunt

Gastrointestinal Bleeding Question 7

A 38-year-old man presents with hematemesis of 2 hours' duration. He has no other history of gastro-intestinal bleeding and no other symptoms. He has been on a strict vegetarian diet for the past 4 weeks for weight control and has abstained from alcohol for the same amount of time.

Physical examination shows a pale, anxious man with a pulse rate of 130/min and a blood pressure of 90/60 mm Hg. Cardiopulmonary examination is normal. Abdominal examination shows a spleen palpable 3 cm below the left costal margin. The liver is not palpable.

Laboratory studies:

Hemoglobin	8.0 g/dL
Mean corpuscular volume	85 fL
Erythrocyte distribution width	14%
Leukocyte count	10,000/μL, with 80 neutrophils, 15% lymphocytes, and 5% monocytes
Platelet count	75,000/μL
Bleeding time	7.5 min
Prothrombin time	28 sec
Activated partial thromboplastin time	50 sec
Serum creatinine	1.1 mg/dL
Serum albumin	2.0 g/dL
Serum globulin	4.8 g/dL
Serum bilirubin	0.8/dL
Serum alkaline phosphatase	140 IU
Serum aspartate aminotransferase	75 U/L
Serum alanine aminotransferase	45 U/L
Fibrinogen	165 mg/dL
D-dimer	Negative

After the above laboratory results were obtained, the following laboratory studies are done:

Activated partial thromboplastin time with 1:1 mix with normal plasma	30 sec
Prothrombin time with 1:1 mix with normal plasma	12 sec

What is the most likely diagnosis?

(A) Vitamin K deficiency
(B) Disseminated intravascular coagulation
(C) Chronic liver disease
(D) Acquired inhibitor of factor V
(E) Systemic fibrinolysis

Gastrointestinal Bleeding Question 8

A 75-year-old woman presents to the Emergency Department because she has had three large-volume, bloody stools in the past 24 hours. She has no previous history of gastrointestinal bleeding or ulcer disease. She had no hematemesis or melena. Her medical history includes hypertension treated with an ACE inhibitor and rheumatoid arthritis treated with an NSAID. She also has a history of diverticulitis and glaucoma.

Her blood pressure is 140/80 mm Hg supine and 90/60 mm Hg sitting. The pulse rate is 110/min supine. The cardiopulmonary examination shows tachypnea. The bowel sounds are hyperactive, but there are no masses or tenderness. She has the joint changes of rheumatoid arthritis. Rectal examination shows no formed stool but fresh blood in the rectal vault. Nasogastric aspirate produces nonbloody bilious material.

The patient most recently passed bright red blood per rectum 6 hours ago. After intravenous volume resuscitation, her blood pressure is 130/86 mm Hg and her pulse rate is 96/min, without orthostatic changes. The hemoglobin concentration is 11 g/dL, but results of other laboratory tests are normal.

In light of her recurrent rectal bleeding, the best management at this time would be:

(A) Rapid colonic lavage and urgent colonoscopy
(B) Left hemicolectomy for presumed diverticular bleeding
(C) Emergency barium enema
(D) Emergency angiography
(E) Radionuclide erythrocyte scan

THE HEALTHY PATIENT

The Healthy Patient Question 1

A 17-year-old girl presents for her college physical. Although she is a new patient in your practice, both of her parents have been your patients. Her 45-year-old father takes niacin and enalapril daily. Her maternal grandmother had breast cancer after menopause. Her mother is closely followed for fibrocystic breast disease and takes levothyroxine.

The patient is appropriate weight for her age and height. Blood pressure is 110/70 mm Hg, and pulse is 66/min. No abnormalities are found on examination.

Which one of the following would you next recommend for this patient?

(A) Measure cholesterol level.
(B) Measure hematocrit.
(C) Order baseline mammography.
(D) Measure thyroid-stimulating hormone.
(E) None of the above.

The Healthy Patient Questions 2-3

A 54-year-old woman presents for an insurance examination that requires HIV testing. Physical examination is normal, and there are no symptoms of HIV disease. She has a monogamous sexual relationship with her husband of 24 years, uses no recreational drugs, and had a single blood transfusion because of trauma from a motor vehicle accident in 1970.

Her HIV ELISA (enzyme-linked immunosorbent assay) test result is positive. Based on available information, you determine that the sensitivity and specificity of HIV ELISA testing at your institution are each 98%. The pretest probability (prevalence) of HIV positivity in similar patients is judged to be about 1 in 10,000.

Question 2

Before confirmation with Western blot testing, what is the post-test probability of this patient having HIV infection?

(A) About 99.5%
(B) About 90%
(C) About 32%
(D) About 1%
(E) About 0.5%

Question 3

Given the same test parameters of 98% sensitivity and specificity, but now a person at high risk whose pretest probability of HIV infection is 50%, the post-test probability of HIV infection following an ELISA test is:

(A) 98% with a positive test result; 98% with a negative test result
(B) 98% with a positive test result; 2% with a negative test result
(C) 90% with a positive test result; 25% with a negative test result
(D) 50% with a positive test result; 50% with a negative test result
(E) 2% with a positive test result; 98% with a negative test result

The Healthy Patient Question 4

A 43-year-old woman plans to travel with her husband and 11-year-old child to Mexico for vacation next year. Her family has no known history of hepatitis or liver disease, and none of the family members has received vaccinations for viral hepatitis. She is interested in learning which vaccinations for hepatitis would be appropriate for her family

Which of the following would you recommend?

(A) Hepatitis A vaccination for both parents and the child
(B) Hepatitis A vaccination for the parents and child and hepatitis B vaccination for the child
(C) Hepatitis A and hepatitis B vaccination for both parents and the child
(D) Screen both parents for previous hepatitis A infection and recommend hepatitis A vaccination for the child
(E) Screen all members of the family for hepatitis A and hepatitis B exposure

The Healthy Patient Questions 5-10

For each patient described below, select the recommended colon cancer surveillance strategy (A-E) (each answer may be used more than once or not at all):

(A) Annual flexible sigmoidoscopy beginning no later than age 25 years.
(B) Flexible sigmoidoscopy every 3 to 5 years beginning at age 50 years.
(C) Colonoscopy every 2 to 3 years beginning at age 20 to 25 years.
(D) Colonoscopy every 2 years with segmental biopsies.
(E) Colonoscopy within 3 to 6 months.

5. A patient with no risk factors for colon carcinoma.

6. A patient with a family history of familial polyposis coli.

7. A patient whose father died at age 48 years of colon cancer and whose brother recently was diagnosed at age 45 years with colon carcinoma.

8. A patient whose father died of colon cancer at age 70 years.

9. A patient who was found to have one hyperplastic polyp on flexible sigmoidoscopic examination.

10. A patient found to have a single 10-mm tubular adenoma on flexible sigmoidoscopic examination.

The Healthy Patient Question 11

A 35-year-old woman requests a routine health assessment. She has no specific medical complaints or past medical history. Her father developed colon cancer at age 54 years but is still living. His brother died of colon cancer at age 41 years. Their father (the patient's grandfather) died in his sixties of colon cancer. His sister died of gastric cancer. The patient's sister was recently diagnosed with endometrial cancer at age 43 years.

The patient has a good appetite and has no nausea, vomiting, or weight loss. She has had no change in her bowel habits or hematochezia, and her menstrual periods are normal. Physical examination is normal. Digital rectal examination is negative for fecal occult blood. A screening complete blood count and biochemical profile are normal.

Which one of the following actions is most appropriate?

(A) Perform annual occult blood tests of three stool specimens. Initiate screening with flexible sigmoidoscopy at age 50 years.
(B) Perform colonoscopy at least every 2 years.
(C) Barium enema now; if normal no further evaluation.
(D) Perform colonoscopy now; if no polyps are seen, no further investigation is necessary.
(E) Perform fecal occult blood testing and flexible sigmoidoscopy now. If no polyps are seen now, the patient should be followed routinely with fecal occult blood testing and flexible sigmoidoscopy beginning at age 50 years.

The Healthy Patient Question 12

A treadmill electrocardiographic (ECG) exercise test would most likely help diagnose the presence or absence of significant coronary artery disease in which of the following patients?

(A) A 62-year-old man who smokes and has atypical chest pain
(B) A 70-year-old man who is asymptomatic 6 months after coronary angioplasty
(C) A 31-year-old sedentary woman who wishes to start an exercise program
(D) A 55-year-old man who has rest angina pectoris associated with transient electrocardiographic changes
(E) An asymptomatic 69-year-old woman who has severe long-standing hypertension

The Healthy Patient Question 13

An 18-year-old female college freshman seeks your advice on her likelihood of having significant heart disease. When she was 10 years old, her pediatrician ordered echocardiography for a possible heart murmur; the findings were normal. She is now worried because an uncle, previously believed to be healthy, recently died suddenly at the age of 38 years. At autopsy, he was found to have severe concentric left ventricular hypertrophy and histopathologic findings consistent with hypertrophic cardiomyopathy. Her father, aged 36 years, had a heart murmur diagnosed in college but denies any limitations on his physical activity.

Physical examination shows a thin, well-appearing young woman. Her pulse rate is 78/min, and blood pressure is 100/60 mm Hg. Carotid upstrokes are 2+ without bisferious character. Her chest is clear. Cardiac examination shows a flat jugular venous pulse. S_1 is normal, and S_2 is split physiologically. There is a grade 2/6 systolic murmur at the left upper sternal border that does not change with isometric or Valsalva's maneuvers. No gallop is noted. Her abdomen and extremities are normal.

What is the most cost-effective method to evaluate this young woman for the presence of asymptomatic hypertrophic disease?

(A) Physical examination
(B) Electrocardiography
(C) Echocardiography
(D) Detailed family pedigree
(E) Genotyping of peripheral blood lymphocytes

The Healthy Patient Questions 14-17

For each patient described below, select the appropriate preventive approach for pneumonia (A-E) (each answer may be used more than once or not at all):

(A) Pneumococcal vaccine
(B) Pseudomonal vaccine
(C) *Haemophilus influenzae* type b vaccine
(D) Influenza vaccine
(E) None of the above

14. A 65-year-old man was hospitalized for an exacerbation of newly diagnosed chronic obstructive pulmonary disease. He was discharged 4 weeks ago and now presents to your office in the early spring. He has never received any adult vaccinations.

15. A 37-year-old woman was in a motor vehicle accident and suffered a ruptured spleen. She had required splenectomy, had an uneventful recovery, and is about to be discharged home. She is taking no chronic medications and has been given *Haemophilus influenzae* type b vaccine.

16. A 68-year-old man with congestive heart failure was admitted to the hospital in late October for an episode of acute pulmonary edema. He has recovered and is about to be discharged. He thinks he got "a pneumonia shot" 4 years ago but cannot remember any other vaccinations.

17. A 45-year-old woman with no significant medical history comes to your office for a routine examination early in November. She is taking no medications. The woman is working as a teacher's aide in a nursery school.

The Healthy Patient Question 18

A 45-year-old man with well-controlled hypertension comes to your office for a routine blood pressure check. He has no other significant medical problems but is moderately overweight. His plasma cholesterol level is 200 mg/dL. He has no family history of heart disease, and he has never smoked. He has been largely sedentary since college but now wants to start an exercise program.

What would you do for the patient?

(A) Suggest that he join a health club and exercise for 30 minutes three times a week.
(B) Order an exercise treadmill test as a screening test before he starts exercising.
(C) Teach him to check his heart rate and advise him to exercise at 75% of his maximum heart rate for 30 minutes 3 times a week.
(D) Help him to plan exercise involving an activity that he enjoys and at a frequency that fits into his lifestyle.
(E) Educate him about the health benefits of exercise and facilitate his exploration of the pros and cons of exercising.

The Healthy Patient Question 19

A 44-year-old man has his blood pressure measured in the 148-158/92-100 mm Hg range on four clinic visits over 3 months. He smokes 1.5 packs of cigarettes a day, drinks four to five cups of coffee per day, and drinks alcohol regularly (but has no positive responses on the CAGE screen). He has no significant medical history and takes no medications. He is a manager of a car dealership and feels pressured when sales are down.

On physical examination, his blood pressure is 150/96 mm Hg, pulse rate is 66/min; he is 182.8 cm (72 in) tall and weighs 77.3 kg (170 pounds). No retinopathy or cardiac abnormalities are present.

Laboratory studies:

Sodium	143 meq/L
Potassium	4.4 meq/L
Blood urea nitrogen	13 mg/dL
Glucose	93 mg/dL
Creatinine	0.8 mg/dL
Cholesterol	214 mg/dL
γ-Glutamyltransferase (GGT)	59 U/L
Urinalysis	Normal
Electrocardiogram	Normal

The patient would like to avoid taking antihypertension medication.

Which one of the following interventions is likely to be the most effective in lowering his blood pressure?

(A) Weight reduction
(B) Smoking cessation
(C) Reducing his alcohol intake to less than two drinks per day
(D) Eliminating caffeine from his diet
(E) Relaxation therapy

The Healthy Patient Question 20

A 54-year-old woman presents for her annual visit. She is postmenopausal but has decided to stop hormone replacement therapy because of side effects. When discussing her calcium requirements, she reports drinking one glass of skim milk and eating one cup of nonfat yogurt each day. Past attempts at increasing her dietary calcium have resulted in bloating and loose stools.

Which one of the following is most appropriate to fulfill this patient's calcium requirement?

(A) Calcium supplementation with 400 mg of dolomite calcium a day
(B) Increase her intake of spinach and other green leafy vegetables
(C) Calcium supplementation with 1500 mg of calcium carbonate a day
(D) Calcium supplementation with 900 mg of calcium gluconate a day
(E) Calcium supplementation with 400 mg of calcium citrate a day

The Healthy Patient Question 21

A 33-year-old woman presents with menometrorrhagia-like symptoms of 2 to 3 months' duration. She had previously been healthy and her only medication is oral contraceptives, which she has taken for the past 6 years.

Physical examination, including pelvic bimanual and speculum examination, shows cervical erosions; urinalysis is normal and examination of stool for occult blood is negative. The Pap smear cytology reports states: "class I negative, no endocervical cells."

The most appropriate course at this time is to:

(A) Schedule the patient for return office visit in 3 months; if the problem persists, perform endometrial biopsy.
(B) Prescribe change in birth control pills for "breakthrough menstrual bleeding."
(C) Repeat Pap smear, review HIV risk factors, and discuss need for culposcopy.
(D) Discontinue oral contraceptives and arrange for dilatation and curettage.
(E) Measure serum CA-125 and request transvaginal ultrasound.

The Healthy Patient Questions 22-26

For each patient described below, select the appropriate diagnostic procedure (A-E) (each answer may be used more than once or not at all):

(A) Observation on a monthly basis
(B) Ultrasound
(C) A breast biopsy procedure
(D) Thermography
(E) Mammogram with magnified views

22. A 56-year-old man with a 1-cm subareolar lump and a negative mammogram

23. A 36-year-old-woman with a 1-cm palpable lump of 2 months' duration and a negative mammogram and negative attempt at cyst aspiration

24. A 53-year-old woman with a new (since previous mammogram 1 year ago) cluster of four irregular microcalcifications and no mass on mammogram or physical examination

25. An 18-year-old woman with a 2-cm breast lump of 1 week's duration

26. An 18-year-old woman with a 2-cm breast lump of 2 months' duration

The Healthy Patient Question 27

During a routine annual physical, a 70-year-old man is found to have an elevation of serum alkaline phosphatase (480 U/L) that has been determined to be of bone origin. A bone scan reveals increased uptake involving the occipital region of the skull. Skull roentgenograms reveal mottled increase of bone density with a cotton-wool appearance in the occipital area. Audiometric testing is normal, and the patient is asymptomatic. All additional laboratory tests are normal except that there is borderline elevation of his urinary hydroxyproline level.

What is the most appropriate therapeutic agent for managing this patient?

(A) Calcitriol
(B) Bisphosphonates
(C) Calcitonin
(D) Mithramycin
(E) No therapy

The Healthy Patient Question 28
Response to 23-valent pneumococcal vaccine is likely to be poor in:

(A) Patients with HIV infection
(B) Elderly patients with vitamin B_{12} deficiency
(C) Patients with common variable immunodeficiency
(D) Post-splenectomy patients
(E) All of the above

The Healthy Patient Question 29
A 19-year-old woman presents with irritation of the vagina that has gradually become worse over the past several weeks. She has had only one sexual partner over the last 8 months and five partners since becoming sexually active at age 16.

Physical examination is normal except for approximately a dozen exophytic lesions 1 to 3 mm in diameter located on both labia minora. Additional perianal lesions are also present.

What diagnostic tests are now indicated?

(A) Serologic test for HIV infection
(B) Serologic test for genital herpes infection
(C) Biopsy of one of the exophytic lesions
(D) Papanicolaou smear
(E) No additional diagnostic test

HIV DISEASE

HIV Disease Question 1

A 27-year-old HIV-positive man presents with multiple purple pedunculated nodules on his skin. He says that these lesions have spread rapidly and have a tendency to bleed. In the previous 2 weeks, he has had intermittent fevers and general malaise.

The most likely diagnosis is:

(A) Kaposi's sarcoma
(B) Pyogenic granulomas
(C) Bacillary angiomatosis
(D) Secondary syphilis
(E) Cutaneous cryptococcosis

HIV Disease Question 2

A 36-year-old man with a history of HIV infection for the past 5 years comes to your office for a second opinion about starting antiretroviral therapy. He had varicella zoster infection 1 year ago. The only medications he is taking are vitamins. Physical examination reveals diffuse adenopathy, which appears unchanged from previous examinations.

Laboratory studies:

Hematocrit	36%
Leukocyte count	2200/μL
Platelet count	125,000/μL
CD4 cell count	660/μL
HIV RNA level	5,000 copies/mL

What is the most appropriate recommended antiretroviral therapy?

(A) No therapy
(B) Zidovudine, 200 mg three times daily
(C) Zidovudine, 200 mg three times daily, in combination with didanosine, zalcitabine or lamivudine
(D) Zalcitabine, 0.75 mg three times daily, plus didanosine, 200 mg twice daily

HIV Disease Question 3

A 48-year-old woman with HIV infection and a CD4 cell count of 150/μL reports the acute onset of fever, odynophagia, retrosternal pain, and nausea. She has a history of recurrent oral and vaginal candidiasis, recurrent herpes labialis, and chronic hepatitis B infection following a blood transfusion. Her medications include zidovudine, didanosine, trimethoprim–sulfamethoxazole, and a multivitamin.

Physical examination is normal. She is treated with fluconazole, 100 mg daily for 7 days, but symptoms persist. An upper gastrointestinal endoscopy shows multiple shallow mucosal esophageal ulcers with overlying patchy exudate. Several mucosal samples are obtained for biopsy and culture.

Her symptoms are most likely to be caused by which one of the following?

(A) *Candida albicans*
(B) Cytomegalovirus
(C) Herpes simplex virus
(D) Retained pills (zidovudine-associated esophageal ulcer)
(E) Idiopathic esophageal ulcers

HIV Disease Question 4

A 35-year-old man who has had HIV infection for at least 6 years and has a CD4 cell count between 400 and 600/μL comes to your office because he has felt fatigued for 3 weeks. He has had three episodes of genital herpes but no AIDS-defining opportunistic infections. He is taking zidovudine, didanosine, and lamivudine.

Physical examination is remarkable only for white plaques consistent with oral candidiasis. Repeat CD4 cell count is 293/μL. Determination of viral load by HIV RNA polymerase chain reaction (PCR) is ordered, and treatment is begun with oral clotrimazole troches.

What additional step should be taken at this visit?

(A) Initiation of *Mycobacterium avium* complex prophylaxis
(B) Initiation of *Pneumocystis carinii* pneumonia prophylaxis
(C) Long-term fungal prophylaxis
(D) Herpes simplex prophylaxis
(E) No additional treatment

HIV Disease Question 5

A 33-year-old man with HIV infection enrolls in a methadone maintenance program where you provide HIV care. On enrollment, he is asymptomatic and has an unremarkable physical examination. His CD4 cell count is 243/µL. Hepatitis B surface antibody and hepatitis C core antibody are positive. Placement of purified protein derivative (PPD) results in 6 mm of induration.

The next step in this patient's management is:

(A) Hepatitis B immunization
(B) Chest radiography
(C) Treatment with isoniazid, 300 mg daily, and pyridoxine, 50 mg daily
(D) Trimethoprim–sulfamethoxazole, 1 double-strength tablet daily
(E) Repeat PPD in 1 week for booster effect

HIV Disease Question 6
A 32-year-old woman comes to your office because she notices easy bleeding when she brushes her teeth. She is taking no medications and has a history of heroin and crack cocaine use. Physical examination reveals posterior cervical adenopathy and moderate gingivitis; there are no other abnormalities. Her leukocyte count is 7600/µL with a normal differential; hemoglobin is 14.2 g/dL; and platelet count is 14,000/µL. She is HIV seropositive, and her CD4 cell count is 645/µL.

The next step in this patient's evaluation and management is:

(A) Prednisone, 60 mg/d
(B) High-dose intravenous immunoglobulin
(C) Splenectomy
(D) An antiviral regimen containing zidovudine, 600 mg/d
(E) Bone marrow biopsy

HIV Disease Question 7
A 43-year-old man with advanced HIV infection (CD4 cell count of 34/µL) is interested in aggressive prophylactic management and asks you for prophylaxis against *Mycobacterium avium* complex (MAC) infection. His viral load has fallen from 135,000 copies/mL to undetectable levels with the institution of a drug regimen of zidovudine, lamivudine, and ritonavir. He takes trimethoprim–sulfamethoxazole, 1 double-strength tablet daily.

What is the best strategy for this patient?

(A) Add rifabutin, 300 mg daily.
(B) Add azithromycin, 1200 mg weekly.
(C) Discontinue ritonavir; begin clarithromycin and ethambutol.
(D) Do not add prophylaxis for MAC infection.

HIV Disease Question 8
A 28-year-old man, HIV-infected for 12 years and with a recent CD4 cell count of 10/µL, comes to your office for a routine follow-up visit. He reports the presence of perianal irritation, which he attributes to hemorrhoids. He reports no painful ulceration, lesions, or rectal discharge. His risk factor for HIV infection is sex with other men, but he denies engaging in any unprotected anal intercourse since his HIV diagnosis. He was treated with benzathine penicillin 12 years earlier for an asymptomatic positive serum rapid plasma reagin test. On physical examination, he is found to have two external, broad-based verrucous lesions resembling warts; neither are obstructing the anal canal, and no irritation or bleeding is noted.

Appropriate management for this patient should include:

(A) No intervention
(B) A repeat rapid plasma reagin test and anoscopy with cytologic screening
(C) A repeated course of benzathine penicillin for treatment of recurrent syphilis
(D) Repeat anal examination in 3 months
(E) Topical corticosteroid for treatment of hemorrhoids

HIV Disease Question 9
An asymptomatic 36-year-old woman comes to your office because she has just learned that she is HIV seropositive. Her CD4 cell count is 827/µL, and her HIV RNA viral load is 1300 copies/mL. Her physical examination is unremarkable. The patient is sexually active.

The following test results are obtained at baseline:

Papanicolaou smear	Atypical squamous cells of uncertain significance
Rapid plasma reagin assay	Nonreactive
Cytomegalovirus antibody	Negative
Toxoplasma antibody	Negative
Serum cryptococcal antigen	Negative
Purified protein derivative	6-mm induration
Hepatitis serologies:	
Hepatitis B surface antibody	Positive
Hepatitis B surface antigen	Negative
Hepatitis C antibody	Negative

Which one of the following studies is required at least annually?

(A) Serum cryptococcal antigen
(B) Hepatitis B surface antibody
(C) Rapid plasma reagin assay
(D) *Toxoplasma* antibodies
(E) Purified protein derivative

HIV Disease Question 10

A 32-year-old man is seen for an initial visit after the diagnosis of HIV infection. The patient believes his infection was sexually acquired. He works at a nursing home, and 2 years ago had a positive tuberculin skin test, for which he received 1 year of isoniazid therapy. His physical examination is unremarkable.

In addition to a CD4 cell count, viral load testing, and blood chemistry profile, what additional clinical and laboratory testing should be ordered?

(A) Rapid plasma reagin
(B) HIV-1 p24 antigen
(C) Hepatitis C antibody
(D) Tuberculin skin testing
(E) β_2-microglobulin

HIV Disease Question 11

A 23-year-old HIV-infected woman comes to your office because she has noticed painless white lesions in her mouth when brushing her teeth. She is taking no medications. Her last CD4 cell count 2 months earlier was 520/μL. On physical examination, she has patches of white, linear, frondlike lesions along both lateral surfaces of the buccal mucosa; the lesions do not scrape off with a tongue blade. Scrapings from the surface of the buccal mucosa reveal a few yeast forms in a microscopic wet mount prepared with potassium hydrochloride.

The likeliest diagnosis is:

(A) Oral hairy leukoplakia
(B) Oral candidiasis
(C) Aphthous stomatitis
(D) Acute necrotizing ulcerative gingivitis

HIV Disease Question 12

A 28-year-old married woman states at the end of a visit for mild knee pain that she would like an HIV test. Brief review of her HIV risk factors confirms that neither she nor her husband uses drugs. She was last sexually active with a man other than her husband in college. She has had no extramarital relationships and believes that her husband also is monogamous.

The best response to this patient's request is to:

(A) Explain that the expense of the HIV test is unjustified given her negligible risk.
(B) Order a CD4 cell count as a proxy for HIV testing.
(C) Order quantitation of viral RNA by polymerase chain reaction (PCR) as a more precise assessment of HIV status.
(D) Order an HIV antibody test by enzyme-linked immunosorbent assay (ELISA) with a confirmatory Western blot.

HIV Disease Question 13

A 34-year-old HIV-seropositive man with a CD4 cell count of 89/μL comes to your office with a 2-week history of progressive headache and subjective fever. Current medications include dapsone, 200 mg orally per day; zidovudine, 100 mg orally three times a day; didanosine, 200 mg twice daily; and nevirapine, 200 mg twice daily. A serologic test for antibodies to *Toxoplasma gondii* obtained 2 years ago was positive (titer of 1:32).

Physical examination is remarkable for mild weakness in his left arm and temperature of 39 °C (102.4 °F). A contrast-enhanced CT scan shows multiple enhancing lesions in the right cerebral hemisphere.

What is the most appropriate next step in management?

(A) Initiate therapy with pyrimethamine–sulfadiazine.
(B) Obtain a magnetic resonance imaging scan.
(C) Consult a neurosurgeon for a brain biopsy.
(D) Obtain a positron emission tomography scan.
(E) Repeat the serologic test for toxoplasmosis to assess change in titer.

HIV Disease Question 14

You are assisting with the medical care of pregnant women in an inner-city neighborhood clinic. Most of the patients are in the second trimester and also in high-risk groups for exposure to HIV. Their single visit may be the only time they receive routine prenatal care. The prevalence of HIV infection in these women is approximately 15%.

Diagnostic evaluation for HIV infection to aid in the decision to start antiretroviral therapy during the pregnancy should include:

(A) ELISA testing for antibodies against HIV, with positive tests confirmed by Western blot
(B) PCR amplification to detect HIV RNA in the serum of all patients
(C) ELISA testing for antibodies against HIV, with PCR amplification to detect HIV RNA in the serum of patients with ELISA-negative results
(D) Measurement of serum p24 antigen levels

HYPERTENSION

Hypertension Question 1

A 28-year-old multiparous woman is seen in a prenatal clinic 3 months after her last menstrual period. Her pregnancy has been uneventful, and she has gained weight progressively. She has had hypertension for 3 years. Because of a strong family history of hypertension and an unrevealing evaluation for secondary hypertension 1 year ago, she is considered to have essential hypertension. She had initially been treated with enalapril, but discontinued the medication 1 year ago. She had been lost to follow-up for a year and currently is not taking any medication. Her last pregnancy was 5 years ago, and she has no history of preeclampsia. Her medical records are not available. Her blood pressure is 150/110 mm Hg, and she has trace edema. One month ago, her blood pressure was 130/90 mm Hg, and she had trace urine protein on dipstick urinalysis.

Laboratory studies:

Hematocrit	36.7%
Leukocyte count	5200/µL
Platelet count	289,000/µL
Serum uric acid	3.2 mg/dL
Blood urea nitrogen	6 mg/dL
Serum creatinine	0.5 mg/dL
Urinalysis	
Microscopic	No hematuria, casts, or pyuria
24-hour urine protein excretion	125 mg
Creatinine clearance	137 mL/min

The most appropriate therapy for this patient's hypertension is:

(A) Atenolol
(B) Diuretic agent
(C) Methyldopa
(D) Enalapril
(E) No treatment with antihypertensive drugs is required.

Hypertension Questions 2-3

A 33-year-old woman has a 12-month history of sustained level 1 hypertension (blood pressure, 138/94 mm Hg) but is otherwise asymptomatic. She is a non-smoker and has no family history of premature atherosclerotic disease. Her physical examination is normal. Her total serum cholesterol concentration is 196 mg/dL, HDL cholesterol is 40 mg/dL, and fasting plasma glucose is 90 mg/dL. An echocardiogram shows no evidence of left ventricular hypertrophy.

Question 2

In addition to regular exercise and appropriate diet, which of the following would you recommend for this patient?

(A) Hydrochlorothiazide and blood pressure monitoring
(B) Hydralazine and blood pressure monitoring
(C) Captopril and blood pressure monitoring
(D) Blood pressure monitoring only

Ten years later, the patient reappears. Despite your prescription her blood pressure has remained in the level 1 range. Laboratory findings are essentially unchanged. However, the echocardiogram shows left ventricular hypertrophy.

Question 3

Which of the following would you recommend for this patient now?:

(A) Hydrochlorothiazide and blood pressure monitoring
(B) Hydralazine and blood pressure monitoring
(C) Captopril and blood pressure monitoring
(D) Blood pressure monitoring only

Hypertension Question 4
Which one of the following medications is contra-indicated for the treatment of hypertension in pregnancy?

(A) Labetalol
(B) Enalapril
(C) Methyldopa
(D) Hydralazine
(E) Propranolol

Hypertension Question 5
A 53-year-old male accountant returns to your office for follow-up of hypertension. He was found to have a blood pressure of 160/104 mm Hg on an employ-ment physical 5 years earlier; the rest of the physical examination and electrolytes had been normal. He has been treated with various regimens, including thiazide diuretics, β-blockers, and calcium-channel antagonists. Most recently, he has been taking nifedipine, 90 mg daily in a sustained-release formulation. Diastolic pressure has varied from 90 to 106, with no consistent relationship to dose or class of drug used. The past history is notable for hyperuricemia, bilateral inguinal herniorrhaphies, esophageal reflux, mild obesity, and allergic rhinitis.

On examination, he appears well. The blood pressure is 158/100 mm Hg; heart and lungs are normal. There is trace pretibial edema bilaterally.

What is the next best step in the management of this patient?

(A) Increase the dosage of the calcium-channel blocker.
(B) Inquire about use of over-the-counter medications.
(C) Advise the patient to lose weight.
(D) Evaluate for renovascular causes of hypertension.
(E) Discuss the importance of compliance in the therapy of hypertension.

Hypertension Question 6
A 20-year-old man is referred to you for evaluation of hypertension. While he was in high school, his blood pressure was found to be elevated, but he was told he did not require any treatment at that time. He acknowledges that he has been unable to com-pete in athletics because he tires easily. Both parents developed hypertension when they were in their 40s. On physical examination, his pulse rate is 75/min and blood pressure is 160/94 mm Hg. There is seborrheic dermatitis of the face. Carotid pulsation is normal. Lungs are clear to auscultation. Cardiac examination shows 1+ left ventricular lift, normal S_1 and S_2, and an S_4 at the apex. A grade 2/6 systolic

ejection murmur is heard along the left sternal border and is audible in the interscapular area. The extremities are thin. Femoral, popliteal, dorsalis pedis, and posterior tibial pulses are palpable but diminished.

Laboratory studies:

Hematocrit	46%
Leukocyte count	7200/μL
Platelet count	210,000/μL
Erythrocyte sedimentation rate	4 mm/h
Blood urea nitrogen	12 mg/dL
Serum creatinine	0.8 mg/dL
Total cholesterol	169 mg/dL
Urinalysis	Normal

Electrocardiogram shows sinus rhythm and voltage criteria for left ventricular hypertrophy.

Which of the following tests is most likely to yield the correct diagnosis?

(A) Renal arteriography
(B) Captopril scintigraphy
(C) Magnetic resonance angiography of the thoracic aorta
(D) Serum catecholamine measurement
(E) Computed tomography of the abdomen

Hypertension Question 7
A 77-year-old woman presents to the Emergency Department with the sudden onset of severe back pain. She describes the instantaneous onset of tear-ing pain between the shoulder blades just seconds after lifting a carton of books. Her history is note-worthy for chronic hypertension and mild obesity. Her only medication is a thiazide diuretic.

On physical examination, she is anxious and in severe pain. Her pulse rate is 85/min, and her blood pressure is symmetrically elevated at 180/102 mm Hg. The examination of her chest, heart, abdomen, and extremities is normal. There is no point tender-ness over the spine. All pulses are full, and bowel sounds are normal.

Laboratory studies show a hematocrit of 33%, blood urea nitrogen of 18 mg/dL, and a serum creatinine of 1.1 mg/dL. The chest radiograph shows media-stinal widening. The electrocardiogram shows left ventricular hypertrophy by voltage.

Which one of the following is the most appropriate next step in managing this patient?

(A) Lower the blood pressure urgently using intravenous medications.
(B) Do transthoracic echocardiography.
(C) Call a cardiovascular surgeon.
(D) Obtain a series of radiographs of the spine to rule out ruptured vertebral disc.
(E) Do abdominal ultrasonography immediately to exclude aortic aneurysm with rupture.

Hypertension Question 8
A 49-year-old woman has blood pressure measured at 162/98, 158/102, and 156/100 mm Hg on three consecutive office visits. Her blood pressure measured by an automated device at her local pharmacy was 132/84 and 126/78 mm Hg. She has been taking estrogen, 0.625 mg/d, after a hysterectomy and bilateral salpingo-oophorectomy 3 years ago. She does not smoke, walks regularly, and maintains a low-fat diet. The physical examination and electrocardiogram are normal.

The next best step in the management of this patient is:

(A) Start therapy with hydrochlorothiazide, 25 mg/d
(B) Closely monitor her blood pressure with repeated clinic visits over a 2-month period
(C) Obtain 24-hour ambulatory blood pressure monitoring
(D) Discontinue the estrogen supplement
(E) Start therapy with lisinopril, 5 mg/d

Hypertension Question 9
A 56-year-old black man is found to have a persistently elevated blood pressure. He smokes and has a history of reflux esophagitis, and his family history is positive for hypertension and stroke. Physical examination reveals a blood pressure of 168/104 mm Hg, a pulse of 72/min, no bruits, and an S_4 gallop.

Laboratory studies:

Serum sodium	141 meq/L
Serum potassium	4.3 meq/L
Blood urea nitrogen	13 mg/dL
Plasma glucose	232 mg/dL
Serum creatinine	1.0 mg/dL
Serum uric acid	9.1 mg/dL
Urinalysis	Normal, no protein
Electrocardiogram	Borderline left ventricular hypertrophy by voltage criteria

The best initial therapy to manage this patient's hypertension is:

(A) Lisinopril, 5 mg once a day
(B) Nifedipine, extended-release 30 mg once a day
(C) Hydrochlorothiazide, 25 mg once per day
(D) Doxazosin, titrated to 2 mg once a day
(E) Atenolol, 50 mg once a day

Hypertension Question 10
A 32-year-old woman with a 12-year history of type 1 diabetes mellitus who has been followed in your office has an increase in her urine microalbumin excretion. The current level is 118 mg/24 h; the level 3 months ago was 64 mg/24 h. On physical examination, her blood pressure is 128/76 mm Hg, and background diabetic retinopathy is present. The hemoglobin A_{1c} is 7.2% and low-density lipoprotein cholesterol concentration is 134 mg/dL.

Which of the following is the most appropriate choice of therapy?

(A) Verapamil, long-acting, 120 mg/d
(B) Lisinopril, 5 mg/d
(C) Hydrochlorothiazide, 25 mg/d
(D) Prazosin, 2 mg/d
(E) Simvastatin, 10 mg every evening

Hypertension Question 11
A 45-year-old black man is found on health screening to have type 2 diabetes mellitus. The patient has a history of asthma; his family history is positive for hypertension in two siblings and his father had a stroke. There is no family history of coronary artery disease. The patient works as a house painter.

On physical examination, the patient is obese and has a blood pressure of 178/108 mm Hg. Funduscopic examination shows grade 1 hypertensive retinopathy but no diabetic changes. A fasting plasma glucose is 162 mg/dL and hemoglobin A_{1c} (HbA_{1c}) is 7.9%. Urine microalbumin is 11 mg/24 h. Total serum cholesterol is 192 mg/dL.

After 3 months of treatment with a hypocaloric low-saturated fat diet plus exercise, he loses 7.3 kg (16 lb). Although his blood pressure has decreased with treatment, it has stabilized at 158/98 mm Hg despite progressive increase of enalapril to a dosage of 20 mg/d. His HbA_{1c} has decreased to 6.5%, and total serum cholesterol has decreased to 178 mg/dL.

Which one of the following additional treatments should be prescribed now?

(A) Lisinopril, 5 mg/d
(B) Propranolol, long-acting, 60 mg/d
(C) Hydrochlorothiazide, 25 mg/d
(D) Prazosin, 2 mg/d
(E) Simvastatin, 10 mg every evening

Hypertension Question 12

A 22-year-old woman in the 32nd week of her first pregnancy is admitted to the hospital because of epigastric pain, nausea, and vomiting. Physical examination shows blood pressure 150/105 mm Hg, puffiness of the eyes, 1+ peripheral edema, and segmental arteriolar narrowing but no hemorrhages or exudates of the fundus; cardiovascular examination is normal.

Laboratory studies:

Hematocrit	40%
Leukocyte count	7000/μL
Platelet count	70,000/μL
Blood urea nitrogen	15 mg/dL
Serum uric acid	8.3 mg/dL
Serum creatinine	1.7 mg/dL
Serum bilirubin	2.7 mg/dL
Serum aspartate aminotransferase	500 U/L
Serum lactate dehydrogenase	500 U/L
Serum haptoglobin	14 mg/dL
Urinalysis	2+ protein, no erythrocytes, no leukocytes

Peripheral smear shows schistocytes and helmet cells. Reticulocyte count is 5%. Plasma fibrin split products level is 20 mg/mL (normal <10 mg/mL).

What is the most likely diagnosis?

(A) Thrombotic thrombocytopenic purpura
(B) Malignant hypertension
(C) Acute glomerulonephritis
(D) Acute pancreatitis
(E) Fulminant preeclampsia

Hypertension Question 13

A 28-year-old woman in the 28th week of her first pregnancy presents with hypokalemia. She has had hypertension both before and during her pregnancy. Her blood pressure is now 230/150 mm Hg. Funduscopic examination is normal. Physical examination shows a heart rate of 80/min with a grade II systolic murmur, clear lung fields, no abdominal bruits, and no peripheral edema. The uterus is appropriate in size for her stage of pregnancy.

Laboratory studies:

Blood urea nitrogen	8 mg/dL
Serum electrolytes	
Sodium	146 meq/L
Potassium	2.5 meq/L
Chloride	108 meq/L
Bicarbonate	24 meq/L
Serum uric acid	4 mg/dL
Serum creatinine	0.8 mg/dL
24-hour urine protein	150 mg

Plasma renin activity, both at 8 AM and noon, is 4 ng/mL per hour. Her plasma aldosterone concentration is 50 ng/dL at 8:00 AM and 22 ng/dL at noon

What is the most likely diagnosis?

(A) Malignant hypertension
(B) Primary aldosteronism secondary to an adrenal adenoma
(C) Renal artery stenosis
(D) Preeclampsia
(E) Primary aldosteronism secondary to bilateral adrenal hyperplasia

Hypertension Questions 14-18

For each of the hypertensive patients described below, select the most appropriate class of drug to use for initial therapy (A-D) (each answer may be used more than once or not at all):

(A) Thiazide diuretics
(B) Calcium channel blockers
(C) Direct vasodilators (hydralazine)
(D) Angiotensin-converting enzyme inhibitors

14. A 55-year-old man with left ventricular hypertrophy and diastolic dysfunction

15. A 43-year-old woman who has had insulin-dependent diabetes mellitus for 20 years and nephrotic range proteinuria and whose serum creatinine level is 1.5 mg/dL

16. A 72-year-old woman with asymptomatic systolic hypertension

17. A 53-year-old man with chronic asymptomatic left ventricular systolic dysfunction

18. A 65-year-old man with unilateral renal artery stenosis

Hypertension Question 19

A 48-year-old black woman presents with edema and hypertension. She has been taking furosemide and labetalol but has fatigue and decreased libido. A renal biopsy done 18 months ago showed focal glomerulosclerosis, but she was unresponsive to trials of corticosteroids and cyclosporine. She is concerned about the possibility of renal failure in the future and asks what she can do to prevent it.

On physical examination, her temperature is 36.6 °C (98 °F) and blood pressure is 165/100 mm Hg. The eyelids are puffy; the chest is clear. Cardiac examination shows a soft S_4 with a grade 1/6 systolic murmur. The abdomen is soft without tenderness to palpation. Extremities show 2+ pedal edema.

Laboratory studies:

Serum electrolytes
Sodium	137 meq/L
Potassium	5.9 meq/L
Chloride	97 meq/L
Bicarbonate	21 meq/L
Blood urea nitrogen	52 mg/dL
Serum creatinine	3.8 mg/dL

The electrocardiogram shows left ventricular hypertrophy with strain.

The best management to slow progression of the renal insufficiency is to:

(A) Lower labetalol dosage to improve compliance.
(B) Provide dietary consultation for advice about a protein-restricted diet.
(C) Advise the patient to drink at least 8 glasses of water a day.
(D) Achieve rigorous control of blood pressure.

JOINT DISEASE

Joint Disease Question 1

A 24-year-old woman presents to the emergency room with a history of a "spider bite" on her toe. She also has vague joint pains and feels warm. She has a temperature of 38.5 °C (101.4 °F), pulse rate of 100/min, and a normal respiration rate and blood pressure. On physical examination, she has a 5-mm pustule with surrounding erythema on her fourth toe. The rest of the skin examination reveals eight other scattered similar skin lesions on her trunk. There is no joint swelling or erythema. There is tenderness adjacent to the metacarpal joints. The rest of the physical examination is normal. Upon further questioning the patient recalls a similar illness 2 years ago.

Which of the following historical clues would be the most important in reaching a diagnosis?

(A) Previous allergy to spider bites
(B) Exposure to a child with varicella
(C) Exposure to a new sexual partner
(D) Exposure to a febrile child with blisters in mouth, on hands, and feet
(E) Determine whether she knows the difference between a spider and a tick

Joint Disease Question 2

A 46-year-old Little League coach pitched batting practice over the course of a 6-week season and his right shoulder became sore. His symptoms persisted for several weeks after the end of the Little League season despite self-treatment with ibuprofen, 600 mg four times a day, and acetaminophen as needed. He presents now, 6 weeks later, with some loss of passive range of motion in external rotation and abduction, and pain with elevation of his arm above the horizontal. Pain and weakness are present when his right shoulder is positioned at 90 degrees of abduction, his elbow flexed, and his forearm pronated (as if emptying a can of soda). Injection of lidocaine, 2 mL, into the subacromial space immediately relieves his symptoms; the passive range of motion loss is still present.

Appropriate management at this time would include:

(A) Plain radiographs of the shoulder
(B) MRI of the shoulder
(C) Subacromial injection of a long-acting anesthetic-corticosteroid and immobilization in a sling
(D) Immobilization in a sling for 2 weeks followed by physical therapy
(E) Subacromial injection of a long-acting anesthetic-corticosteroid followed by physical therapy

Joint Disease Question 3

A 36-year-old female business executive is diagnosed as having seropositive rheumatoid arthritis after 3 months of symmetric polyarthritis and fatigue. Because of her joint pains and fatigue, she has had to leave work. Physical examination shows symmetric swelling, warmth, and tenderness of the wrists, metacarpophalangeal (MCP) joints, and proximal interphalangeal joints (PIP) of the hands, and similar joints in the feet. She also has bilateral knee, ankle, and elbow inflammation.

Laboratory studies:

Hematocrit	32%
Leukocyte count	9500/μL
Platelet count	560,000/μL
Erythrocyte sedimentation rate	60 mm/h

Anteroposterior and lateral radiographs of the right hand show juxta-articular osteoporosis about the MCP and PIP joints with radial marginal joint erosion of the second PIP joint.

The most appropriate treatment for this patient is:

(A) Nonsteroidal anti-inflammatory drugs (NSAIDs) and radiography of the hand in 3 months to look for the development of more erosions
(B) Prednisone, 40 mg/d orally, until joint inflammation is controlled and then taper to a maintenance dose of 10 mg/d
(C) NSAIDs; methotrexate, 7.5 mg per week orally; and physical therapy
(D) NSAIDs and minocycline, 100 mg twice daily orally
(E) Acetaminophen as needed, wrist splints, and short courses of prednisone

Joint Disease Question 4

A 66-year-old woman has mild osteoarthritis of her hips and knees. Her symptoms have been relieved with acetaminophen. Recently, she has developed pain and tenderness well localized extra-articularly several inches below the left knee joint and medial to the knee. She has stiffness in the morning, after prolonged sitting, and when climbing stairs. Sleeping with a pillow between her knees provides some relief. Physical examination shows mild, fine crepitation of both knees without instability, synovitis, or swelling; tenderness with puffiness is detected 5 cm (2 in) below the medial aspect of the left knee.

What is the most likely diagnosis?

(A) Patellar tendinitis
(B) Osteonecrosis
(C) Anserine bursitis
(D) Prepatellar bursitis
(E) Flare of osteoarthritis

Joint Disease Question 5

A 41-year-old woman presents because she "hurts all over." She has fatigue, loss of energy, and stiffness on awakening in the morning, along with pain at her wrists, elbows, shoulders, neck, hips, and knees; she says that her joints feel "swollen"; she sleeps poorly. These symptoms have progressed over the past 3 years. She has a history of tension-type headaches for many years and was told by another physician that she has irritable bowel syndrome. She works as an executive secretary in a stressful office. She was recently divorced and cares for her chronically ill mother in her home.

Physical examination shows tender points at the elbows, shoulder and hip girdles, wrists, and knees. Complete blood count, chemistry panel, and thyroid stimulating hormone are normal. Erythrocyte sedimentation rate is 21 mm/h.

Which of the following management programs is most appropriate?

(A) Doxycycline, 100 mg twice daily for 4 weeks
(B) A nonsteroidal anti-inflammatory drug; plaquenil, 400 mg/d; and, if needed, methotrexate, 7.5 mg weekly
(C) Tricyclic antidepressants and an aerobic exercise program
(D) Plaquenil, 400 mg/d, and prednisone, 10 mg/d
(E) Gammaglobulin, 0.75 mg/kg intravenously for 3 doses

Joint Disease Question 6

A 49-year-old third-grade schoolteacher presents with marked stiffness. About 8 months ago she began to notice swelling in her knees, particularly in the morning and lasting an hour. Six months ago she also developed marked morning stiffness and visible swelling in her wrists and the proximal interphalangeal joints of both hands. The results of laboratory tests were obtained by her family doctor 6 months ago and are shown below.

Laboratory studies:

Hemoglobin	10.5 g/dL
Hematocrit	35%
Leukocyte count	6800/μL, with a normal differential
Erythrocyte sedimentation rate	30 mm/h
Repeat erythrocyte sedimentation rate	45 mm/h (2 months ago)
Urinalysis	Normal
Latex agglutination test	Negative
Serum antinuclear antibody test	Negative

Treatment with ibuprofen, 600 mg three times daily, produced only moderate relief. The patient's joint symptoms increased, and she was having trouble standing up to teach her class.

Physical examination at this time shows definite synovial tenderness and swelling in both wrists as well as swelling in the proximal interphalangeal joints and metacarpophalangeal joints of both hands. The left knee shows fluid and synovial thickening.

Roentgenograms of the hands, wrists, and knees show periarticular osteopenia in the wrists, metacarpophalangeal joints, and proximal interphalangeal joints of both hands. There is also narrowing of the joint space medially in the left knee. Aspiration of fluid from the left knee produces 20 mL of thick, viscous, clear yellow synovial fluid containing 15,000 cells, of which 70% are polymorphonuclear neutrophil leukocytes and 30% are lymphocytes. Polarizing light examination shows no crystals either in the fluid or within polymorphonuclear neutrophil leukocytes.

What is the most likely diagnosis?

(A) Osteoarthritis
(B) Rheumatoid arthritis
(C) Chondrocalcinosis
(D) Septic arthritis
(E) Reactive arthritis

79

Joint Disease Question 7

A 62-year-old man has aching in the left lateral hip and thigh, which is worse when lying on his left side.

What is the most likely diagnosis?

(A) Hip osteoarthritis
(B) Pseudoclaudication syndrome of spinal stenosis
(C) Leriche's syndrome
(D) Trochanteric bursitis
(E) Early osteonecrosis of the femoral neck

Joint Disease Question 8

A 42-year-old woman presents with pain and swelling of the third and fourth toe of the left foot. Her symptoms have been present for 3 weeks and have not responded to acetaminophen or ibuprofen. She denies fever and chills or trauma. Her medical history is remarkable for psoriasis, which is being treated with topical agents.

Physical examination reveals psoriatic plaques involving extensor surfaces of the elbows and localized patches on her back and lower abdomen. There is pitting of multiple fingernails and toenails. The third and fourth toes are diffusely swollen and painful to palpation along their length (see Figure below). Radiograph reveals no bony changes.

What is the most appropriate therapy to institute at this time?

(A) Dicloxacillin, 500 mg four times daily
(B) Indomethacin, 50 mg two times daily with food
(C) Methylprednisolone, 4 mg/d
(D) Colchicine, 6 mg twice daily
(E) Nafcillin, 2 g every 6 hours intravenously

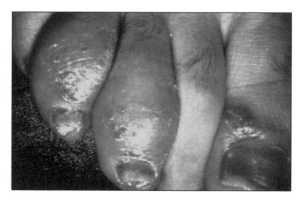

Joint Disease Question 9

A 75-year-old healthy woman has medial knee pain that occurs after prolonged standing. There is no morning stiffness or joint effusion. Walking upstairs and downstairs does not affect the pain. The physical examination is unremarkable. Her right knee shows no effusion, ligamentous laxity, or patellar crepitus. Her right foot is pronated. Radiographs of the knee taken while the patient is standing show narrowing of the medial joint space, subchondral bone cysts, and eburnation.

Which of the following would be appropriate initial management?

(A) Transcutaneous electrical stimulation
(B) Indomethacin, 50 mg four times daily
(C) Knee brace
(D) Limiting walking to 20 minutes per day
(E) Acetaminophen, 650 mg four times daily

Joint Disease Question 10

A 55-year-old woman presents to your office because of pain in her left hand. Four weeks ago she underwent a left modified radical mastectomy. All axillary nodes were negative. Three weeks ago she had pain with motion of the left shoulder that has gradually worsened; she now finds it difficult to comb her hair or do tasks such as empty the dishwasher. One week ago her left hand felt stiff and swollen and has gradually become so painful that she is unable to sleep.

Physical examination is normal except for the healing surgical wounds and pain in the left shoulder. The shoulder is limited in motion to approximately 45 degrees of flexion, 15 degrees of extension, 30 degrees of abduction, and 15 degrees of internal and external rotation. Palpation of the shoulder is normal. The left hand is diffusely puffy, has a mottled cyanotic appearance, and is slightly warm and moist. She holds her left hand in her lap with the fingers flexed at about 30 degrees and prefers not to move it.

Which of the following is the most likely diagnosis?

(A) Lymphangitis
(B) Subclavian vein obstruction
(C) Streptococcal cellulitis
(D) Reflex sympathetic dystrophy syndrome
(E) Hypertrophic osteoarthropathy

Joint Disease Question 11

You are called to consult about a 69-year-old man who has just undergone a cholecystectomy and is having severe pain and swelling in both knees that began shortly after the surgical procedure. He states that he has had swelling in his knees previously, as well as in his wrists and elbows.

The patient's blood pressure is 150/95 mm Hg, pulse is 80/min, and temperature is 37 °C (98.6 °F). Physical examination shows swelling of both knees with large effusions. You have ordered a serum rheumatoid factor test, serum antinuclear antibody test, and erythrocyte sedimentation rate study, but the results are not yet available.

Laboratory studies:

Leukocyte count	25,000/µL, with 85% neutrophils, 12% lymphocytes, and 3% monocytes
Blood urea nitrogen	24 mg/dL
Plasma glucose	60 mg/dL
Serum creatinine	0.9 mg/dL

Arthrocentesis of his knee shows a negative Gram stain and intracellular and extracellular weakly positively birefringent crystals in the synovial fluid.

The most likely diagnosis is:

(A) Calcium pyrophosphate dihydrate deposition disease
(B) Calcium oxalate deposition disease
(C) Basic calcium phosphate deposition disease
(D) Gout
(E) Septic arthritis

Joint Disease Question 12
A 64-year-old man presents because of the acute onset of pain, tenderness, and swelling of the right ankle. He has occasional pain and stiffness at the knees that have been controlled with acetaminophen. He successfully underwent renal transplantation 18 months ago for end-stage, inactive lupus nephropathy. He has been taking prednisone, 15 mg/d, azathioprine, 100 mg/d, and cyclosporine, 350 mg/d.

On physical examination, his temperature is 38.4 °C (101.1 °F).

Laboratory studies:

Hematocrit	33%
Leukocyte count	12,800/µL, with 80% neutrophils and 20% lymphocytes
Platelet count	180,000/µL
Blood urea nitrogen	22 mg/dL
Serum creatinine	1.4 mg/dL

Radiography of the joints shows changes of mild osteoarthritis.

Synovial fluid aspiration and analysis is most likely to show:

(A) Hemorrhagic fluid
(B) Needle-shaped, strongly negatively birefringent intra- and extracellular crystals
(C) Gram-positive organisms
(D) Rhomboidal, weakly positively birefringent intra- and extracellular crystals
(E) Noninflammatory fluid

Joint Disease Question 13
A 19-year-old woman presents with acute onset of severe pain overlying the dorsum of her left foot. The left ankle is not swollen, but passive flexion and extension of the left great toe induces severe pain over the dorsum of the midfoot and ankle. Additional physical findings include inability to fully extend the right elbow, which is swollen and mildly tender to palpation. The rest of the examination is unremarkable and notable for the absence of fever or skin lesions. Arthrocentesis of the left elbow produces several drops of synovial fluid; Gram stain indicates the presence of neutrophils in the fluid, but no organisms are seen.

What is the most appropriate medication to initiate at this time?

(A) Nafcillin sodium, intravenously, 1 g every 6 hours
(B) Ceftriaxone sodium, 1 g every 24 hours
(C) Ampicillin, orally, 3 g, with probenecid, 1000 mg
(D) Indomethacin, orally, 50 mg three times daily
(E) Aspirin, 975 mg four times daily, with penicillin V potassium, 500 mg four times daily

LIPID DISORDERS

Lipid Disorders Question 1

A 57-year-old man presents to the Emergency Department with a 2-hour history of substernal chest pain. He is subsequently diagnosed as having had an acute anterior myocardial infarction. A fasting lipid profile done on admission reveals a total serum cholesterol of 220 mg/dL, high-density lipoprotein (HDL) cholesterol of 40 mg/dL, and triglycerides of 100 mg/dL.

What is this patient's estimated low-density lipoprotein (LDL) cholesterol?

(A) 100 mg/dL
(B) 120 mg/dL
(C) 140 mg/dL
(D) 160 mg/dL
(E) 180 mg/dL

Lipid Disorders Question 2

A 53-year-old woman presents with concerns about coronary risk and questions regarding estrogens. She underwent a hysterectomy at age 48 years. Menopausal symptoms were bothersome 3 years ago but not any longer. Her father had a high serum cholesterol value and died of a myocardial infarction at age 52 years; her mother is well at 75 years. There is no family history of cancer or diabetes mellitus. She is a nonsmoker, consumes no alcohol, stopped using butter a few years ago, and does not exercise.

On physical examination, she is 163 cm (64 in) tall and weighs 75 kg (165 lb). Pulse rate is 80/min, and blood pressure is 160/90 mm Hg in the right and left arms. The fundi are normal. Carotid and jugular venous pulses are normal. The lungs are clear. The breasts are normal. The apical impulse is not palpable, but the left border of cardiac dullness is 8 cm from the midsternal line in the fourth intercostal space. The heart sounds are normal. The abdomen is moderately obese, with no organomegaly or bruits. The extremities are normal, with good pulses.

Her nonfasting serum cholesterol level is measured at 307 mg/dL, and high-density lipoprotein (HDL) cholesterol is 38 mg/dL. She returns the following morning for a fasting lipid profile and thyroid-stimulating hormone assay. A repeat blood pressure taken at this time is 140/94 mm Hg.

Laboratory studies:

Serum cholesterol (fasting)	245 mg/dL
Serum triglycerides	305 mg/dL
Serum HDL-cholesterol	34 mg/dL
Calculated low-density lipoprotein cholesterol	150 mg/dL
Serum thyroid stimulating hormone	1.2 µU/mL

Which of the following is the best advice for this woman?

(A) Begin dieting and exercising
(B) Begin estrogen replacement therapy
(C) Begin therapy with an HMG-CoA reductase inhibitor
(D) Begin therapy with gemfibrozil
(E) Begin therapy with niacin

Lipid Disorders Question 3

A 72-year-old woman presents 6 weeks after sustaining an inferior myocardial infarction that was without complications. She was treated with aspirin, 325 mg/d, and metoprolol, 25 mg twice daily. The predischarge echocardiogram showed an akinetic inferior wall and left ventricular ejection fraction of 51%, and on exercise electrocardiogram she achieved 6 minutes on the Bruce protocol with a normal hemodynamic response and no ST-T abnormalities. Two weeks postdischarge, she began cardiac rehabilitation.

On presentation, she is doing well. She has been healthy and is 18 years postmenopausal. There is no family history of breast cancer, but her mother died of ovarian cancer. She is 168 cm (66 in) tall and weighs 64 kg (141 lb). Her pulse rate is 80/min, and blood pressure is 140/82 mm Hg. Findings on fasting lipid profile are cholesterol, 198 mg/dL; triglycerides, 235 mg/dL; high-density lipoprotein (HDL) cholesterol, 33 mg/dL; and calculated low-density lipoprotein (LDL) cholesterol, 118 mg/dL. You recommend estrogen and progesterone for this woman. She is following a low-fat diet.

Which one of the following is also most appropriate?

(A) Pravastatin
(B) Niacin
(C) Bile resin
(D) Discontinuation of the β-blocker
(E) Gemfibrozil

Lipid Disorders Question 4

A 52-year-old black man wants to do everything possible to prevent a myocardial infarction and requests advice about the use of antioxidant vitamins. He exercises and follows a low-fat diet. His father died of a myocardial infarction at 46 years of age. His pulse rate is 56/min, blood pressure is 120/74 mm Hg, and the physical examination is normal. Random serum cholesterol is 199 mg/dL and high-density lipoprotein (HDL) cholesterol is 45 mg/dL. Because of the family history you obtain other studies.

Laboratory studies:

Cholesterol (fasting)	196 mg/dL
Triglycerides	120 mg/dL
HDL cholesterol	46 mg/dL
Calculated low-density lipoprotein cholesterol	126 mg/dL
Lipoprotein(a)	50 mg/dL

Which of the following recommendations is most appropriate?

(A) Vitamin A, 25,000 IU
(B) β-carotene, 25 mg
(C) Vitamin C, 500 mg
(D) Vitamin E, 800 IU
(E) None of the above

Lipid Disorders Question 5

A 62-year-old accountant presents with severe right foot pain that has been present for 3 weeks. This pain has been preventing him from sleeping comfortably, so he sits in a chair most of the night for relief. For the past 6 months, he has had right calf discomfort when he walks one block. He has hypertension and type 2 diabetes mellitus. He smokes two packs of cigarettes per day. Medications include lisinopril, glyburide, and aspirin.

On physical examination, his pulse rate is 78/min, and blood pressure is 150/90 mm Hg. The lungs are clear to auscultation. A grade 2/6 early-peaking systolic ejection murmur is heard along the left sternal border. There is a periumbilical bruit. Examination of the extremities shows a cool and swollen right foot. When the foot is elevated, it becomes pale; when it is dependent, rubor develops. The right femoral pulse is diminished. The right popliteal, dorsalis pedis, and posterior tibial pulses are absent. The left femoral pulse is present and normal. The left popliteal pulse is diminished. The left dorsalis pedis and posterior tibial pulses are absent. There is decreased sensation to pin prick in both feet in a stocking distribution.

Laboratory studies:

Hematocrit	41%
Leukocyte count	9800/μL
Platelet count	241,000/μL
Blood urea nitrogen	31 mg/dL
Serum creatinine	1.3 mg/dL
Total cholesterol	224 mg/dL
Triglycerides	350 mg/dL

Electrocardiogram shows sinus rhythm, left atrial enlargement, and left ventricular hypertrophy.

What diagnostic test will confirm this patient's diagnosis and guide the appropriate treatment decision?

(A) Echocardiography
(B) Arteriography of the aorta and peripheral arteries
(C) Pulse volume recording (PVR)
(D) Venous ultrasonography
(E) Nerve conduction study

Lipid Disorders Question 6

A 76-year-old woman presents because she had a cholesterol level of 290 mg/dL by finger stick in the local mall. She has not been taking estrogens and does not like the idea of doing so. She and her husband have been avoiding butter and eggs for years. On physical examination, her pulse rate is 70/mm, and blood pressure is 130/70 mm Hg. Her carotid pulses are normal, without bruits. The lungs are clear. Her breasts are atrophied and without masses. The heart sounds and apical impulse are normal, and the abdomen and extremities are normal, with adequate pulses. She agrees to your suggestion of a fasting lipid profile with the following results: cholesterol, 294 mg/dL; triglycerides, 120 mg/dL; HDL cholesterol, 84 mg/dL; and calculated LDL cholesterol, 186 mg/dL.

Which of the following strategies is most appropriate?

(A) Diet and exercise
(B) A bile resin with psyllium
(C) An HMG-CoA reductase inhibitor
(D) Aspirin
(E) Estrogen with progestin

Lipid Disorders Question 7

The National Cholesterol Education Panel recommends which of the following treatment goals for patients with established coronary artery disease?

(A) Lower low-density lipoprotein (LDL) cholesterol to 70 mg/dL
(B) Lower LDL cholesterol to 100 mg/dL
(C) Lower LDL cholesterol to 130 mg/dL
(D) Raise high-density lipoprotein (HDL) cholesterol to 45 mg/dL
(E) Raise HDL cholesterol to 55 mg/dL

Lipid Disorders Question 8

A 51-year-old man is found on routine health examination to have plasma fasting glucose of 285 mg/dL and urine negative for ketones. On questioning, he says he has had frequent urination and increased thirst for at least 1 year. Family history is positive for coronary artery disease before age 50 years in his father and two paternal uncles but is negative for diabetes mellitus. There is no history of excessive alcohol intake. He is 30% above ideal body weight.

Initial laboratory studies:

Hemoglobin A_{1c} (HbA_{1c})	11.5%
Plasma total cholesterol	258 mg/dL
Plasma high-density lipoprotein (HDL) cholesterol	28 mg/dL
Serum triglycerides	550 mg/dL
Thyroid-stimulating hormone	2.2 µU/mL

After 6 months of treatment with a sulfonylurea drug, diet of 1800 calories (25% saturated fat), and exercise, he has lost 14.5 kg (32.0 lb) and is now at ideal body weight.

Current laboratory studies:

HbA_{1c}	6.1%
Plasma fasting glucose	110 mg/dL
Plasma total cholesterol	212 mg/dL
Plasma HDL cholesterol	34 mg/dL
Serum triglycerides	350 mg/dL

The best next step in treatment is:

(A) Add gemfibrozil.
(B) Change the diabetes drug from glyburide to metformin.
(C) Add nicotinic acid.
(D) Add lovastatin.
(E) Add cholestyramine.

Lipid Disorders Question 9

A 45-year-old woman presents to your office because of concern over her serum cholesterol level. She is otherwise healthy, and has no other risk factors for atherosclerotic cardiovascular disease. Her total serum cholesterol after a 12-hour fast is 260 mg/dL.

Your next step should be to:

(A) Repeat total cholesterol measurement after an 18-hour fast
(B) Perform a fasting lipoprotein analysis
(C) Refer to a dietitian for dietary intervention
(D) Recommend an exercise program
(E) Request other family members to undergo cholesterol testing

Lipid Disorders Question 10

Which one of the following statements about lipid abnormalities in patients with the nephrotic syndrome is true?

(A) Total serum cholesterol is usually increased; LDL cholesterol is usually normal.
(B) Using ACE inhibitors to reduce proteinuria leads to a decrease in total serum cholesterol concentrations.
(C) HMG-CoA reductase inhibitors should not be used because they bind to serum albumin and cause side effects in hypoalbuminemic patients.
(D) Lowering elevated cholesterol concentrations in patients with the nephrotic syndrome has been shown to reduce the risk for cardiovascular disease.

LIVER DISORDERS

Liver Disorders Question 1

A 38-year-old woman has received 6 months of interferon alfa therapy for chronic hepatitis due to infection by the hepatitis C virus. The infection presumably occurred from a blood transfusion 15 years ago. The hepatitis was documented by histopathologic examination before initiation of treatment, and no other causes of chronic hepatitis were identified. Her constitutional symptoms have dramatically improved during the course of therapy, and the serum aminotransferases have remained below the upper limits of normal.

Further evaluation to determine the need for a longer course of therapy might include:

(A) Determination of the titer of serum anti–hepatitis C antibodies
(B) Quantification of serum viral load by either polymerase chain reaction (PCR) or branched DNA amplification
(C) Percutaneous liver biopsy for histopathologic reevaluation
(D) Percutaneous liver biopsy for PCR amplification to determine if viral RNA is still present
(E) Stop therapy and follow for clinical signs of hepatitis

Liver Disorders Question 2

A 36-year-old woman presents to the outpatient clinic with a 3-week history of fatigue and vague intermittent right upper quadrant discomfort, which has partially responded to two or three 500-mg acetaminophen tablets per day. She denies past parenteral blood exposure, high-risk sexual behavior, alcohol use, or recent exposure to persons with known hepatitis. She has no known family history of liver disease. She was diagnosed as having hypothyroidism 5 years ago, and her only medication is thyroid hormone replacement.

Physical examination shows a well-developed, slender, anicteric woman with a pulse rate of 88/min and a blood pressure of 110/60 mm Hg. There is evidence of palmar erythema and spider angiomata; the abdomen is flat and soft with active bowel sounds; the liver span percusses to 10 cm in the mid-clavicular line with a vague edge palpated 2 cm below the xiphoid process on deep inspiration. No spleen tip is palpable.

Laboratory studies:

Serum aspartate aminotransferase (AST)	720 U/L
Serum alanine aminotransferase (ALT)	850 U/L
Serum alkaline phosphatase	126 U/L
Serum total bilirubin	0.8 mg/dL
Serum direct bilirubin	0.2 mg/dL
Serum albumin	4.0 g/dL
Serum total protein	8.5 g/dL
Anti-HCV (ELISA II)	Positive
Serum antinuclear antibody (ANA)	Positive, 1:360

Liver biopsy specimen shows cirrhosis with severe inflammatory activity.

The most likely diagnosis is:

(A) Hepatitis C
(B) Autoimmune hepatitis
(C) Acetaminophen hepatotoxicity
(D) Nonalcoholic steatohepatitis
(E) Autoimmune cholangiopathy

Liver Disorders Question 3

A 43-year-old woman who has consumed a pint of 80-proof whiskey daily for 18 years presents with right upper quadrant pain. The pain began approximately a week ago and has been transiently relieved by her taking two extra-strength acetaminophen tablets every 4 hours for the past 4 days. She has had some nausea and vomiting but no fever. There is no history of jaundice or cholelithiasis. The patient used intravenous drugs and shared needles during her late teen years. There is no history of recent exposure to hepatitis.

The physical examination reveals an enlarged, tender liver that percusses to 17 cm in the right midclavicular line and a tattoo on the right buttock. The results of liver tests are as follows: bilirubin, 2 mg/dL; aspartate aminotransferase (AST), 3800 U/L; and γ-glutamyltransferase (GGT), 984 U/L. The prothrombin time is normal.

The most likely diagnosis is:

(A) Alcoholic hepatitis
(B) Acute cholecystitis
(C) Acetaminophen hepatotoxicity
(D) Acute viral hepatitis B
(E) Acute viral hepatitis C

Liver Disorders Question 4

A 54-year-old asymptomatic man volunteers to donate blood and is found to have elevated aminotransferase levels. He has no known medical problems and no history of hepatitis. He drinks no alcohol, takes no medications, and has not seen a physician in more than 10 years. He is active, works as a truck driver, and has noted no change in his physical condition. He has no family history of liver disease.

The physical examination is remarkable for obesity. He is 5 feet 10 inches tall and weighs 100 kg (220 pounds).

Laboratory studies:

Complete blood count	Normal
Aspartate aminotransferase	45 U/L
Alanine aminotransferase	85 U/L
Alkaline phosphatase	90 U/L
γ-Glutamyltransferase	125 U/L
Hepatitis serologies (anti-hepatitis A, hepatitis B surface antigen and antibody, anti-hepatitis B core antibody, and hepatitis C antibody)	Negative
Erythrocyte sedimentation rate	Normal
Antinuclear antibody	Negative
Anti–smooth-muscle antibody	Negative
Total cholesterol	260 mg/dL
Low-density lipoprotein cholesterol	225 mg/dL
Triglycerides	830 mg/dL

A liver biopsy specimen shows large-droplet steatosis without significant inflammatory reaction and no fibrosis. Ultrasonography shows a mildly enlarged fatty liver.

The appropriate management of this patient would be:

(A) Interferon therapy for presumed chronic non-B, non-C hepatitis
(B) Alcohol rehabilitation and counseling
(C) Weight loss and therapy for hyperlipidemia
(D) Endoscopic retrograde cholangiopancreatography (ERCP) to evaluate the biliary tree
(E) Corticosteroid therapy

Liver Disorders Question 5

A 72-year-old man is found to have multiple gallstones on ultrasonography performed to evaluate a suspected abdominal aortic aneurysm. He has no history of jaundice or abdominal pain. He has long-standing hypertension, diabetes mellitus, occasional angina, and hypercholesterolemia.

The physical examination is remarkable for a palpable, pulsatile, 3-cm abdominal aortic aneurysm, which is confirmed by the ultrasonography. He has no other abdominal tenderness or masses. Except for a serum cholesterol of 260 mg/dL, the results of laboratory tests are normal.

The best approach to this patient's gallstones would be:

(A) Dissolution therapy with ursodeoxycholic acid
(B) Endoscopic retrograde cholangiopancreatography (ERCP) with stone extraction
(C) Open cholecystectomy
(D) Laparoscopic cholecystectomy
(E) No therapy at this time

Liver Disorders Question 6

A 30-year-old man received blood transfusions 5 years ago after an automobile accident. Evaluation of modest alanine aminotransferase (ALT) elevation yielded a positive anti-HCV antibody. The patient is interested in considering treatment for hepatitis C.

Which one of the following statements is true with respect to counseling about treatment for hepatitis C:

(A) Interferon therapy for hepatitis C prevents cirrhosis and the risk for development of hepatocellular carcinoma.
(B) Approximately 75% of patients with chronic hepatitis C treated with interferon experience a sustained normalization of elevated aminotransferases after treatment.
(C) In patients who have normalized aminotransferases with treatment, prolonged therapy of 12 to 18 months results in improved sustained response rates compared with 6 months of treatment
(D) Response to interferon therapy is independent of the duration of infection or the presence of fibrosis on liver biopsy.

Liver Disorders Question 7

During evaluation of an elevated alanine amino-transferase (ALT), a 45-year-old alcoholic man is found to have a serum iron concentration of 245 mg/dL, a total iron-binding capacity of 290 mg/dL, 84% transferrin saturation, and a serum ferritin concentration of 2120 ng/mL. The physical examination shows no evidence of chronic liver or cardiac disease.

Which one of the following would be appropriate management for this patient?

(A) Biopsy to make a definitive diagnosis
(B) Magnetic resonance imaging (MRI) evaluation for iron overload
(C) Weekly phlebotomy
(D) HLA typing

Liver Disorders Question 8

A 40-year-old married man with two teenage children was recently evaluated for fatigue and elevations of liver enzymes and was found to have chronic hepatitis B. Physical examination reveals a few scattered spider angiomata over the chest and upper extremities.

Laboratory studies:

HBsAg	Positive
HBeAg	Positive
HBV DNA	90 pg/mL (hybridization assay, low value)
Serum alanine aminotransferase	156 U/L
Serum albumin	3.8 g/dL
International normalized ratio (INR)	1.5

A liver biopsy specimen shows cirrhosis with moderate inflammatory activity.

The most appropriate recommendation for this patient is:

(A) He should receive hepatitis A vaccine.
(B) His wife and children should receive hepatitis B vaccine.
(C) He should be treated with interferon alfa.
(D) All of the above

Liver Disorders Questions 9-12

For each patient described below, select the appropriate serologic pattern (A-E) (each answer may be used more than once or not at all):

	HbsAg	Anti-HBs	IgM anti-HBc	Total anti-HBc	HBe Ag	Anti-HDV	Anti-HCV
(A)	+	–	–	+	+	–	+
(B)	–	+	–	–	–	–	+
(C)	–	+	–	+	–	–	+
(D)	+	–	–	+	–	+	–
(E)	+	–	+	+	+	+	–

9. An asymptomatic 50-year-old businessman experimented with injection drugs briefly in his early 20s. He was told 2 years ago that he had abnormal liver tests because of hepatitis C and that he had hepatitis B exposure in the remote past.

10. A 32-year-old dialysis nurse who had hepatitis B vaccination while in nursing school, suffered a needle-stick from a known hepatitis C virus (HCV)–positive patient 6 months ago and has an elevated alanine aminotransferase (ALT).

11. A 45-year-old man with a 5-year history of injection drug use and known to have chronic hepatitis B virus (HBV) infection for 2 years recently developed a rise in his serum ALT concentration accompanied by jaundice and ascites, which is attributed to hepatitis D virus (HDV) superinfection.

12. A 59-year-old man has chronic hepatitis B, which is believed to have been acquired in childhood. He also received blood transfusions at the time of coronary artery bypass grafting in 1985. When he presents for initiation of interferon therapy for the replicative form of HBV infection, he is also found to be infected with HCV.

Liver Disorders Questions 13-16
For each patient described below, select the most likely cause of the cholestasis (A-D) (each answer may be used more than once or not at all):

(A) Primary biliary cirrhosis
(B) Primary sclerosing cholangitis
(C) Drug-induced cholangiopathy
(D) Infectious cholangiopathy

13. A 35-year-old man with AIDS presents with right upper quadrant abdominal pain and a temperature of 38.1 °C (100.6 °F). Laboratory values are as follows: alanine aminotransferase, 95 U/L; aspartate aminotransferase, 70 U/L; alkaline phosphatase, 450 U/L; and total bilirubin 4.5 mg/dL. He is taking multiple medications, including zidovudine and trimethoprim-sulfamethoxazole. Endoscopic cholangiography shows multifocal strictures of the extrahepatic biliary tree.

14. A 45-year-old man with a 20-year history of ulcerative colitis presents with recurrent fever and right upper quadrant pain. His colitis has been quiescent for 5 years while he has been taking sulfasalazine. A colonoscopy 3 months ago with multiple biopsies was negative for neoplasia and dysplasia. The physical examination is remarkable for a temperature of 38.1 °C (100.5 °F) and right upper quadrant abdominal tenderness. Laboratory values are as follows: leukocyte count, 400/µL; alanine aminotransferase, 104 U/L; aspartate aminotransferase, 98 U/L; alkaline phosphatase, 620 U/L; and total bilirubin, 3.2 mg/dL. Endoscopic retrograde cholangiopancreatography (ERCP) shows multifocal strictures of the extrahepatic biliary tree.

15. A 52-year-old woman is found to have abnormal liver enzymes on a screening examination. She complains of dry skin that causes her to scratch frequently. She takes estrogen and progesterone. The physical examination is normal. Laboratory values are as follows: leukocyte count, 8200/µL; alanine aminotransferase, 50 U/L; aspartate aminotransferase, 42 U/L; alkaline phosphatase, 843 U/L; γ-glutamyltransferase, 430 U/L; and total bilirubin, 0.9 mg/dL.

16. A 60-year-old schizophrenic man presents with the onset of painless jaundice. He has taken multiple psychotropic medications, including chlorpromazine, for 10 years. The physical examination is normal except for his jaundice. Laboratory values are as follows: aspartate aminotransferase, 60 U/L; alanine aminotransferase, 86 U/L; alkaline phosphatase, 422 U/L; γ-glutamyltransferase, 280 U/L; and total bilirubin, 7 mg/dL. ERCP is normal. Liver biopsy specimen shows a paucity of bile ductules in the portal areas.

Liver Disorders Question 17
A 63-year-old Native American woman comes to the emergency room because of nausea, vomiting, shaking chills, fever, and abdominal pain of 4 hours' duration. Physical examination reveals a temperature of 39.2 °C (102.5 °F), scleral icterus, and epigastric tenderness.

Laboratory studies:

Hematocrit	35%
Leukocyte count	8,000/µL with 80% polymorphonuclear leukocytes, 4% band forms, 12% lymphocytes, 4% monocytes
Serum creatinine	1.8 mg/dL
Serum alanine aminotransferase	250 U/L
Serum alkaline phosphatase	350 IU
Serum bilirubin	4.5 mg/dL
Serum amylase	1280 U/L
Serum lipase	920 U/dL

Ultrasonography of the abdomen reveals gallstones and dilatation of the common bile duct. Intravenous antibiotic therapy is begun.

Which of the following treatment plans would you recommend?

(A) Laparotomy with cholecystectomy, common duct exploration, and T-tube drainage of common bile duct within 12 hours
(B) Endoscopic retrograde cholangiopancreatography (ERCP) and papillotomy within 12 hours
(C) Continued administration of intravenous antibiotics and supportive care with elective surgery in the future
(D) Lithotripsy of gallstones
(E) Laparoscopic cholecystectomy

Liver Disorders Question 18

A 43-year-old woman complains of itching that keeps her awake at night. Physical examination is normal except for the liver, which is felt 7 cm below the right costal margin.

The blood count is normal; the results of serum chemistry tests are as follows:

Creatinine	0.8 mg/dL
Bilirubin	0.6 mg/dL
Alanine aminotransferase	78 U/L
Albumin	4.2 g/dL
Alkaline phosphatase	450 U/L

Which test would you order next to diagnose the underlying disorder?

(A) Serum protein electrophoresis
(B) Anti–smooth-muscle antibody
(C) Antimitochondrial antibody
(D) Technetium-99m liver-spleen scan
(E) Endoscopic retrograde cholangiopancreatography (ERCP)

Liver Disorders Questions 19-22

For each pregnant woman with jaundice described below, select the most likely cause of the jaundice (A-D) (each answer may be used more than once or not at all):

(A) Acute viral hepatitis
(B) Intrahepatic cholestasis of pregnancy
(C) The HELLP syndrome
(D) Acute fatty liver of pregnancy

19. A 24-year-old woman with a history of injection drug abuse presents in the second month of pregnancy with the acute onset of jaundice, dark urine, and light stools. She has no medical problems, other than the ongoing drug use. There is no family history of jaundice or liver disease. She takes no prescription medications. Her physical examination is remarkable only for jaundice and mild hepatomegaly.

Laboratory values:

Alanine aminotransferase	900 U/L
Aspartate aminotransferase	750 U/L
Alkaline phosphatase	250 U/L
Total bilirubin	14 mg/dL

The complete blood count is normal, without evidence of hemolysis on the smear.

20. A 35-year-old woman presents in the eighth month of her first pregnancy with jaundice and encephalopathy. She has no history of liver disease or hypertension, and she takes no medications. The physical examination shows jaundice, asterixis, and normal fetal heart sounds. The mental status examination reveals abnormalities in concentration and cognition.

Laboratory values:

Alanine aminotransferase	150 U/L
Aspartate aminotransferase	123 U/L
Total bilirubin	13 mg/dL
Prothrombin time	24 seconds (INR, 4.1)

21. A 25-year-old woman presents in the seventh month of pregnancy with mild jaundice, hypertension, and proteinuria. The physical examination is remarkable only for tender hepatomegaly and normal fetal heart sounds.

Laboratory values:

Alanine aminotransferase	220 U/L
Aspartate aminotransferase	150 U/L
Lactate dehydrogenase	753 U/L
Total bilirubin	5.0 mg/dL
Direct bilirubin	3.0 mg/dL
Platelet count	80,000/μL
Hemoglobin	10 mg/dL with evidence of hemolysis on the smear
Prothrombin time	Normal

22. A 23-year-old woman presents in the eighth month of pregnancy with pruritus and mild jaundice. The physical examination shows only mild scleral icterus and normal fetal heart sounds.

Laboratory values:

Alanine aminotransferase	90 U/L
Aspartate aminotransferase	85 U/L
Alkaline phosphatase	480 U/L
Total bilirubin	4.0 mg/dL

The complete blood count is normal, as is the prothrombin time.

Liver Disorders Question 23

A 39-year-old nurse presents with abdominal swelling. She works in the tuberculosis clinic of a large city hospital and has been taking birth control pills for 20 years. Her mother and older sister both died of ovarian cancer. Physical examination shows only obvious ascites with shifting dullness and a fluid wave.

Complete blood count, serum electrolytes, blood urea nitrogen (BUN), and creatinine are normal. Other serum chemistry studies show:

Alanine aminotransferase	40 U/L
Aspartate aminotransferase	140 U/L
Bilirubin	2.8 mg/dL
Alkaline phosphatase	140 U/L
Protein	5.8 g/dL
Albumin	2.9 g/dL

A diagnostic paracentesis is performed, and analysis of ascitic fluid shows:

Leukocyte count	190/μL with 90% lymphocytes
Protein	5.8 g/dL
Albumin	2.9 g/dL

The most likely diagnosis is:

(A) Budd-Chiari syndrome
(B) Ovarian cancer
(C) Alcoholic cirrhosis
(D) Tuberculous peritonitis
(E) Primary biliary cirrhosis

MYOCARDIAL INFARCTION

Myocardial Infarction Question 1

A 60-year-old man presents to the emergency room of a small rural hospital with a 4-hour history of shortness of breath, diaphoresis, and "just not feeling well." Physical examination reveals a pulse rate of 110/min, blood pressure of 90/60 mm Hg, and rales halfway up the lung fields. Electrocardiogram reveals 6 mm of ST-segment elevation in the anterior chest leads.

The patient is treated with oxygen, intravenous diuretics, nitrates, heparin, and accelerated dosing of tissue plasminogen activator (tPA). Over the next several minutes his pulse rate increases to 130/min with a sinus tachycardia, systolic blood pressure decreases to 75 mm Hg, and he continues to be short of breath. Arterial blood gases reveal a pH of 7.29, a P_{CO_2} of 30 mm Hg, and an oxygen saturation of 90% on 6 liters of oxygen by nasal cannula. The patient is transferred to the cardiac care unit, where Swan-Ganz catheterization reveals a pulmonary capillary wedge pressure of 25 mm Hg, a cardiac output of 2.0 L/min, and a systemic vascular resistance of 2000. The systolic blood pressure is now 70 mm Hg. The hospital does not have facilities for doing a percutaneous transluminal coronary angioplasty.

The most appropriate treatment at this time is:

(A) Intravenous digoxin
(B) Intravenous furosemide
(C) Intravenous dopamine
(D) Intubation and mechanical ventilation
(E) Intra-aortic balloon pump placement and transfer for emergency cardiac catheterization

Myocardial Infarction Question 2

A 45-year-old man with no prior cardiac history is admitted to the hospital with an acute inferior myocardial infarction. He is treated with tissue plasminogen activator (tPA) within 2 hours of the onset of his symptoms. He develops a Q-wave myocardial infarction with a peak creatine kinase of 2500 U/L (normal is less than 250 U/L). With the exception of short runs of ventricular tachycardia during the first 24 hours, the patient otherwise does well. He has no evidence of congestive heart failure, and an echocardiogram reveals inferior severe hypokinesis with an estimated ejection fraction of 50%. A 24-hour Holter monitor recording obtained at day 5 demonstrates rare premature ventricular contractions but no runs of ventricular tachycardia. At day 6, submaximal exercise thallium test produces no chest pain or electrocardiographic changes. However, the thallium scan shows an inferior perfusion defect with partial redistribution versus artifact due to diaphragmatic attenuation.

The appropriate management at this point is:

(A) Discharge on medical therapy
(B) Exercise multiple gated image acquisition analysis (MUGA) scan
(C) Catheterization, with angioplasty if a significant lesion is present
(D) Continued hospitalization to monitor for recurrent ischemia

Myocardial Infarction Questions 3-5

For each of the following outcomes in patients with acute Q-wave myocardial infarctions, select the drug most likely related to that outcome (A-D) (each answer may be used more than once or not at all):

(A) Aspirin
(B) Calcium channel blocker
(C) Beta-blocker
(D) Angiotensin-converting enzyme (ACE) inhibitor

3. Increases subsequent mortality if given to patients with congestive heart failure

4. Reduces ventricular dilatation

5. Reduces the incidence of subsequent sudden death

Myocardial Infarction Question 6

A 47-year-old man presents to the emergency room with 2 hours of central chest pressure. He is a heavy smoker and has not seen a physician in several years. He frequently uses antacids for epigastric burning.

On physical examination, he is diaphoretic and pale; his pulse rate is 60/min, and blood pressure is 104/72 mm Hg. The jugular venous pressure is approximately 12 cm H_2O. The lung fields are clear.

The heart sounds are soft; there is no murmur. Examination of the stool for occult blood is negative. The remainder of the examination is normal.

The electrocardiogram shows a normal sinus rhythm with 4-mm ST-segment elevations in leads 2, 3, and aVF, and 1- to 2-mm horizontal ST-segment depressions in leads V_1 and V_2. He is given nitroglycerin, 0.3 mg sublingually. His systolic blood pressure decreases to 80 mm Hg.

The most likely diagnosis is:

(A) Hypovolemic shock
(B) Cardiogenic shock from primary left ventricular pump failure
(C) Papillary muscle rupture
(D) Inferior posterior myocardial infarction with right ventricular involvement
(E) Anterior myocardial ischemia

Myocardial Infarction Question 7

A 66-year-old woman presents for follow-up after sustaining an acute myocardial infarction 2 years ago. Her exercise capacity is limited by fatigue, but she has no angina. She is taking diltiazem, aspirin, and simvastatin.

On physical examination, her pulse rate is 82/min, and respiration is normal. Blood pressure is 160/90 mm Hg. The carotid arteries are firm and tortuous without bruits, and the upstroke is brisk. The apical impulse is displaced to the left in the fifth intercostal space, 9 cm from the midsternal line and slightly sustained. S_1 is mildly decreased, S_2 is paradoxically split, and an S_4 is audible. A faint crescendo-decrescendo murmur is heard at the apex. There is no hepatomegaly or peripheral edema. Peripheral pulses are palpable but sclerotic.

The electrocardiogram shows sinus rhythm, a broad terminal P wave in lead V_1, and left bundle branch block. You obtain a multiple gated image acquisition analysis (MUGA). The left ventricular ejection fraction is 34%, the upper septum and anterior walls are akinetic, and right ventricular ejection fraction is 49%. You discontinue the diltiazem and add an angiotensin-converting enzyme (ACE) inhibitor.

Which one of the following is also indicated?

(A) Amlodipine
(B) β-blocker
(C) Nitrates
(D) Diuretic agent
(E) Digoxin

Myocardial Infarction Question 8

A 42-year-old man presents for routine follow-up 4 weeks after he developed an acute inferior myocardial infarction while playing basketball. At that time, he received thrombolytic therapy, and 3 days later he underwent cardiac catheterization. The left ventriculogram showed an ejection fraction of 55% and akinetic inferior wall. The right coronary artery was totally occluded, with good collaterals. The left anterior descending and circumflex arteries were large, with mild luminal irregularities. On the day of discharge, his nonfasting serum cholesterol was 180 mg/dL, and high-density lipoprotein (HDL) cholesterol was 48 mg/dL. He was prescribed a β-blocker and aspirin.

In your office 4 weeks later, he feels fine. There is no history of coronary artery disease, diabetes, or lipid disorders in first-degree relatives. On physical examination, he appears well; he is 170 cm (65 in) tall and weighs 74 kg (163 lb). Pulse rate is 82/min, and blood pressure is 120/80 mm Hg. The fundi are normal, and there is no corneal arcus. Cardiac examination is normal, and all pulses are full. The abdomen and extremities are normal.

What is the most important laboratory test for assessing this patient 4 weeks after the acute myocardial infarction?

(A) Fibrinogen concentration
(B) Lipoprotein(a) concentration
(C) Platelet count
(D) Fasting homocysteine concentration
(E) Lipid profile

Myocardial Infarction Question 9

A 52-year-old man presents to the emergency department with crushing substernal chest pain. His electrocardiogram shows a 3-mm ST-segment elevation across the anterior precordial leads. He receives thrombolytic therapy and is admitted to the coronary care unit. He is diagnosed with a myocardial infarction and develops Q waves across the anterior precordium. Six hours later, he develops ventricular fibrillation and is successfully defibrillated. An echocardiogram shows hypokinesis of the anterior wall with an estimated ejection fraction of 50%.

What recommendation would you make regarding long-term arrhythmia management?

(A) Placement of an implantable defibrillator
(B) Electrophysiology study with subsequent therapy based on the results
(C) Amiodarone
(D) Atenolol
(E) Procainamide

Myocardial Infarction Question 10

A 52-year-old sedentary accountant had an acute myocardial infarction 2 years ago and was treated with lytic therapy. Because of postinfarction angina on day 2, coronary arteriography was done. Percutaneous transluminal coronary angioplasty (PTCA) reduced a 95% stenosis of the proximal left anterior descending coronary artery to 20%. There was an 80% heavily calcified and concentric stenosis of the mid-right coronary artery, 40% stenosis of the distal left anterior descending coronary artery, and 40% to 60% stenosis in the circumflex artery and each of two branches. He was treated with aspirin, a β-blocker, and an HMG-CoA reductase inhibitor for a low-density lipoprotein (LDL) cholesterol of 180 mg/dL.

Six weeks after discharge, the patient's LDL cholesterol was 120 mg/dL. A thallium stress test using single-photon emission computed tomography (SPECT) was done. He was limited by fatigue at the end of stage III of the Bruce protocol. There was 1-mm horizontal ST-segment depression in the inferior leads at peak exercise. A small, fixed defect was present in the mid septum and a moderate reversible defect in the inferior wall. He has been well for 2 years with medical therapy. This morning, crushing chest pain developed during exercise, and the patient was rushed to the emergency department. The electrocardiogram showed an acute injury, and he underwent coronary arteriography.

Which of the following is most likely to be found?

(A) Thrombus occluding the right coronary artery
(B) Restenosis in the left anterior descending coronary artery at the site of previous PTCA
(C) Thrombus occluding the circumflex artery or one of its branches
(D) Partial occluding thrombus in the left main coronary artery
(E) Nonthrombotic occlusion of the right coronary artery

Myocardial Infarction Question 11

A 42-year-old man presents to the emergency department with substernal chest pressure and dyspnea. He reports experiencing mild chest pain while walking his dog yesterday and the sudden onset of 10/10 chest pain 2 hours ago. He denies any prior cardiac illness. His cardiac risk factors include a 60–pack-year smoking history, moderate hypertension, and positive family history.

Physical examination shows an obese, mildly dyspneic man in moderate distress. His pulse rate is 106/min and regular, and blood pressure is 145/90 mm Hg. Lung examination reveals fine crackles at both bases. There is a prominent S_4 but no murmur. Jugular venous pressure is 4 cm H_2O. The extremities are cool and clammy.

Chest radiograph shows normal heart size and increased interstitial markings consistent with mild congestive heart failure. Electrocardiogram shows sinus tachycardia, left atrial enlargement, and borderline left ventricular hypertrophy. There are 4-mm ST-segment elevations noted in leads V_1 through V_4; 3-mm Q waves are evident in V_1 through V_3. T waves are inverted deeply in leads V_1 through V_6.

Initial management consists of intravenous tissue plasminogen activator (tPA), metoprolol, and furosemide. Within 90 minutes, the patient's ST-segment elevations have decreased to less than 1 mm in leads V_1 through V_4. An echocardiogram done at 72 hours shows a mildly dilated left ventricle, with a left ventricular end-diastolic dimension of 55 mm. There is anteroapical akinesis and 1+ mitral regurgitation. The left ventricular ejection fraction is assessed at 38%.

Which of the following treatment plans best describes the most useful timing and duration of angiotensin-converting enzyme (ACE) inhibitor therapy in this patient?

(A) Intravenous enalapril in the emergency room followed by 12 months of oral enalapril.
(B) Oral enalapril begun within 48 hours
(C) Oral enalapril begun at approximately 3 weeks as an outpatient and continued for 12 months.
(D) An ACE inhibitor is not needed.

Myocardial Infarction Question 12

A 56-year-old man develops recurrent chest discomfort 5 days after an anterior ST-segment elevation myocardial infarction, which was managed initially with accelerated-dose tissue plasminogen activator. The pain is described as sharp and is somewhat positional but different in quality than that associated with his infarction. The pain radiates toward both clavicles. He is afebrile and there is no rub despite careful listening in three positions. An electrocardiogram shows mild PR-segment depression in lead 2, but no significant change in the evolutionary pattern of his Q-wave anteroseptal myocardial infarction.

The most appropriate therapy for this patient is:

(A) Salicylates
(B) Indomethacin
(C) Corticosteroids
(D) Colchicine

Myocardial Infarction Question 13

An 81-year-old woman presents to the emergency department for evaluation of a rapid, irregular pulse, diaphoresis, and dyspnea. She has eaten poorly for the past 2 days and did not eat breakfast this morning. She has a history of a left hemispheric stroke 4 years ago (from which she made a near complete recovery), hypertension, hypothyroidism, urinary incontinence, and a left hip fracture. Her medications include warfarin, enalapril, furosemide, thyroid hormone replacement, and nitrofurantoin.

On physical examination, she appears weak and short of breath. Her temperature is 38 °C (100.4 °F), pulse rate is 122/min and irregularly irregular, respiratory rate is 25/min (O_2 saturation of 84% on 2 L of oxygen), and blood pressure is 144/80 mm Hg. She is able to answer questions appropriately. There is a slight weakness of right hand grip. The venous pressure is difficult to estimate because of her short, full neck. There are bilateral carotid and subclavian bruits. The breath sounds are diminished at the bases. There is a grade 3/6 ejection-type murmur at the base, which is well transmitted to the apex. The abdomen is large and soft without masses. She is incontinent of urine; there is no stool in the rectum. She has evidence of chronic venous stasis changes bilaterally, with 2+ edema on the right and 3+ on the left.

A chest radiograph shows a large heart with low lung volumes, blunted costophrenic angles, and pulmonary vascular redistribution. An electrocardiogram shows rapid atrial fibrillation, right bundle branch block, left ventricular hypertrophy, and 2- to 4-mm ST-segment elevations in leads V_1 and V_2. The hematocrit is 38%, leukocyte count is 12,800/µL, and international normalized ratio is 1.9. The blood urea nitrogen is 41 mg/dL, plasma glucose is 223 mg/dL, potassium is 5.6 meq/L, and creatinine is 2.3 mg/dL.

She is given intravenous furosemide and nitroglycerin.

Which of the following would be the strongest contraindication to thrombolytic therapy in this patient?

(A) Age greater than 80 years
(B) Stroke 4 years previously
(C) Warfarin use
(D) Uncertainty about the timing of the onset of symptoms
(E) Hypertension

Myocardial Infarction Questions 14-18

For each of the following patients, select the most appropriate treatment strategy (A-E) (each answer may be used more than once or not at all):

(A) Primary percutaneous transluminal coronary angioplasty
(B) Thrombolytic therapy
(C) Cardiac surgery
(D) Conservative management with risk stratification

14. A 64-year-old man presents to the emergency room with sudden shortness of breath and cough. He had felt generally unwell over the preceding week and had intermittent epigastric pain, nausea, and anorexia. He has no cardiac history. On physical examination, he is slightly sweaty and in mild respiratory distress. His temperature is 38 °C (100.4 °F); pulse rate is 85/min and regular; respiration rate is 24/min; and blood pressure is 132/90 mm Hg. His jugular venous pressure is 8 cm H_2O. The carotid upstrokes are of full volume without delay. There are crackles at both lung bases. The left ventricular impulse is not displaced. There is a grade 3 murmur, which is loudest at the lower left sternal border. The abdomen is soft and nontender without mass or aneurysm. A guaiac test for stool occult blood is negative. The extremities are slightly cool. The pulses are intact. There is no peripheral edema. A chest radiograph shows a normal heart size, mild pulmonary vascular redistribution, and a small right pleural effusion. An electrocardiogram shows a normal sinus rhythm with small Q waves and T-wave inversions in the inferior leads and prominent R waves in V_1 and V_2. The hematocrit is 41%, leukocyte count is 9400/µL, and platelet count is 232,000/µL. Serum electrolytes are normal. The blood urea nitrogen is 24 mg/dL, and creatinine is 1.2 mg/dL. The initial creatine kinase level is not elevated; an MB determination is not done.

15. A 55-year-old man presents to the hospital on his way home from work after the night shift. Two nights previously, he had experienced lower retrosternal chest discomfort of a steady but low-grade nature with radiation to the neck for 6 hours. Last night, the symptoms returned at approximately 10 PM and persisted continuously for the next 8½ hours. The discomfort abated approximately 30 minutes ago, but he now feels generally weak and exhausted. He is a heavy cigarette smoker and is aware of an untreated high cholesterol

level. He was adopted. Currently, he is in no acute distress. The pulse rate is 71/min and regular, and blood pressure is 116/82 mm Hg in both arms. There are xanthelasmas around both eyes. The venous pressure and carotid upstrokes are normal. There are scattered wheezes in both lung fields posteriorly. The left ventricular impulse is not displaced. There is an apical S_4 but no audible murmur. The abdomen and extremities are normal. A chest radiograph shows a normal heart size with clear lung fields. An electrocardiogram shows Q waves with T-wave inversions in leads 1, aVL, V_5, and V_6. The RS ratio is greater than 1 in lead V_1 with an upright T wave.

16. An active and independent 81-year-old woman presents to the hospital 35 minutes after the onset of severe, retrosternal chest discomfort accompanied by ST-segment elevation in an anteroseptal distribution. She had recognized the warning symptoms. Her pulse rate is 82/min and regular, and blood pressure is 160/90 mm Hg initially but decreases to 134/70 mm Hg after administration of sublingual nitroglycerin. There are no findings to suggest heart failure. She has a grade 1 murmur of aortic stenosis and an apical S_4. Her abdomen is soft and nontender. The neurologic examination is unremarkable. The initial laboratory studies are normal. Her stool guaiac test for occult blood is negative. Catheterization facilities are not available within the next hour.

17. A 60-year-old man presents to the emergency room with clinical and radiographic evidence of pulmonary edema. This morning, while on an errand, he had been overcome by waves of nausea and breathlessness. He is being managed for coronary artery disease, hypertension, peripheral vascular disease, and type 1 diabetes mellitus. He had an inferior myocardial infarction 6 years ago, which was managed conservatively. His inferior myocardial infarction developed in the setting of an upper gastrointestinal bleed. Following this event, his ejection fraction was estimated at 0.45 with posterobasal, inferior, and apical severe hypokinesis. He has never had chest discomfort or claudication. His medications include aspirin, atenolol, enalapril, and insulin. On physical examination, his pulse rate is 110/min and regular, and blood pressure is 80/60 mm Hg. The heart tones are inaudible. His electrocardiogram shows anterolateral ST-segment elevations and Q waves in an inferior distribution. The hematocrit is 36%, leukocyte count is 14,800/μL, and platelet count is 174,000/μL, His plasma glucose is 354 mg/dL, blood urea nitrogen is 38 mg/dL, and creatinine is 2.1 mg/dL. An arterial blood gas study drawn on 100% oxygen by face mask shows a Po_2 of 71 mm Hg, Pco_2 of 56 mm Hg, and pH of 7.21.

18. A 52-year-old man is brought by ambulance to the emergency room with 2 hours of constricting central chest discomfort and a "smothering" sensation. He had been an exercise enthusiast until 6 months ago when he required arthroscopic surgery of his right knee for a meniscal tear. The knee never healed properly so he has been unable to pursue his favorite pastimes of singles tennis, jogging, and long-distance cycling. He had been under a great deal of stress at work for the last 6 months. At his last doctor's visit, he was diagnosed with mild hypertension and admonished to consider lifestyle changes. He quit smoking 4 years ago, but he has not had his cholesterol level rechecked, which was last measured at 210 mg/dL the previous year. His pulse rate is 95/min and regular, respiration rate is 20/min, and blood pressure is 140/90 mm Hg. There are no signs of heart failure. The left ventricular impulse is slightly dyskinetic. S_2 is widely split, and there is an S_4 and a grade 1 midsystolic murmur along the left sternal border. The right knee has a small effusion and lacks full range of motion. Pulses are normal throughout. An electrocardiogram shows a sinus rhythm with borderline left atrial enlargement, right bundle branch block, and 3-mm ST-segment elevations in leads V_2 toV_4.

NOSOCOMIAL INFECTION

Nosocomial Infection Question 1

A 72-year-old diabetic man with hypertension was admitted to the hospital after a right hemispheric stroke; he developed seizures, suffered cardiorespiratory arrest, and required intubation. He never regained full consciousness and has required ventilatory assistance for the past 3 weeks. This patient has a gastrostomy tube, tracheostomy, a left subclavian catheter, and a Foley catheter in place.

On physical examination, his temperature is 39.2 °C (102.5 °F), and pulse rate is 110/min and regular. On chest examination there are scattered, diffuse rhonchi bilaterally, but a chest radiograph shows no infiltrate. There is a stage 1 sacral decubitus ulcer. The patient's urine is hazy in the collection bag. Laboratory studies show a leukocyte count of 14,000/μL and serum creatinine of 1.0 mg/dL. The patient's sputum cultures grow methicillin-resistant *Staphylococcus aureus,* and his urine culture grows vancomycin-resistant enterococci *(Enterococcus faecium).*

Which of the following measures is the most appropriate?

(A) Treatment with vancomycin, 750 mg intravenously every 12 hours
(B) Treatment with ciprofloxacin, 400 mg intravenously every 12 hours
(C) Placing the patient in a room with another patient with methicillin-resistant *Staphylococcus aureus*
(D) Placing a dedicated stethoscope and thermometer in the patient's room
(E) Placing the patient in a laminar flow room

Nosocomial Infection Question 2

A 64-year-old man with acute myeloid leukemia fails to achieve remission despite high-dose idarubicin and cytarabine therapy. His treatment has been complicated by granulocytopenic fever that responded to ceftazidime and gentamicin therapy. Ceftazidime and gentamicin have been continued because his absolute granulocyte count never rose above 200/μL before he received additional chemotherapy. Ongoing antibiotic prophylaxis has consisted of oral ciprofloxacin, fluconazole, and acyclovir.

On the patient's 40th hospital day a dry cough and fever with temperature to 38 °C (100.4 °F) develop. Physical examination reveals a dozen discrete, nodular skin lesions on his abdomen and extremities. His lungs are clear to auscultation.

Laboratory studies:

Hemoglobin	8.0 g/dL
Leukocyte count	300/μL, with 100% lymphocytes
Platelet count	8000/μL
Serum creatinine	2.1 mg/dL

A chest radiograph shows two nodules, 1 cm in diameter, located peripherally in the right upper lobe that were not present on a radiograph taken 2 weeks earlier.

The best immediate action in the management of this patient is:

(A) Add vancomycin to the antibiotic regimen.
(B) Change ceftazidime to imipenem-cilastatin.
(C) Change ceftazidime to aztreonam.
(D) Do a skin biopsy of one of the nodules and initiate amphotericin B therapy.
(E) Arrange for bronchoscopy with transbronchial biopsy and initiate isoniazid and rifampin therapy.

Nosocomial Infection Question 3

A 42-year-old woman with acute myelogenous leukemia develops fever with temperature to 39 °C (102.2 °F) 9 days after admission for induction chemotherapy. She has nausea, sore throat, and heartburn. She notes that her Hickman catheter has become painful during the last 2 days. She has been compliant with antibiotic prophylaxis, consisting of ciprofloxacin, 500 mg orally twice a day; fluconazole, 200 mg orally once a day; and acyclovir, 400 mg orally three times a day. During the physical examination, she experiences a shaking chill. She has severe oropharyngeal mucositis, and the Hickman catheter exit site shows an area of redness and tenderness 1.5 cm in diameter. Her leukocyte count is 100/μL with 100% lymphocytes. The chest radiograph is normal.

The best empiric antibiotic regimen for this patient is:

(A) Ceftazidime and gentamicin
(B) Vancomycin and ceftazidime
(C) Piperacillin-tazobactam and tobramycin
(D) Ceftazidime and amphotericin B
(E) Imipenem-cilastatin

Nosocomial Infection Question 4
In which one of the following situations is the use of vancomycin considered acceptable?

(A) Routine empiric antimicrobial prophylaxis for the febrile neutropenic patient
(B) The primary treatment of antibiotic-associated colitis
(C) Home intravenous antibiotic treatment for *Staphylococcus aureus* sensitive to oxacillin
(D) Routine surgical prophylaxis for total knee replacement
(E) Treatment of serious infections caused by β-lactam–resistant staphylococci

Nosocomial Infection Question 5
Which one of the following statements is true regarding management of infections related to use of long-term, tunneled central venous catheters (for example, Hickman or Broviac catheter)?

(A) Catheters should always be removed when bacteremia is present.
(B) Catheters should always be removed promptly when candidemia is present.
(C) Catheter tunnel infections (defined as inflammation extending more than 2 cm proximally from the catheter exit site) can almost always be controlled with antibiotic therapy alone and do not require removal of the catheter for cure.
(D) Catheters should always be removed in neutropenic patients (absolute granulocyte count <1000/µL) when bacteremia is present.
(E) Because staphylococci are commonly associated with catheter-related infection, empiric antibiotic therapy should always include nafcillin or cefazolin, unless drug allergies preclude their use.

Nosocomial Infection Question 6
A 50-year-old woman was hospitalized following a gunshot wound to her abdomen. Penetrating wounds of the liver, small bowel, and pancreas were noted at surgery. The patient was treated with piperacillin-tazobactam during surgery and through her time in the recovery room. After surgery she became febrile and did not improve during the first postoperative week, despite the change of antibacterial medication to imipenem 4 days after surgery.

The patient was unable to eat and required intravenous fluid feeding for 2 weeks after surgery.

On physical examination, the patient's temperature is 38.9 °C (102 °F), pulse rate is 105/min, respiration rate is 18/min, and blood pressure is 120/75 mm Hg. In addition, erythema and mild tenderness are present at the site of a central venous catheter insertion.

Laboratory studies (10 days after surgery):

Hematocrit	35%
Leukocyte count	2500/µL, with 55% polymorphonuclear neutrophils, 25% band forms, 10% lymphocytes, and 10% monocytes
Serum creatinine	1.4 mg/dL
Serum albumin	1.5 g/dL
Serum bilirubin	1.8 mg/dL
Serum alkaline phosphatase	145 U/L
Serum aspartate aminotransferase	230 U/L
Serum alanine aminotransferase	286 U/L
Serum amylase	230 U/L

Urinalysis is normal, with no leukocytes or organisms seen on Gram's stain. One of four blood cultures on days 7 and 8 after surgery is positive for *Candida*. Chest radiograph is normal, as are abdominal radiographs in flat and upright views. Abdominal computed tomographic scan reveals no abnormal fluid collections or masses and no gas outside the intestines.

Which of the following is the most appropriate next step in the management of this patient?

(A) Repeat the blood cultures and initiate treatment only if they are positive.
(B) Replace the catheter in a new site and advise the patient and family that the positive culture for *Candida* represents a trivial problem that does not require further therapy.
(C) Change the catheter over a J wire and culture the tip.
(D) Place the catheter in a new site and initiate treatment with fluconazole, 400 mg/d.
(E) Initiate treatment with amphotericin B lipid complex (Abelcet), 5 mg/kg per day.

Nosocomial Infection Questions 7-11

For each of the diseases listed, select the best type of isolation precaution (A-E) (each answer may be used more than once or not at all):

(A) Standard precautions alone
(B) Airborne and contact precautions
(C) Droplet precautions
(D) Contact precautions
(E) Airborne precautions

7. Disseminated varicella-zoster

8. Measles

9. *Neisseria meningitidis* sepsis and disseminated intravascular coagulation

10. *Clostridium difficile*–associated diarrhea

11. AIDS

Nosocomial Infection Question 12

A 48-year-old man is admitted to the hospital with an acute hemorrhagic stroke, requiring mechanical ventilation. On the third hospital day a fever develops, and the nurse notes that the patient has increased respiratory secretions, which are now thick and green. In addition to having an oral endotracheal tube in place, the patient has a small-bore feeding tube inserted through the nose for administering enteral feeding. He is not receiving any antibiotic therapy. Laboratory data show a leukocyte count of 21,000/µL, and a chest radiograph shows a new left lower lobe infiltrate.

What diagnostic test, if any, is most appropriate for this patient before the start of antibiotic therapy?

(A) Endotracheal aspiration of sputum for culture and sensitivity
(B) No further testing
(C) Bronchoscopy with quantitative cultures
(D) Nonbronchoscopic bronchoalveolar lavage for quantitative cultures
(E) Aspiration and culture of the maxillary sinuses

Nosocomial Infection Question 13

A 30-year-old woman develops fever with a temperature of 39 °C (102.2 °F). She had induction therapy for myeloid leukemia and has been aplastic for 5 days. A chest radiograph shows several patchy infiltrates. Cultures of blood and urine are negative. Treatment with ceftazidime and tobramycin is initiated through her Hickman catheter.

Three days later she is afebrile, but a second chest radiograph shows persistence of infiltrates.

The best treatment option for this patient is:

(A) Add amphotericin B to the treatment regimen because she may have an opportunistic fungal infection.
(B) Continue current antibiotic therapy for at least 1 week and stop only if she is still afebrile.
(C) Continue current antibiotic therapy until the peripheral polymorphonuclear leukocyte count increases to more than 500/µL to 1000/µL and the patient remains afebrile.
(D) Add vancomycin to the treatment regimen because staphylococci are not covered.
(E) Add intravenous gamma globulin to the treatment regimen.

PNEUMONIA

Pneumonia Question 1

A 38-year-old alcoholic man is seen because of a 6.8-kg (15-lb) weight loss over a 6-week period, during which he has had a cough with occasional blood-streaked sputum. The patient was treated several years ago for tuberculosis; he took two drugs for about 6 months but acknowledges that he sometimes forgot to take his medicine.

A chest roentgenogram shows a right upper lobe infiltrate with a possible small cavity and a left mid-lung infiltrate. A sputum acid-fast bacillus smear shows a few acid-fast organisms.

An appropriate approach to this patient is:

(A) Defer treatment until results of bacteriologic studies are available.
(B) Prescribe twice-weekly, directly observed therapy with isoniazid and rifampin pending drug susceptibility test results.
(C) Prescribe twice-weekly, directly observed therapy with isoniazid, rifampin, and ethambutol pending drug susceptibility test results.
(D) Prescribe twice-weekly, directly observed therapy with isoniazid, rifampin, ethambutol, pyrazinamide, and streptomycin pending drug susceptibility test results.
(E) Prescribe twice-weekly, directly observed therapy with isoniazid, rifampin, and pyrazinamide pending drug susceptibility test results.

Pneumonia Question 2

A 22-year-old woman who is 36 weeks pregnant presents to your office with community-acquired pneumonia. The patient has purulent sputum and is moderately toxic. She has a chest radiograph showing a lobar pneumonia. Her sputum Gram's stain is negative for any organism predominance, but many neutrophils are seen. Blood and sputum cultures are pending.

Which of the following antibiotics would be the most appropriate for this patient?

(A) No antibiotic
(B) Ofloxacin
(C) Tetracycline
(D) Chloramphenicol
(E) Cefuroxime

Pneumonia Question 3

A 73-year-old man who has had chronic lymphocytic leukemia for 2 years is hospitalized with a 1-week history of increasing dry cough, shortness of breath, fevers, chills, myalgias, and anorexia. His leukemia has been treated with chlorambucil (Leukeran), 8 mg/d, and prednisone, 20 mg twice a day. He has been admitted to the hospital twice in the previous 4 months for pneumonia and has improved with ceftriaxone therapy. On physical examination, he is pale and mildly dyspneic at rest. His temperature is 38.8 °C (101.8 °F). A few bibasilar rales are present, but the lungs are otherwise clear. A chest radiograph shows diffuse interstitial infiltrates. He is given ceftriaxone, 1 g/d intravenously, and erythromycin, 500 mg 4 times per day intravenously, but he worsens clinically over the next 2 days. Blood cultures are negative.

The best course of action is to:

(A) Change the antibiotic treatment to imipenem-cilastatin and vancomycin.
(B) Order a high-resolution computed tomographic scan of the chest.
(C) Ask for a pulmonary medicine consultation for bronchoscopy and transbronchial biopsy.
(D) Place tuberculin and control skin tests, and add isoniazid and rifampin to the antibiotic regimen.
(E) Order a bone marrow biopsy with acid-fast and fungal stains and culture.

Pneumonia Question 4

A 33-year-old Kansas farmer interrupts his winter wheat harvest because he develops the sudden onset of fever and chills. He has experienced coryza, mild facial headache, and sore throat for the last 5 days, but he continued to work. In the 4 hours it takes for his wife to get him to the emergency department, he becomes obtunded. His medical history is remarkable for a motor vehicle accident 2 years ago that resulted in placement of a prosthetic hip and a splenectomy. His wife provides day care in their home for five children, ranging in age from 6 months to 4 years.

On initial physical examination, the patient is moaning softly and does not follow commands. Temperature is 39.5 °C (103.1 °F), pulse rate is 130/min, respiration rate is 32/min, and blood pressure is 80/45 mm Hg. He has widespread petechiae and ecchymoses. Gangrenous changes are developing on multiple fingers and toes of all extremities. He has modest posterior pharyngeal inflammation, nuchal rigidity, and diminished breath sounds in both lower lung fields. Laboratory studies show a peripheral leukocyte count of 1400/μL with 15% polymorphonuclear neutrophils, 45% band forms, 30% lymphocytes, and 10% monocytes. Chest radiograph shows dense alveolar infiltrates in the left lower lobe, lingula, and right lower lobe.

Which of the following pathogens is the most likely cause of this patient' disease?

(A) *Rickettsia rickettsii*
(B) *Pseudomonas aeruginosa*
(C) *Staphylococcus aureus*
(D) Hantavirus
(E) *Streptococcus pneumoniae*

Pneumonia Question 5

A 30-year-old woman presents with the acute onset of fever, pleuritic chest pain, and a productive cough. The patient's history is unremarkable except for recurrent cystitis, for which she takes trimethoprim-sulfamethoxazole. She smokes cigarettes. On physical examination her temperature is 40 °C (104 °F), pulse rate is 120/min, respiration rate is 36/min, and blood pressure is 130/80 mm Hg. Abnormalities are localized to the right lung, where rales, rhonchi, and egophony are heard. Oxygen saturation is 85% by pulse oximetry. Chest radiograph shows a right lower lobe lobar pneumonia. Sputum Gram's stain is purulent with few epithelial cells and a predominance of gram-positive diplococci.

Which of the following antimicrobial agents would be the best initial therapy for this patient?

(A) Ciprofloxacin
(B) Vancomycin
(C) Trimethoprim-sulfamethoxazole
(D) Ceftriaxone
(E) Ceftazidime

Pneumonia Question 6

A 24-year-old male college student with cystic fibrosis presents to your office with a 4-week history of increasing dyspnea and decreasing exercise tolerance. In contrast to 1 month ago, he can no longer ride his bicycle 3 miles without stopping to rest. His appetite has decreased. His chronic cough productive of 90 mL of greenish sputum each day is somewhat increased. He denies fever or chest pain. He was hospitalized 2 years ago for a right pneumothorax. Current medications include pancreatic enzyme replacement, a multiple vitamin, and inhaled β-agonists as needed. He admits to some noncompliance with his daily chest physiotherapy regimen.

On physical examination, the patient appears well nourished and not in any respiratory distress. He weighs 60 kg (132 lb), a 2.5 kg (5.5 lb) weight loss from 2 months ago, and is 170 cm (67 in) tall. He is afebrile, with a pulse rate of 86/min, respiration rate of 24/min, and blood pressure of 106/78 mm Hg. Chest examination reveals diffuse, coarse, early inspiratory crackles and expiratory rhonchi with occasional wheezes over both upper lung fields. Fingers and toes are clubbed. There is no cyanosis or peripheral edema.

Laboratory studies:

Hematocrit	41%
Leukocyte count	11,400/μL, with 78% neutrophils, 16% lymphocytes, 4% band forms, and 2% eosinophils

Pulmonary function studies (percent of predicted):

	6 Months Ago	Current
Forced vital capacity (FVC)	74%	62%
Forced expiratory volume in 1 sec (FEV_1).	48%	40%
Ratio of FEV_1 to FVC	70%	62%
Percentage of oxyhemoglobin saturation	92%	93%

The chest radiograph is unchanged from 1 year ago, showing hyperinflation; a small, vertical heart shadow; peribronchial cuffing; and increased upper lobe bronchovascular markings.

The most efficacious management option is:

(A) Initiate intensive inhaled bronchodilator therapy with ipratropium and β-agonists.
(B) Initiate antibiotic therapy with ticarcillin and tobramycin pending sputum culture and sensitivity results.
(C) Initiate long-term continuous inhaled antibiotic therapy with high-dose tobramycin.
(D) Initiate regular once-daily therapy with inhaled recombinant human deoxyribonuclease (DNase).
(E) Reinstitute twice-daily chest physiotherapy with postural drainage and use of an airway oscillator.

Pneumonia Question 7

A 66-year-old woman presents with a history of cough and sputum production of 3 weeks' duration, with some blood tinging of the sputum, and a 2.3-kg (5-lb) weight loss. The woman has a history of multiple episodes of childhood pneumonia. She has not been a smoker but reports a 5-year history of chronic cough, present throughout the day, with sputum production on a daily basis. Several times per year she has an episode of purulent sputum and requires antibiotic therapy. Her tuberculin skin test has been positive for the past 20 years, according to her history, but she does not remember any tuberculosis exposure.

A chest radiograph shows increased markings at the lung bases, with "tram-tracks" and dilated bronchial shadows, and an infiltrate with a 1-cm thin-walled cavity in the right lower lobe. Acid-fast bacilli staining of a sputum sample is positive.

The next best step in the management of this patient is:

(A) Collect more sputum samples for acid-fast bacilli smear and mycobacterial culture before starting therapy.
(B) Collect more sputum samples for acid-fast bacilli smear and mycobacterial culture and await final culture results before starting therapy.
(C) Arrange for immediate bronchoscopy with transbronchial biopsy before starting therapy.
(D) Start therapy with isoniazid and ethambutol.
(E) Start therapy with isoniazid and pyrazinamide while awaiting final culture and sensitivity patterns.

Pneumonia Question 8

A 47-year-old woman comes to your office with a 3-day history of fever, shortness of breath, and cough with mucoid sputum. On physical examination she is alert but slightly confused. Her temperature is 40 °C (104 °F), respiration rate is 34/min, and blood pressure is 110/50 mm Hg. Examination of the chest shows bibasilar crackles, and her chest radiograph confirms the presence of pneumonia, showing bilateral lower lobe infiltrates. Arterial blood gases on room air are Pao$_2$, 46 mm Hg; Paco$_2$, 28 mm Hg; and pH, 7.45. The patient is admitted to the hospital and started on therapy with erythromycin, ceftriaxone, and gentamicin.

There has recently been a documented case of *Legionella pneumophila* pneumonia (not a serogroup I infection) in your community, and you suspect this diagnosis in your patient.

Which, if any, of the following tests is likely (> 50% chance) to confirm the diagnosis at this time?

(A) Sputum for direct fluorescent antibody testing for *Legionella*
(B) A urinary antigen test for *Legionella*
(C) Sputum culture for *Legionella* on selective medium
(D) Testing for *Legionella* antibodies in serum obtained at the time of admission
(E) None of the above

Pneumonia Question 9

A 45-year-old male smoker presents with symptoms of cough, fever with temperature to 39 °C (102.2 °F), and yellow sputum of 2 days' duration. He denies shortness of breath and has no chest pain. His symptoms were of gradual onset but have steadily worsened since they first appeared.

On physical examination, the patient is alert, oriented, and not obviously dyspneic. His temperature is 39.2 °C (102.6 °F), pulse rate is 88/min, respiration rate is 22/min, and blood pressure is 110/75 mm Hg. His skin has normal turgor and his mucosae are moist. Examination of the chest shows crackles at the right lung base posteriorly. A chest radiograph shows a patchy right lower lobe infiltrate; no effusion is present.

What is the most appropriate drug therapy for this patient?

(A) Oral azithromycin
(B) Oral cefuroxime
(C) Oral penicillin G
(D) Intravenous ceftriaxone in your office, followed by oral cefpodoxime
(E) Oral tetracycline

Pneumonia Question 10

A 44-year-old man with a history of injection drug use is hospitalized critically ill after a week-long illness. An HIV test is negative, and a chest radiograph shows bilateral pulmonary infiltrates. Sputum Gram's stain and culture show 4+ *Streptococcus pneumoniae*. Blood cultures are also positive for this organism, which is sensitive to penicillin when tested on an oxacillin disc.

High-dose intravenous penicillin is administered to the patient, but his respiratory symptoms worsen, and a second chest radiograph shows increased infiltrates. He remains septic, with blood cultures again positive for penicillin-sensitive *S. pneumoniae* 4 days after admission.

101

Appropriate management would include which one of the following?

(A) Change high-dose penicillin to vancomycin.
(B) Obtain indium-labeled leukocyte scan.
(C) Do computed tomography of the chest.
(D) Change antibiotics to imipenem for broad-spectrum coverage.

SMOKING

Smoking Question 1

A 50-year-old healthy man presents with concerns about his risk of having a heart attack. His father died of a myocardial infarction at 60 years of age. As a city bus driver he is inactive, has job stress, and is depressed about the future. He has not watched his diet — "I eat bacon and eggs every morning" — and is a 30–pack-year smoker.

On physical examination, he is 168 cm (66 in) tall and weighs 87 kg (191 lb). His pulse rate is 72/min, and blood pressure is 160/100 mm Hg. The fundi show increased arteriole light reflex. There are no carotid bruits. The lungs are clear. Cardiac examination reveals a normal S_1 and S_2 and an S_4 gallop. The abdomen is obese. The peripheral pulses are normal.

Laboratory studies include serum cholesterol, 240 mg/dL; triglycerides, 230 mg/dL; high-density lipoprotein (HDL) cholesterol, 46 mg/dL; and calculated low-density lipoprotein (LDL) cholesterol, 148 mg/dL.

Elimination of which risk factor has the greatest chance of reducing the risk of an acute myocardial infarction?

(A) Smoking
(B) Dietary saturated fat
(C) Hypertension
(D) Physical inactivity
(E) Stress and depression

Smoking Question 2

A 37-year-old man presents with severe pain of the toes of the right foot. For approximately 1 year he has felt his toes become very numb during cold exposure. On one occasion, he removed his socks and observed that the toes were white. Six months ago, several red lumps developed on his right calf. He saw a dermatologist, and a biopsy was done of one of the affected areas. Now the toes burn persistently; yet, when felt, they are cold to touch. A painful ulcer has developed at the tip of the right third toe. He is unable to walk because of the pain. He has had two episodes of bronchitis in the past year. He drinks three beers and smokes one pack of cigarettes each day. His family history is significant for hypertension.

On physical examination, his pulse rate is 90/min, and blood pressure is 138/84 mm Hg. Auscultation of the lungs reveals scattered expiratory rhonchi. Diminished heart sounds are present; no murmurs are heard. Abdominal examination is negative. The Allen's test of the left hand is abnormal. On examination of the lower extremities, the right foot is cool. The toes of the right foot are cyanotic. A 4-mm ulcer with a pale base is present at the tip of the third toe. The right and left femoral, popliteal, and dorsalis pedis pulses are palpable on each side, but the posterior tibial pulses are not present.

Laboratory studies:

Hematocrit	47%
Leukocyte count	10,100/μL
Platelet count	367,000/μL
Serum creatinine	0.9 mg/dL
Total cholesterol	210 mg/dL
Triglycerides	280 mg/dL
Antiphospholipid antibody	Negative
Factor V Leiden	Negative
Homocysteine concentration	9.6 μmol/L

Skin biopsy specimen shows venulitis.

The most appropriate treatment for this patient's problem is:

(A) Smoking cessation
(B) Pentoxifylline
(C) Nifedipine
(D) Simvastatin
(E) Percutaneous transluminal angioplasty of the right tibioperoneal trunk

Smoking Question 3

A 40-year-old man comes to your office and asks about quitting smoking. He has smoked for 20 years and currently smokes two and a half packs per day. He has never tried to quit before but has experienced feelings of agitation on long airplane flights. He is currently out of work and concerned about finances.

The best recommendation for this patient is to:

(A) Negotiate a quit date and start the nicotine patch at 21 mg/day on the quit date.
(B) Negotiate a quit date and start the nicotine patch at 14 mg/day on the quit date.
(C) Negotiate a quit date and start use of nicotine gum, one piece three times a day for 4 weeks, on the quit date.
(D) Advise him to taper his smoking and start the nicotine patch at 21 mg/day while he tapers his smoking.

Smoking Question 4

A 55-year-old woman presents for her yearly physical. She has no chronic medical conditions but has smoked one and a half packs of cigarettes per day for 35 years. She has a family history of early coronary artery disease in her father and paternal uncles. The physical examination shows decreased breath sounds bilaterally but is otherwise unremarkable.

When discussing her smoking, she tells you that she enjoys it and dismisses the health risks. Smoking helps her relax, and she is not prepared to quit.

What approach would be the most appropriate to help this patient quit smoking?

(A) Prescribe the nicotine patch and encourage her to quit smoking.
(B) Refer her to a smoking cessation program.
(C) Facilitate her making a plan to quit smoking and have her follow up in 2 weeks.
(D) Educate her about her health risks and explore her reasons for smoking.
(E) Facilitate her making a plan to cut down on her smoking.

Smoking Question 5

A 63-year-old man presents with a 4-day history of cough, yellow sputum production, and fever. He had a similar illness approximately 2 months earlier, when he was told he had a right upper lobe pneumonia. He has smoked 2 packs of cigarettes per day for 40 years but stopped smoking when he had the recent pneumonia.

On physical examination, his temperature is 38.9 °C (102 °F). Chest examination shows decreased breath sounds in the anterior part of the right upper lung field.

Laboratory evaluation shows a leukocyte count of 15,800/μL. Sputum Gram's stain shows more than 25 polymorphonuclear leukocytes and rare epithelial cells per high-power field. There are multiple morphologic types of both gram-positive cocci and gram-negative rods. Chest radiograph shows right upper lobe consolidation with upward displacement of the minor fissure. Cytologic examination of sputum is negative for malignant cells.

The patient is treated with antibiotics. Which of the following diagnostic plans would be most appropriate?

(A) Needle aspiration of the right upper lobe
(B) Fiberoptic bronchoscopy
(C) Computed tomography
(D) Thoracoscopy with wedge biopsy of the right upper lobe
(E) No further evaluation at this time

SUBSTANCE ABUSE

Substance Abuse Question 1

A 33-year-old man with a long history of alcohol abuse presents to the Emergency Department with abdominal pain. He has had nausea and some vomiting over the past 48 hours. His last alcohol intake was 12 hours ago. He reports a history of alcohol withdrawal seizures in the past. On physical examination, his blood pressure is 140/100 mm Hg, and his pulse is 100/min. He has right upper quadrant tenderness with mild hepatomegaly. The results of laboratory studies are as follows: serum aspartate aminotransferase (AST), 60 U/L; serum alanine aminotransferase (ALT), 25 U/L; hemoglobin, 13 g/dL; hematocrit, 39%; mean corpuscular volume (MCV), 101 fL; amylase, 80 U/L; blood alcohol, 200 mg/dL; and bilirubin, 2.0 mg/dL.

What would be the most appropriate therapy for this patient?

(A) Chlordiazepoxide
(B) Alprazolam
(C) Chlorpromazine
(D) Intravenous ethyl alcohol
(E) Propranolol

Substance Abuse Question 2

A 31-year-old man with a 12-year history of injection heroin use is brought to the Emergency Department comatose and cyanotic. The patient's friend reports that the patient was fine last night.

On physical examination, he has a temperature of 36.5 °C (97.7 °F), pulse rate of 120/min, respiration rate of 8/min, blood pressure of 80/60 mm Hg. He has constricted pupils, bilateral crackles, and marked cyanosis of his fingertips and lips. He is tachycardic without an S_3 gallop, and an electrocardiogram shows sinus tachycardia without ST-segment changes. Oxygen saturation is 50%. Chest radiograph reveals a normal cardiac silhouette and bilateral infiltrates. He is intubated and placed on a ventilator with high concentrations of oxygen.

What would be the most appropriate management for this patient?

(A) Intravenous dopamine
(B) Intravenous digitalis
(C) Intravenous flumazenil
(D) Intravenous furosemide
(E) Intravenous naloxone

Substance Abuse Question 3

A 46-year-old woman with a 20-year history of alcohol abuse presents to the Emergency Department with abdominal discomfort, nausea, and vomiting. She states she had been drinking heavily (15 to 20 beers/day and a fifth of vodka every 2 days) and stopped yesterday morning when she noticed worsening right upper quadrant pain and nausea. She has noticed some mild abdominal pain for the past week. She has been vomiting frequently. She has not eaten a full meal for 7 days and had very little oral intake of any kind yesterday.

Physical examination reveals a thin, pale woman with a marked tremor. Her temperature is 36.8 °C (98.2 °F), pulse rate is 120/min, and blood pressure is 90/60 mm Hg. Her liver is palpable 6 cm below the right costal margin, with a span of 14 cm in the right midclavicular line, and the edge is tender.

Laboratory studies:

Hemoglobin	10 g/dL
Hematocrit	30%
Leukocyte count	12,000/µL
Mean corpuscular volume	104 fL
Serum electrolytes	
Sodium	136 meq/L
Potassium	3.6 meq/L
Chloride	94 meq/L
Bicarbonate	16 meq/L
Serum aspartate aminotransferase (AST)	60 U/L
Serum alanine aminotransferase (ALT)	22 U/L
Plasma glucose	150 mg/dL
Serum amylase	80 U/L
Blood alcohol	10 mg/dL

Abdominal ultrasound reveals an enlarged liver, a gallbladder without stones, and no dilated bile ducts. She receives intravenous thiamine, multivitamins, and benzodiazepines in the Emergency Department.

What further intravenous therapy is indicated?

(A) Sodium bicarbonate
(B) Glucose and saline
(C) Insulin
(D) β-blockers
(E) Corticosteroids

Substance Abuse Question 4

A 38-year-old man is found to have a serum alanine aminotransferase (ALT) concentration of 55 U/L with an otherwise normal chemistry panel on a screening insurance examination. He drinks two to three mixed alcohol drinks per night. He takes no medications and denies risk factors for viral hepatitis. His family history is negative for liver disease. Physical examination shows normal vital signs, no cutaneous stigmata of chronic liver disease, no hepatosplenomegaly, and no peripheral edema. The patient is 9 kg (20 lb) over ideal body weight.

The most appropriate current recommendation would be:

(A) Discontinue alcohol use and return for recheck of laboratory results in 1 month
(B) Obtain hepatitis B and C serology, and measure serum iron/iron-binding capacity, ferritin, ceruloplasmin, antinuclear antibody, and anti–smooth muscle antibody
(C) Refer for gastroenterology consultation
(D) Obtain abdominal ultrasound
(E) Obtain percutaneous liver biopsy

Substance Abuse Question 5

A 21-year-old male known cocaine user is brought to the Emergency Department because of agitation and confusion. He most recently used intravenous cocaine 10 hours ago. At that time, he had limb and back pains. No seizures were reported.

Physical examination shows an alternatively agitated and drowsy male with a temperature of 38.8 °C (101.8 °F), a pulse rate of 110/min, and a blood pressure of 175/100 mm Hg. There are multiple venipuncture sites in the skin of the left forearm. The oropharynx is clear; there is no murmur or rub on cardiac examination. Abdominal examination shows no hepatosplenomegaly. There is tenderness to palpation over all muscle groups.

Laboratory studies

Hematocrit	48%
Leukocyte count	10,750/μL
Blood urea nitrogen	25 mg/dL
Serum creatinine	3.8 mg/dL
Serum potassium	4.9 meq/L
Serum creatine kinase	10,350 U/L
Urinalysis	
pH	5.0
Specific gravity	1.012
Protein	Trace
Blood	4+
Microscopic	1 to 2 erythrocytes per high-power field (hpf), 1 to 3 leukocytes/hpf with many brown pigmented casts

In this patient, the urinalysis is most consistent with which one of the following diagnoses?

(A) Prerenal azotemia
(B) Chronic glomerulonephritis
(C) HIV nephropathy
(D) Rhabdomyolysis
(E) Acute interstitial nephritis

Substance Abuse Question 6

A 38-year-old woman with a 15-year history of heavy alcohol use presents to the Emergency Department with severe abdominal pain exacerbated by meals. An abdominal radiograph reveals diffuse calcifications in the pancreas.

Which one of the following tests is necessary to confirm the diagnosis of chronic pancreatitis in this patient?

(A) Endoscopic retrograde cholangiopancreatography (ERCP)
(B) Secretin stimulation test
(C) N-benzoyl tyrosine (bentiromide) para-aminobenzoic acid (NBT-PABA) test
(D) Ultrasound of the abdomen
(E) No further testing required

Substance Abuse Question 7

A 33-year-old salesman admits to weekend use of freebase cocaine ("crack"). Which one of the following pulmonary complications of habitual cocaine smoking is he most likely to develop?

(A) Atelectasis
(B) Hemoptysis
(C) Emphysema
(D) Eosinophilic pneumonitis
(E) Pulmonary embolism

Substance Abuse Question 8

A 48-year-old man visits your primary care practice 3 weeks after being evaluated in a local Emergency Department for palpitations. He had no history of cardiovascular disease. A diagnosis of new-onset atrial fibrillation was made in the Emergency Department, and he was prescribed digoxin, 0.125 mg orally every day. He has had no further symptoms suggestive of a rapid ventricular rate. A two-dimensional echocardiogram was normal, as was measurement of serum thyroid-stimulating hormone.

At this time, you obtain a history of more than 10 years of regular alcohol use, including the loss of two jobs and a revoked driving license. He mentions that the recent hospital visit was preceded by a week of heavy drinking. He states that he has not had any alcohol in the past 2 weeks, and would like help to stop drinking. Physical examination is normal. The serum total bilirubin, alanine aminotransferase, and aspartate aminotransferase concentrations are normal. An electrocardiogram shows normal sinus rhythm, without evidence of prior myocardial infarction.

Which one of the following would you do at this time?

(A) Begin treatment with naltrexone, 50 mg orally every day, and see the patient in your office on a regular basis.
(B) Explain to the patient he has an alcohol use disorder and that you will help monitor his alcohol use while you provide his primary medical care.
(C) Provide regular primary care for the patient and refer him to a drug rehabilitation program.
(D) Encourage the patient to enroll in Alcoholics Anonymous.
(E) Begin treatment with coumadin, with the goal of an international normalized ratio (INR) at 1.5 to 2.0, and refer the patient to a drug rehabilitation program.

Substance Abuse Question 9

Which one of the following statements regarding infective endocarditis in injection drug users is true?

(A) Streptococci account for most cases of infective endocarditis in injection drug users.
(B) Transesophageal echocardiography offers no advantages over transthoracic echocardiography in the diagnosis and management of infective endocarditis in injection drug users.
(C) Septic pulmonary embolization is rare (< 5%) in injection drug users with right-sided endocarditis.
(D) Injection drug users with right-sided endocarditis due to methicillin-susceptible *Staphylococcus aureus* may be treated successfully with a 2-week course of nafcillin and gentamicin.
(E) Injection drug users with enterococcal endocarditis can be treated successfully with a 2-week course of vancomycin and gentamicin.

Answers, Critiques, and Bibliographies

ABDOMINAL PAIN

Abdominal Pain Question 1
Answer: A

EDUCATIONAL OBJECTIVE: Manage a ruptured abdominal aortic aneurysm.

Abdominal aortic aneurysms are usually asymptomatic. On occasion they may cause abdominal, back, or flank pain radiating to the left thigh or scrotum. The abdominal computed tomographic (CT) scan in this patient indicates a leaking abdominal aortic aneurysm. This is an indication for emergent repair, because rupture is fatal in most cases.

Coronary artery disease is present in many patients with abdominal aortic aneurysms. In this time of duress and consequent increased blood pressure and heart rate, it is not surprising that this patient's electrocardiogram shows ST-segment depression. The electrocardiographic changes may reflect myocardial ischemia resulting from increased myocardial oxygen demand. However, the clinical presentation is atypical for myocardial infarction, and transfer to the cardiac catheterization laboratory for potential coronary revascularization would delay definitive and timely treatment of the abdominal aortic aneurysm. There is no indication for percutaneous transluminal coronary angioplasty (PTCA) in this patient.

The clinical and radiologic features of this patient are not suggestive of scrotal hemorrhage. Intravenous metoprolol and nitroglycerin are useful agents to reduce blood pressure; however, the clinical situation in this patient should not be confused with that of an aortic dissection, in which metoprolol and sodium nitroprusside would be indicated if hypertension were present. Analgesics would be useful to treat this patient's pain while preparations are being made for surgery. Medical therapy should not delay prompt surgical repair.

Bibliography
1. **Lederle FA, Parenti CM, Chute EP.** Ruptured abdominal aortic aneurysm: the internist as diagnostician. Am J Med. 1994;96:163-7.

Abdominal Pain Question 2
Answer: E

EDUCATIONAL OBJECTIVE: Recognize the need for abdominal angiography in a patient with potential intestinal ischemia.

This patient should have an abdominal angiogram. The patient has evidence of atherosclerotic disease, atrial fibrillation, and recent cardiac decompensation. Treatment with digoxin may increase the risk for intestinal ischemia. The differential diagnosis is between an embolic event and acute ischemia due to progressive disease of the mesenteric vessels. An angiogram should be diagnostic and assist the surgeons in defining an appropriate operation. The patient should be well hydrated before and after the dye load.

The elevated pancreatic amylase is nonspecific and consistent with impending small bowel infarction. Delaying the diagnostic examination could lead to infarction and perforation. Invasive endoscopic studies are contraindicated with progressive abdominal pain.

Bibliography
1. **Goldman L, Bennett JC, eds.** Cecil Textbook of Medicine. 21st ed. Philadelphia: WB Saunders Co; 1999.

Abdominal Pain Question 3
Answer: A

EDUCATIONAL OBJECTIVE: Recognize and evaluate irritable bowel syndrome.

This patient has classic irritable bowel syndrome. The absence of weight loss, bleeding, inflammatory symptoms, and negative prior examinations exclude a pathologic explanation of her symptoms. The association of symptoms of irritable bowel syndrome with menstrual cycle complaints is common. Additional invasive or costly diagnostic studies are unnecessary until a careful psychosocial interview has been completed.

This patient's story is typical of a woman with a history of sexual abuse: note the clues—symptoms since childhood, hints of a dysfunctional family, sister with similar complaints, and fear of intimate relations with her fiancé (symptoms are worse in his presence).

Bibliography

1. **Camilleri M, Prather CM.** The irritable bowel syndrome: mechanisms and a practical approach to management. Ann Intern Med. 1992;116:1001-8.

2. **Drossman DA, Leserman J, Nachman G, Li ZM, Gluck H, Toomey TC, et al.** Sexual and physical abuse in women with functional or organic gastrointestinal disorders. Ann Intern Med. 1990;113:828-33.

3. **Drossman DA, Thompson WG.** The irritable bowel syndrome: review and a graduated multicomponent treatment approach. Ann Intern Med. 1992;116:1009-16.

Abdominal Pain Question 4
Answer: E

EDUCATIONAL OBJECTIVE: Diagnose acute colonic pseudo-obstruction and intervene before perforation occurs.

This patient has acute pseudo-obstruction. Medications such as narcotics that might slow intestinal transit should be discontinued in such patients, and electrolyte abnormalities, especially hypokalemia, should be corrected. Nasogastric suction may help decompress the patient's colon. Turning the patient from side to back to side to stomach may passively move air to the distal colon.

Colonoscopy would be the next maneuver to attempt colon decompression if more conservative measures (for example, increasing colon diameter) were unsuccessful. Cecostomy and/or colectomy might be indicated if colonoscopy were not therapeutic. A cecal diameter greater than 10 cm is considered highly susceptible to perforation.

Bibliography

1. **Sleisenger MH, Fordtran JS.** Gastrointestinal Disease. Philadelphia: WB Saunders; 1993:1551-2.

2. **Laine L.** Management of acute colonic pseudo-obstruction. N Engl J Med. 1999;341:192-3

Abdominal Pain Question 5
Answer: C

EDUCATIONAL OBJECTIVE: Evaluate a patient with an elevated serum gastrin concentration.

Although a serum gastrin test was not indicated in this patient because she did not have any of the features of the Zollinger-Ellison syndrome (recalcitrant peptic ulcers and/or diarrhea), the finding of a high serum gastrin concentration is not infrequently a reason for referral for tests to diagnose Zollinger-Ellison syndrome. The first test that should be done is to assess whether the patient has hyperchlorhydria or hypochlorhydria by inserting a nasogastric tube and measuring basal acid secretion. The other tests are appropriate only if hyperchlorhydria is detected or until a gastrinoma has been diagnosed. In gastrinoma the parietal cells are constantly driven to secrete acid by a pancreatic or duodenal gastrin-secreting tumor. However, some of the highest serum gastrin concentrations are found in patients with achlorhydria or hypochlorhydria due to gastric atrophy (for example, in pernicious anemia or after the prolonged use of antisecretory drugs, particularly proton-pump inhibitors). In the latter, the high gastrin concentration is due to the lack of feedback inhibition from acid bathing the antrum, resulting in uncontrolled gastrin secretion.

In the present case, had the patient been tested for acid secretion, she would have been found to be achlorhydric and the other tests would not have been done. Antisecretory drugs, especially proton-pump inhibitors, should be stopped for at least 5 days before repeating the serum gastrin measurement if hypergastrinemia is found in a patient receiving such therapy.

Bibliography

1. **Frucht H, Howard JM, Slaff JI, Wank SA, McCarthy DM, Maton PN, et al.** Secretin and calcium provocative tests in patients with Zollinger-Ellison syndrome. A prospective study. Ann Intern Med. 1989;111:713-22.

2. **Metz DC, Weber HC, Orbach M, Strader DB, Lubensky IA, Jensen RT.** *Helicobacter pylori* infection. A reversible cause of hypergastrinemia and hyperchlorhydria which may mimic Zollinger-Ellison syndrome. Dig Dis Sci. 1995;40:153-9.

Abdominal Pain Question 6
Answer: B

EDUCATIONAL OBJECTIVE: Recognize alcohol as the cause of pancreatic calcification.

There are relatively few causes of calcific pancreatitis. By far the most common in Western countries is alcohol-induced pancreatitis, with most such patients consuming at least 75 g of alcohol per day for 5 to 15 years. (In India and other tropical countries, nonalcoholic tropical pancreatitis of unknown cause predominates.) The mechanism of calcification with prolonged alcohol use appears to be oversecretion of enzymes that precipitate in the pancreatic duct; these protein plugs become the nidus for calcium deposition due possibly to a deficiency of a protein (lithostatin) that usually keeps pancreatic calcium in solution. Therefore, despite the fact that the patient has three other possible causes of pancreatitis, none of them is likely to produce calcific pancreatitis. About 6% of patients with Crohn's disease taking 6-mercaptopurine develop mild reversible pancreatitis, and calcification has not yet been reported in such patients. The role of corticosteroids as a cause of acute pancreatitis is at best speculative, and corticosteroid therapy has also not been incriminated in promoting calcification.

Although hypercalcemia may produce calcific pancreatitis, particularly in patients with hyperparathyroidism, it is extremely unlikely to occur with excessive oral calcium intake, especially if the serum calcium concentration remains in the normal range. For all practical purposes then, the common causes of calcific pancreatitis are alcohol and tropical pancreatitis.

Rare causes are hyperparathyroidism, familial-hereditary, fibrocystic disease of the pancreas, and juvenile or senile idiopathic calcific pancreatitis. Even rarer almost anecdotal causes are following severe necrotic pancreatitis (gallstones or hyperlipemia), pancreatic duct obstruction (for example, pancreas divisum), calcification in tumors, and calcified ascaris remnants.

Bibliography

1. **Ammann RW, Heitz PU, Kloppel G.** Course of alcoholic chronic pancreatitis: a prospective clinicomorphological long-term study. Gastroenterology. 1996;111:224-31.

2. **Lankisch PG, Droge M, Gottesleben F.** Drug induced acute pancreatitis: incidence and severity. Gut. 1995;37:565-70.

Abdominal Pain Question 7
Answer: B

EDUCATIONAL OBJECTIVE: Treat cholangitis in an elderly patient with acute pancreatitis.

This patient most likely has both acute obstructive pancreatitis and acute cholangitis due to a stone impacted in a "common channel" type of ampulla, with common entry of the pancreatic duct and common bile duct into the duodenum. This latter anatomic arrangement occurs in about 70% of persons. In this patient,

the dominant feature is the cholangitis, as evidenced by the high fever, tachycardia, and low blood pressure, suggesting the onset of shock. As these latter features may occur in acute pancreatitis due to any cause, other signs have to be evaluated to make a diagnosis of a possible gallstone.

The presence of jaundice and the abnormal liver function test results are highly suggestive of an impacted gallstone, which is unlikely to resolve until the obstruction is relieved. Therefore, the treatment of choice in this situation is broad-spectrum antibiotics (preferably not vancomycin, which does not enter the biliary system well) and endoscopic retrograde cholangiopancreatography (ERCP) to detect and remove stones in the common bile duct before the patient develops septic shock. Although intravenous antibiotics alone may resolve the septic state and the evaluation for the cause can be done later, this is a risky approach in a septic older patient; the common bile duct should therefore be cleared. Although octreotide has been used in acute pancreatitis to reduce pancreatic secretion, clinical trials are few and the results not entirely convincing. In any event, the cholangitis is the dominating disease requiring attention initially.

The question as to whether early ERCP should be undertaken in all severely ill patients with acute pancreatitis to exclude common bile duct stones even though the blood tests do not suggest cholangitis or common bile duct obstruction is controversial and requires further evaluation.

Bibliography

1. **Fan ST, Lai EC, Mok FP, Lo CM, Zheng SS, Wong J.** Early treatment of acute biliary pancreatitis by endoscopic papillotomy. N Engl J Med. 1993;328:228-32.

2. **Folsch UR, Nitsche R, Ludtke R, Hilgers RA, Creutzfeldt W.** Early ERCP and papillotomy compared with conservative treatment for acute biliary pancreatitis. The German Study Group on Acute Biliary Pancreatitis. N Engl J Med. 1997; 336:237-42.

Abdominal Pain Question 8
Answer: A

EDUCATIONAL OBJECTIVE: Recognize indications for inpatient therapy for pelvic inflammatory disease.

This young woman has pelvic inflammatory disease as indicated by lower abdominal pain, cervical motion pain, and adnexal tenderness. She has three indications for admission to the hospital for intravenous cefoxitin and doxycycline (or clindamycin and gentamicin) therapy. First, she has an adnexal mass that may represent a tubo-ovarian abscess. Second, she shows evidence by physical examination that she is dehydrated and may not tolerate oral medications. Third, adolescents have had a significant rate of noncompliance with outpatient therapy in a number of studies.

The regimen of ceftriaxone, 125 mg intramuscularly, and doxycycline, 100 mg orally twice a day for 7 days, is appropriate treatment for cervicitis but not for pelvic inflammatory disease. Giving a larger dose of ceftriaxone (250 mg) is an unnecessary addition to an otherwise standard regimen for outpatient treatment of mild pelvic inflammatory disease. Ofloxacin, 400 mg orally twice a day for 14 days, is an accepted therapy for mild pelvic inflammatory disease only. Azithromycin, 1 g orally, is an excellent treatment for chlamydial cervicitis but is incompletely effective against gonorrhea. A 2-g dose is required for treatment of gonorrhea.

Bibliography

1. **McCormack WM.** Pelvic inflammatory disease. N Engl J Med. 1994;330:115-9.

2. **Lawson MA, Blythe MJ.** Pelvic inflammatory disease in adolescents. Pediatr Clin North Am. 1999;46:767-82

Abdominal Pain Question 9
Answer: B

EDUCATIONAL OBJECTIVE: Identify the association of hepatitis C virus infection with cryoglobulinemia.

This patient's mononeuritis multiplex, renal insufficiency, hypertension, abdominal angina, and palpable purpura strongly suggest polyarteritis. Either hepatitis B virus (HBV) or hepatitis C virus (HCV) infection or both are found in many patients with polyarteritis. This man had HCV and cryoglobulinemia. Cryoglobulinemia should be suspected in patients who have purpura, glomerulonephritis, and abdominal pain. This case illustrates that polyarteritis can be associated with cryoglobulinemia and that both can be caused by chronic HCV infection.

Three types of cryoglobulins are recognized, based on whether the cryoglobulin is monoclonal and whether the cryoglobulin has rheumatoid factor activity. Different types of cryoglobulins cause different syndromes and are associated with different diseases. Type I cryoglobulins are monoclonal, do not have rheumatoid factor activity, cause hyperviscosity syn-

drome (rather than vasculitis), and are associated with malignancies. Types II and III both have rheumatoid factor activity and cause vasculitis and are therefore called mixed cryoglobulins. The cryoglobulin in type II is monoclonal and seen primarily with rheumatic diseases (such as Sjögren's syndrome) and malignancies. Type III cryoglobulins are polyclonal and seen primarily in patients with rheumatic diseases.

In the past, many cases of mixed (type II or III) cryoglobulinemia were thought to be essential, having no known cause. Studies now show that most essential cases are caused by HCV infection. This patient's transfusion 20 years ago was the presumed source of his HCV infection. For reasons not yet clear, most HCV-associated cryoglobulins are monoclonal IgM kappas with rheumatoid factor activity (type II). Antiviral therapy with interferon may help some patients with HCV-associated cryoglobulinemia.

Antibodies to double-stranded DNA are specific for systemic lupus erythematosus, which is virtually excluded by the negative test for antinuclear antibody. Parvovirus B19 infection can produce polyarthralgia and rash but not this pattern of vasculitis. Antineutrophil cytoplasmic antibodies (ANCAs) are found in two types of patterns. The cytoplasmic ANCA (C-ANCA) is strongly associated with Wegener's granulomatosis, whereas the perinuclear ANCA (P-ANCA) is seen in patients with various conditions, including those with pauci-immune glomerulonephritis and in 10% to 20% of patients with polyarteritis. Polyarteritis rarely complicates HIV infection.

Bibliography

1. **Agnello V, Chung RT, Kaplan LM.** A role for hepatitis C virus infection in type II cryoglobulinemia. N Engl J Med. 1992;327:1490-5.

Abdominal Pain Questions 10-11
Answers: 10(B); 11(A)

EDUCATIONAL OBJECTIVE: Identify common causes of acute pancreatitis, and choose appropriate initial therapy for severe pancreatitis.

The most common causes of acute pancreatitis are alcohol ingestion and biliary tract disease. In the United States, alcohol ingestion is the most common cause, whereas in other countries such as the United Kingdom, gallstone pancreatitis occurs with higher frequency. In this patient, the lack of dilated ducts, cholelithiasis, or elevated alkaline phosphatase and bilirubin makes gallstone pancreatitis unlikely.

Infectious pancreatitis can be caused by viral illnesses or bacteria such as *Mycoplasma, Campylobacter,* or *Mycobacterium avium* complex. However, without a history of antecedent infection, this would be unlikely. Although connective tissue diseases with vasculitis, such as systemic lupus erythematosus, can cause pancreatitis, this patient has no symptoms, examination findings, or laboratory studies making this diagnosis likely.

This patient has early signs of severe acute pancreatitis. Severe disease occurs in about 15% of patients with pancreatitis. There are many classification schemes for acute pancreatitis. Ranson described five presentation criteria predictive of worse prognosis in 1979.

Ranson's Early Prognostic Signs of Severity of Acute Pancreatitis	
At presentation	
Age*	> 55 years
Leukocyte count	> 16,000/µL
Blood glucose	> 200 mg/dL
Lactate dehydrogenase	> 350 U/L
Aspartate aminotransferase	> 250 U/L
At 48 hours	
Hematocrit	Decrease by 10%
Blood urea nitrogen	Increase by 5 mg/dL
Calcium	< 8 mg/dL
Pao$_2$	< 60 mm Hg
Base deficit	> 4 meq/L
Fluid sequestration	> 6000 mL

*For gallstone pancreatitis, age greater than 70 years.

Patients possessing three or more of these criteria have a worse prognosis. This patient had hyperglycemia, and elevated lactate dehydrogenase level, and leukocytosis, meeting the criteria. He also had hypoxemia with examination signs of possible noncardiogenic pulmonary edema as well as tachycardia and oliguria despite vigorous intravenous hydration. These factors also portend a worse prognosis.

Admission to the intensive care unit is appropriate because of the high likelihood of multiorgan dysfunction. The mainstays of therapy for acute pancreatitis include analgesics for pain, intravenous fluids, and bowel rest. Because the patient has no signs of biliary obstruction, endoscopic retrograde cholangiopancreatography (ERCP) would not help and could lead to worsened pancreatitis iatrogenically. Outpatient resuscitation is clearly inappropriate in a patient with a condition of this severity. Ward hospitalization would not provide sufficient monitoring. Nasogastric suction showed no survival benefits in the treatment of mild-to moderate-severity pancreatitis in a recent randomized controlled trial but could be considered for symptom relief in a patient with refractory nausea.

Bibliography

1. **Ranson JH, Rifkind KM, Roses DF, Fink SD, Eng K, Spencer FC.** Prognostic signs and the role of operative management in acute pancreatitis. Surg Gynecol Obstet. 1974;139:69-81.

2. **Bank S, Wise L, Gersten M.** Risk factors in acute pancreatitis. Am J Gastroenterol. 1983;78:637-40.

3. **Steinberg W, Tenner S.** Acute pancreatitis. N Engl J Med. 1995;330:1198-210.

ACID–BASE

Acid–Base Question 1
Answer: C

EDUCATIONAL OBJECTIVE: Recognize the importance of providing sufficient electrolyte-free water to elderly febrile patients with increased insensible water loss.

Hypernatremia in hospitalized patients occurs in two relatively distinct populations; those who have hypernatremia on admission and those who develop hypernatremia in hospital. This patient obviously belongs to the first group. Such patients are typically 20 years older than patients in the second group and most are transferred from nursing homes. In one study (Palevsky, 1996), 15 of 18 patients with hypernatremia on admission to the hospital had serious concomitant infections. The elevated temperature increases insensible water loss, while the dulled sensorium decreases both thirst and the ability to drink water. Moreover, bed-bound and chair-bound nursing home patients also frequently have limited access to electrolyte-free fluids.

Osmotic diuresis would be unlikely given the normal plasma glucose. There was no history of diuretic use and, particularly in this age group, hyponatremia is more likely to result from diuretic agents. Hypernatremia from hypertonic sodium administration usually is seen in adults who are given excess amounts of sodium bicarbonate during cardiopulmonary resuscitation. Nephrogenic diabetes insipidus in adults can have many causes, ranging from intrinsic renal disease to lithium administration, but the urine specific gravity of 1.020 negates that possibility in this patient.

Bibliography

1. **Himmelstein DU, Jones AA, Woolhandler S.** Hypernatremic dehydration in nursing home patients: an indicator of neglect. J Am Geriatr Soc. 1983;31:466-71.

2. **Snyder NA, Feigal DW, Arieff AI.** Hypernatremia in elderly patients. A heterogeneous, morbid, and iatrogenic entity. Ann Intern Med. 1987;107:309-19.

3. **Palevsky PM, Bhagrath R, Greenberg A.** Hypernatremia in hospitalized patients. Ann Intern Med. 1996;1 24:197-203.

Acid–Base Question 2
Answer: B

EDUCATIONAL OBJECTIVE: Recognize and manage mixed respiratory acidosis and metabolic alkalosis, a common mixed acid–base disorder.

This 28-year-old woman with cystic fibrosis presents (from an acid-base perspective) with hypercapnia. Although the patient may have had mild hypercapnia at baseline, the rapidity of the progression of her respiratory distress suggests that the hypercapnia was predominantly acute. The finding of a P_{CO_2} of 69 mm Hg establishes the presence of respiratory acidosis. The finding of normal pH, which is not seen in patients with either acute or chronic respiratory acidosis, immediately establishes the presence of an offsetting (as far as pH is concerned) metabolic alkalosis. Therefore, this patient has mixed metabolic alkalosis and respiratory acidosis.

In patients with acute respiratory acidosis, the hydrogen concentration (in neq/L) increases by approximately 0.7 times the increase in P_{CO_2} (that is, in this patient, $0.7 \times [69 - 40]$), or by approximately 20.3 neq/L (from 40 neq/L to 60 neq/L, or to a pH of about 7.22). Similarly, the increase in serum bicarbonate concentration is predictable for patients with acute hypercapnia, that is, the bicarbonate increases by approximately 1.0 meq/L for each 10 mm Hg increase in P_{CO_2}, or 1.0 $\times$ 3 in this patient, that is, only a 3-meq/L increment in serum bicarbonate.

The presence of the elevated P_{CO_2} excludes the possibilities of mixed metabolic acidosis and metabolic alkalosis and mixed metabolic alkalosis and respiratory alkalosis. The presence of a normal pH and elevated serum bicarbonate concentration excludes the possibility of mixed metabolic acidosis and respiratory acidosis. The normal pH excludes the possibility of acute respiratory acidosis.

Bibliography

1. **Brackett NC Jr, Cohen JJ, Schwartz WB.** Carbon dioxide titration curve of normal man. Effect of increasing degrees of acute hypercapnia on acid-base equilibrium. N Engl J Med. 1965;272:6-12.

2. **Cohen JJ, Schwartz WB.** Evaluation of acid-base equilibrium in pulmonary insufficiency. An approach to a diagnostic dilemma. Am J Med. 1966;41:163-7.

Acid–Base Questions 3-5
Answers: 3(C); 4(B); 5(A)

EDUCATIONAL OBJECTIVE: Distinguish the appropriate set of chemical values and examine both acid-base status and urine electrolytes in patients with hypokalemia.

The 46-year-old man with new-onset hypertension was found to have hypokalemia on initial examination. The diagnosis of primary hyperaldosteronism (due to adrenal hyperplasia or adenoma) must be considered. This disorder is often associated with metabolic alkalosis and high urine chloride concentration, in contrast to the alkalosis of vomiting, which is associated with low urine chloride concentration. There is no reason for acidosis in this patient.

The 32-year-old female dancer is emaciated and her blood pressure is low, suggesting weight loss or bulimia. Surreptitious vomiting is often denied by these patients, although many of them have weakness due to hypokalemia and have an associated metabolic alkalosis. The patient had no diarrhea, no findings associated with renal tubular acidosis, and no other obvious cause for acidosis, which would make the presence of hypokalemia and acidosis (the values in option A) incorrect. The low urine chloride concentration and absence of hypertension supports the diagnosis of vomiting and volume contraction, making the values in option C incorrect.

In the 35-year-old woman with recurrent stone formation, it is essential to consider the diagnosis of type 1 distal renal tubular acidosis. In patients with this disease, serum bicarbonate concentration is decreased because of acidosis. Renal potassium wasting occurs with chronic hypokalemia. The alkaline-rich urine, in association with acidosis-induced hypercalciuria, predisposes these patients to recurrent calcium phosphate stones. Without a history of vomiting, diuretic use, or hypertension, there is no obvious reason for alkalosis in this patient, making the values in options B and C incorrect.

Bibliography

1. **Mitchell JE, Seim HC, Colon E, Pomeroy C.** Medical complications and medical management of bulimia. Ann Intern Med. 1987;107:71-7.
2. **Coe FL, Parks JH, Asplin JR.** The pathogenesis and treatment of kidney stones. N Engl J Med. 1992;327:1141-52.
3. **Arruda JA, Cowell G.** Distal renal tubular acidosis: molecular and clinical aspects. Hosp Prac (Off Ed). 1994;29:75-8.

Acid–Base Question 6
Answer: D

EDUCATIONAL OBJECTIVE: Identify the optimum diagnostic approach to suspected adrenal insufficiency.

This 24-year-old woman has a clinical picture compatible with adrenal insufficiency. Because untreated adrenal insufficiency is fatal, she requires treatment before the diagnosis of adrenal insufficiency can be firmly established. Treatment of adrenal insufficiency will distort the normal hypothalamic–pituitary–adrenal response to provocative stimuli in a matter of days; therefore, delaying the test could lead to a false-positive result and incorrect assessment of adrenal dysfunction. An immediate test of adrenal function is indicated.

The most appropriate test for this patient is the cosyntropin stimulation test. This test is done by administering 250 µg of synthetic adrenocorticotropin as an intravenous bolus and measuring serum cortisol 30 to 45 minutes later. Serum cortisol of less than 18 µg/dL confirms the diagnosis of adrenal dysfunction. The insulin tolerance and metyrapone tests are too time-consuming for this situation and are far less discriminating for the diagnosis of adrenal insufficiency than is the cosyntropin stimulation test. Urine free cortisol is not a suitable test for this purpose because the normal range for the test overlaps the extinction point of the assay; therefore, no value for urine free cortisol can be interpreted as too low.

Bibliography

1. **Oelkers W.** Adrenal insufficiency. N Engl J Med. 1996;335:1206-12.

Acid–Base Question 7
Answer: D

EDUCATIONAL OBJECTIVE: Identify priorities in the treatment of hyperglycemic hyperosmolar nonketotic coma.

Patients with hyperglycemic hyperosmolar nonketotic coma are often profoundly dehydrated on admission, as evidenced by this patient's low blood pressure, high pulse rate, and elevated blood urea nitrogen/creatinine ratio. These patients may suffer myocardial infarction, stroke, mesenteric thrombosis, and other life-threatening events as a result of a low circulating volume, high plasma viscosity, and low cardiac output. Hence, the most important initial maneuver is to restore the intravascular volume and improve cardiac output with isotonic fluid. Although the patient's coma is most likely a result of his hyperosmolarity, the latter will decrease gradually as insulin reduces glucose concentrations, permitting time for brain cells to rehydrate gradually. In addition, isotonic saline is slightly hypotonic (300 mosm/kg) relative to this patient's high calculated osmolality of approximately 380 mosm/kg, so that he does not require 0.45% sodium chloride initially.

The patient's measured serum sodium concentration is normal, but this does not indicate isotonic dehydration. In fact, it indicates profound hypertonic dehydration with a marked deficit of free water, because the patient's extremely high plasma glucose concentration has caused a shift of water from the intracellular to the extracellular space, a shift that would normally lower the sodium concentration in the extracellular fluid by dilution. When corrected for this effect of a plasma glucose of 1900 mg/dL, the patient's serum sodium is 169 meq/L (corrected sodium = 1.6 × [(plasma glucose – 100)/100] + measured sodium), indicating a profound deficit of free water. Therefore, once central volume has been restored, hypotonic fluid should be given. Lowering the glucose concentration rapidly with a pharmacologic dose of insulin will result in a shift of water back from the extracellular space to the intracellular space and a further reduction in intravascular volume with possible shock. Insulin should not be administered before fluid resuscitation has begun.

Bibliography

1. **DeFronzo RA, Matsuda M, Barrett EJ.** Diabetic ketoacidosis: a combined metabolic-nephrologic approach to therapy. Diabetes Metab Rev. 1994;2:209-38.

2. **Lorber D.** Nonketotic hypertonicity in diabetes mellitus. Med Clin North Am. 1995;79:39-52.

3. **Matz R.** Hyperosmolar nonacidotic uncontrolled diabetes: not a rare event. Clin Diabetes. 1988;6:25.

Acid–Base Question 8
Answer: D

EDUCATIONAL OBJECTIVE: Manage the patient with acute, symptomatic hypercalcemia.

The combination of moderate hypercalcemia and hypophosphatemia in this 64-year-old man suggests a process mediated by parathyroid hormone (PTH) itself or a PTH-like peptide substance. A new hilar mass (and presumably postobstructive pneumonia) in a smoker strongly suggests a lung malignancy, with squamous cell carcinoma being a common neoplasm in this setting. These tumor cells produce PTH-related peptide, resulting in most of the metabolic features of primary hyperparathyroidism.

Several treatments are available for this condition, with the intravenous bisphosphonate pamidronate ultimately the most effective. However, the current clinical presentation of azotemia and an inappropriately normal hematocrit suggests dehydration, which always results in additional impairment of renal calcium excretion. Intravenous sodium chloride is likely to substantially reduce the serum calcium by increasing distal renal tubular sodium delivery and urine flow. Correction of volume depletion should be the first therapy in any patient with significant acute hypercalcemia, because an element of decreased vascular volume is frequently present.

Pamidronate, which may take several days for peak effect, is certainly appropriate if hypercalcemia persists once the volume status has been corrected.

This patient's serum calcium will also be lowered by calcitonin injections, perhaps even more quickly than by pamidronate. However, the amount of decrease is usually not as great, and loss of responsiveness to this drug frequently occurs, as a result of desensitization at a molecular level. Calcitonin should also be administered after volume repletion.

Furosemide may enhance calcium excretion in a hydrated patient, but it will worsen volume status if not coadministered with intravenous fluids. Because of toxic renal, hepatic, and bone marrow effects, plicamycin is rarely given and should be reserved for volume-repleted patients who have failed to respond to both pamidronate and calcitonin.

Bibliography

1. **Chisholm MA, Mulloy AL, Taylor AT.** Acute management of cancer-related hypercalcemia. Ann Pharmacother. 1996;30:507-13.

2. **Edelson GW, Kleerekoper M.** Hypercalcemic crisis. Med Clin North Am. 1995;79:79-92.

Acid–Base Question 9
Answer: C

EDUCATIONAL OBJECTIVE: Identify the clinical manifestations of the syndrome of inappropriate secretion of antidiuretic hormone and select the test most likely to confirm the diagnosis.

The likely cause of hyponatremia in this 17-year-old boy with head trauma is the syndrome of inappropriate secretion of antidiuretic hormone (SIADH). This diagnosis should be confirmed as soon as possible by simultaneously measuring urine and plasma osmolality. First, the calculated osmolality should be compared with the measured value to exclude an otherwise unmeasured osmol such as mannitol, which is always a possibility in patients with head trauma. If unmeasured osmols are not detected, a urine osmolality greater than plasma osmolality confirms the diagnosis of SIADH.

Measuring the urine sodium is of limited diagnostic utility. (The patient has been receiving intravenous normal saline and the urinary sodium concentration will reflect this.) Profound hypothyroidism can be associated with SIADH, but this could not have happened in 3 days, and thyroid function tests are often misleading in the setting of a grave illness. The plasma renin activity, along with a cortisol response to cosyntropin, will be useful tests once the diagnosis of SIADH is confirmed.

Bibliography

1. **Robertson GL.** The use of vasopressin assays in physiology and pathophysiology. Semin Nephrol. 1994;14:368-83.
2. **Soupart A, Decaux, G.** Therapeutic recommendations for management of severe hyponatremia: current concepts on pathogenesis and prevention of neurologic complications. Clin Nephrol. 1996;46:149-69.

Acid–Base Question 10
Answer: B

EDUCATIONAL OBJECTIVE: Identify the homeostatic mechanisms involved in nonparathyroid hormone–mediated hypercalcemia.

This 49-year-old woman's hypercalcemia probably results from increased circulating levels of parathyroid hormone–related peptide (PTHrP), which is associated with tumors of epidermal derivation, in this case, recurrent or persistent squamous carcinoma of the cervix.

Although nothing in this patient's presentation necessarily excludes the coexistence of primary hyperparathyroidism, the normal serum calcium 1 year ago makes this chronic condition unlikely. Indeed, because of the hypercalcemia, endogenous PTH production will most certainly be suppressed now.

As they interact with the same receptor, the effects of PTHrP are similar to those of PTH. Therefore, urine calcium excretion will be elevated, with most of this liberated from the skeleton. In patients with PTH-mediated hypercalcemia, 1,25-dihydroxyvitamin D levels are usually high. Increased urine calcium derives from two sources: enhanced gastrointestinal absorption and mobilized calcium from bone stores. For an unclear reason, patients with PTHrP-mediated hypercalcemia typically have decreased serum 1,25-dihydroxyvitamin D levels.

There is no reason for the measured level of serum 25-hydroxyvitamin D to be low in this patient if dietary intake or sunlight exposure is intact, because this value reflects overall body stores of vitamin D.

Because of increased bone turnover, biochemical markers of bone resorption such as urine collagen cross-links are elevated in patients with hyperparathyroidism and PTHrP-mediated hypercalcemia.

Bibliography

1. **Dunbar ME, Wysolmerski JJ, Broadus AE.** Parathyroid hormone-related protein: from hypercalcemia of malignancy to developmental regulating molecule. Am J Med Sci. 1996;312:287-94.
2. **Eriksen EF, Brixen K, Charles P.** New markers of bone metabolism: clinical use in metabolic bone disease. Eur J Endocrinol. 1995;132:251-63.
3. **Ikeda K, Ogata E.** Humoral hypercalcemia of malignancy: some enigmas in the clinical features. J Cell Biochem. 1995;57:384-91.

ACUTE RENAL FAILURE

Acute Renal Failure Question 1
Answer: A

EDUCATIONAL OBJECTIVE: Manage acute renal failure in patients with neoplasms of the genitourinary tract.

A renal ultrasound is the correct test to obtain in a patient with newly discovered renal insufficiency. Signs suggestive of ascites may suggest the diagnosis of volume overload and prerenal azotemia, but the elevated fractional excretion of sodium (FE_{Na}) of 4.1% is inconsistent with this diagnosis. Obstructive uropathy must be considered in this 75-year-old woman with acute renal failure, high FE_{Na}, and a relatively unremarkable microscopic urinalysis before evaluating causes of intrinsic renal disease, which usually present with a characteristic urinalysis

Obstructive uropathy should be excluded before renal biopsy is contemplated. Without evidence of volume depletion, a fluid trial would be inappropriate. Continuous arteriovenous hemofiltration is indicated for hemodynamically compromised, volume overloaded patients in whom fluid administration, usually for parenteral hyperalimentation, is contemplated. Other renal replacement therapies might be more useful in this patient if the cause of her confusion is determined to be uremia. However, there is no acute indication for renal replacement therapy in this patient at the time of evaluation. Without hypertension, and with an ultrasound showing normal equally-sized kidneys, renal scintigraphy is unlikely to yield valuable information.

Bibliography
1. **Klahr S.** New insights into the consequences and mechanisms of renal impairment in obstructive nephropathy. Am J Kidney Dis. 1991;18:689-99.

Acute Renal Failure Question 2
Answer: C

EDUCATIONAL OBJECTIVE: Recognize that numerically small increases in serum creatinine concentration often represent real and significant changes in glomerular filtration rate.

In most clinical laboratories, the precision of the serum creatinine method is ± 10% for measurements in the range of 1 to 2 mg/dL and falls to ± 2% for serum creatinine measurements in the range of 9 to 10 mg/dL. Rhabdomyolysis may cause increased serum creatinine concentration secondary to increased release of creatinine concentration from injured muscle. However, this usually occurs only in certain clinical situations such as crush injuries, cocaine overdose, malignant hyperthermia, and after prolonged or repetitive grand mal seizures. Catheter-induced bacteriuria, in the absence of clinical urinary tract infection, would not cause a decline in renal function.

Bibliography
1. **Levey AS.** Nephrology Forum. Measurement of renal function in chronic renal disease. Kidney Int. 1990;38:167-84.

Acute Renal Failure Question 3
Answer: C

EDUCATIONAL OBJECTIVE: Recognize the clinical pattern of myeloma-induced renal disease.

This patient has renal disease of unknown cause at presentation. In his evaluation, calculation of the anion gap shows it to be low (138 – [113 +22] = 3). There is severe anemia for the degree of renal insufficiency, and there is a large amount of protein on 24-hour urine collection despite the dipstick recording only 1+. In myeloma, positively charged monoclonal protein often offsets the negative charge of serum chloride and bicarbonate, causing a low anion gap. The anemia is due to marrow suppression and plasma cell infiltration. Urine light chains (Bence-Jones proteins) are not well-detected by the urine dipsticks, which are much more sensitive to albumin. Hence the dipstick may read only trace or 1+ in the presence of a large amount of protein. All features point to a diagnosis of myeloma in this patient.

Membranous nephropathy and amyloidosis are both typically associated with large amounts of albuminuria and a 4+ positive urine dipstick. Lead nephropathy gives a picture of tubulointerstitial disease but not anemia disproportionate to the renal function or heavy proteinuria.

Bibliography

1. **Winearls CG.** Acute myeloma kidney. Kidney Int. 1995;48:1347-61.

Acute Renal Failure Question 4
Answer: B

EDUCATIONAL OBJECTIVE: Recognize the absolute indications for initiating emergency dialysis.

This 36-year-old man has dyspnea and findings on physical examination and chest radiograph that suggest incipient pulmonary edema. The absence of fever and presence of pleural effusions make congestive heart failure more likely than an opportunistic infection in this patient. Although blood urea nitrogen of 80 mg/dL and serum creatinine of 9.0 mg/dL suggest this patient will need dialysis soon, emergency dialysis is not indicated in the absence of a serious uremic complication such as seizure or pericarditis. Unresponsiveness to diuretic agents constitutes an absolute indication to initiate emergency dialysis in a patient with end-stage renal disease. Hyperkalemia unresponsive to medical management is also an absolute indication to initiate immediate dialysis but only when it is more severe than in this patient (such as serum potassium >6.5 meq/L). Metabolic acidosis is rarely a reason to initiate chronic dialysis, because the acidosis of renal failure (serum bicarbonate >12 to 15 meq/L) results from underexcretion of daily acid production, rather than over-production, and is therefore usually not severe.

Bibliography

1. **Klahr S.** Chronic renal failure: management. Lancet. 1991;338:423-7.

Acute Renal Failure Questions 5-6
Answers: 5(D); 6(A)

EDUCATIONAL OBJECTIVE: Evaluate diagnostic markers of hypercalcemic nephropathy, and treat hypercalcemia presenting with azotemia.

Hypercalcemic nephropathy comprises discrete diagnoses in which acute renal failure coexists with hypercalcemia, a relatively uncommon finding.

Although hypocalcemia is the more common finding, hypercalcemia may be associated with renal insufficiency for several reasons. However, hypercalcemia from any cause can be associated with renal vasoconstriction, diminution in glomerular ultrafiltration and renal tubular defects in reabsorption of sodium and water (nephrogenic diabetes insipidus), worsening of volume depletion, and amplification of the hypercalcemia. This sequence may lead to a vicious circle of volume depletion and increasing hypercalcemia, in the absence of intrinsic renal disease. This is particularly evident in the uncommon milk-alkali syndrome, a triad of metabolic alkalosis, hypercalcemia, and renal insufficiency. Ingestion of large amounts of oral alkali, leading to metabolic alkalosis, limits tubular excretion of calcium.

In the presence of ingestion of large amounts of elemental calcium, hypercalcemia develops, causing renal insufficiency and occasionally resulting in soft tissue calcification within the kidneys and other organs. Vitamin D–fortified milk can worsen positive calcium balance, and renal insufficiency limits renal excretion of bicarbonate. Patients with primary hyperparathyroidism may also present rarely with renal insufficiency because of nephrolithiasis, obstruction, or nephrocalcinosis. The milk-alkali syndrome can be differentiated from primary hyperparathyroidism by the presence of alkalosis, and the findings of low or normal N-terminal parathyroid hormone (PTH) and 1,25 dihydroxyvitamin D concentrations. The PTH and 1,25 dihydroxyvitamin D concentrations in this patient are in the low-normal range, thereby arguing against primary hyperparathyroidism and vitamin D intoxication. Chronic renal insufficiency is unlikely in a patient with a normal renal ultrasound and hematocrit and severe diminution in renal function, but hypercalcemia can develop in such patients treated with calcium supplementation and vitamin D analogues. Although this patient's history, high plasma bicarbonate level, and low-normal PTH and vitamin D levels are consistent with the milk-alkali syndrome, malignancy is always a consideration in patients with hypercalcemia, and neoplasia must be ultimately excluded as a diagnostic consideration. Granulomatous diseases such as sarcoidosis may present with renal disease and hypercalcemia. Multiple myeloma should be ruled out in all patients with acute renal failure, particularly those presenting with hypercalcemia. However, multiple myeloma is unlikely in a patient with a normal hematocrit.

Thiazide diuretic agents, which increase calcium reabsorption in the distal convoluted tubule, are contraindicated in patients with hypercalcemia, such as this 71-year-old woman. The hypercalcemia and renal insufficiency characterizing the milk-alkali syndrome are reversible with volume repletion, cessation of calcium supplements and alkali, and treatment of hypercalcemia, although residual renal insufficiency may persist. Furosemide may be used to increase urine calcium excretion (by blocking its reabsorption in the thick ascending limb of the loop of Henle) when volume stores are repleted. The patient's hypernatremia suggests excessive loss of hypotonic fluid, through both insensible and urinary routes, as is supported by the relatively hypotonic urine. In such patients, sodium and water deficits should be repleted, usually with sequential administration of isotonic and hypotonic fluids. Calcitonin is effective and may be used in the initial treatment of hypercalcemia, but resistance to its effects often develops, especially when the drug is used without concurrent administration of corticosteroids.

Bibliography

1. **Abreo K, Adlakha A, Kilpatrick S, Flanagan R, Webb R, Shakamuri S.** The milk-alkali syndrome. A reversible form of acute renal failure. Arch Intern Med. 1993;153:1005-10.
2. **Bilezikian JP.** Management of acute hypercalcemia. N Engl J Med. 1992;326:1196-203.

Acute Renal Failure Question 7
Answer: C

EDUCATIONAL OBJECTIVE: Treat acute interstitial nephritis.

For this 50-year-old woman, the most reasonable course of action would be to discontinue cimetidine and observe her renal function and results of urinalysis. The findings on the physical examination suggest volume depletion, and isotonic saline should be administered, rather than hypotonic solutions that can cause the development of hyponatremia. The formed elements seen in the urinalysis in this patient, however, are inconsistent with a unifying diagnosis of prerenal azotemia. Appropriate urine cultures should be obtained in patients with sterile pyuria to rule out nonbacterial infections.

There is no indication for administering antibiotics in this patient without clear evidence of infection. To the extent the renal insufficiency is a result of prerenal azotemia, renal function will improve, and the serum creatinine concentration will diminish. If there is no improvement or if there is worsening of renal function in the absence of infection, obtaining renal ultrasonography and doing a renal biopsy is reasonable. Corticosteroid therapy should be used only if the biopsy specimen shows interstitial nephritis and renal function is not improving after cessation of the suspected agent in the absence of infection.

Acute interstitial nephritis clinically comprises a constellation of renal insufficiency and sterile pyuria, often in the setting of signs of systemic hypersensitivity such as fever, rash, leukocytosis, and eosinophilia. However, systemic signs may be absent in patients with acute interstitial nephritis. Cessation of the initiating drug usually results in improvement of renal function. Renal biopsy should be considered in cases where there is no obvious response to discontinuation of the suspected offending agent after several days. Renal histology shows an acute interstitial infiltrate composed of mononuclear cells, and less often, eosinophils. The therapeutic efficacy of corticosteroid therapy in such patients has not been subjected to rigorous clinical trials. The use of cimetidine has been associated with acute interstitial nephritis, and the drug interferes with proximal tubular secretion of creatinine but not with its measurement in blood. Cimetidine is not the sole reason for the elevation of the serum creatinine concentration in this patient, because the level of blood urea nitrogen is also abnormal.

Bibliography

1. **Neilson EG.** Nephrology Forum. Pathogenesis and therapy of interstitial nephritis. Kidney Int. 1989;35:1257-70.

Acute Renal Failure Question 8
Answer: B

EDUCATIONAL OBJECTIVE: Recognize the factors that may cause a sudden deterioration in renal function in patients with chronic renal insufficiency.

In patients with chronic renal insufficiency who have a sudden deterioration of glomerular filtration rate, reversible causes must always be sought. The most common of these include volume contraction or overload, worsening hypertension or hypotension, nephrotoxic drugs, infection, and obstruction.

In this 46-year-old man, prerenal azotemia is most likely, because the patient had symptoms of syncope and was taking two classes of agents (ACE inhibitors and diuretic agents) that can alter glomerular hemodynamics and result in reversible renal insufficiency. The combination of bumetanide and metolazone is particularly potent and frequently leads to episodes of prerenal azotemia in patients maintained on these agents long-term. ACE inhibitors can also lead to reversible renal insufficiency in patients whose glomerular filtration rate is angiotensin-dependent, such as those with renal artery stenosis or low renal perfusion related to low cardiac output, as in this patient. Renal artery stenosis is less likely in this setting without worsening hypertension. Progression of renal failure from polycystic kidney disease does not usually occur this quickly. Acute pyelonephritis is also unlikely in the absence of fever, flank pain, or significant pyuria. Allergic interstitial nephritis from over-the-counter nonsteroidal anti-inflammatory drugs is also less likely in the absence of significant hematuria or pyuria.

Bibliography

1. **Klahr S.** Chronic renal failure: management. Lancet. 1991;338: 423-7.

2. **Toto RD, Mitchell HC, Lee HC, Milam C, Pettinger WA.** Reversible renal insufficiency due to angiotensin converting enzyme inhibitors in hypertensive nephrosclerosis. Ann Intern Med. 1991;115:513-9.

Acute Renal Failure Questions 9-13
Answers: 9(A); 10(C); 11(E); 12(B); 13(D)

EDUCATIONAL OBJECTIVE: Recognize the usefulness of the urinalysis in diagnosing various renal diseases.

The usefulness of urinalysis in diagnosing various renal diseases partially depends on careful microscopic examination of the spun sediment of a freshly voided urine specimen. Erythrocyte casts, renal tubular cell casts, pigmented casts, or large numbers of renal tubular cells will not usually be found or reported by routine laboratory studies. Furthermore, identification of eosinophils requires special staining, which is not done unless specifically ordered. Therefore, urinalysis is most valuable when done by the clinician most familiar with the diagnostic possibilities for the patient.

About 50% to 70% of patients with acute tubular necrosis have urine sediment showing features of renal tubular cell injury, including renal tubular cells, renal tubular cell casts, and muddy brown casts. Eosinophiluria exceeding 5% of urine leukocytes suggests acute interstitial nephritis, but it may also be seen in atheroembolic renal disease and urinary tract infection. Clumped leukocytes, especially when accompanied by bacteria, in a fresh, clean-voided urine specimen are highly suggestive of urinary tract infection. Leukocyte casts suggest intrarenal infection with pyelonephritis. Erythrocyte casts are most commonly found in patients having some form of inflammatory glomerulonephritis. In obstructive uropathy, the urine is characteristically bland without significant cellular elements or proteinuria.

Bibliography

1. **Ruffing KA, Hoppes P, Blend D, Cugino A, Jarjoura D, Whittier FC.** Eosinophils in urine revisited. Clin Nephrol. 1994;41:163-6.

2. **Wilson DM, Salazer TL, Farkouh ME.** Eosinophiluria in atheroembolic renal disease. Am J Med. 1991;91:186-9.

ALTERED MENTAL STATUS

Altered Mental Status Question 1
Answer: D

EDUCATIONAL OBJECTIVE: Diagnose and evaluate the acute onset of agitation in a nursing home resident with dementia and multiple medical problems.

The sudden change in the behavior of this 86-year-old woman is among the most common situations presented to on-call physicians covering a nursing home. Although behavioral disorders such as disruptive vocalizations and physical aggression are common among nursing home residents with dementia, a sudden change in a patient's behavior may be the manifestation of the onset of delirium, which requires a thorough medical evaluation. Thus, the most appropriate response in this situation is to transfer the resident to the emergency room and request that the emergency room physician exclude such conditions as acute infection (for example, pneumonia, urinary tract infection) or acute cardiovascular event (for example, myocardial infarction, congestive heart failure, stroke).

These conditions may present without specific symptoms and may manifest as an acute behavioral change or delirium. This patient may also have an iatrogenic illness, such as electrolyte imbalance or dehydration related to diuretic therapy, digoxin toxicity, or an adverse reaction to nortriptyline. It is inappropriate simply to prescribe a sedative (such as lorazepam) or an antipsychotic (such as haloperidol) or simply to increase the antidepressant dose before a medical evaluation has been done. Similarly, it is inappropriate to call the consultant psychiatrist before a medical evaluation has excluded an acute condition.

Bibliography

1. **Francis J, Kapoor WN.** Delirium in hospitalized elderly. J Gen Intern Med. 1990;5:65-79.
2. Psychotherapeutic medications in the nursing home. Board of Directors of the American Association for Geriatric Psychiatry, Clinical Practice Committee of the American Geriatrics Society, and Committee on Long-Term Care and Treatment for the Elderly, American Psychiatric Association. J Am Geriatr Soc. 1992;40:946-9.

Altered Mental Status Question 2
Answer: C

EDUCATIONAL OBJECTIVE: Select the most appropriate mechanism for detecting cognitive impairment.

The first step in assessing an older person such as this 86-year-old woman who presents with forgetfulness for the first time is to do a complete history and physical examination. However, the standard history and physical and neurologic examinations are usually not sufficiently sensitive to detect mild and possibly even moderate cognitive disorders. A history from a reliable family member is probably the most sensitive means of detecting early onset of a cognitive disorder in older persons. However, sensitivity of the physician's examination can be greatly enhanced by administering a standard mental status examination directly to the patient.

The Folstein Mini-Mental State examination takes only 5 to 10 minutes to administer and assesses memory, attention, calculations, naming, and constructional abilities. Therefore, the first step for the physician is to do an in-depth structured mental status examination to increase the likelihood of detecting a cognitive disorder.

For skilled physicians, clues from the interview process may be as important as a structured mental status examination. Simply listening to the patient's conversational style (detection of disorders of language) or observing the patient's dress and appearance may provide helpful clues.

Bibliography

1. **Applegate WB, Blass JP, Williams TF.** Instruments for the functional assessment of older patients. N Engl J Med. 1990;322:1207-14.

Altered Mental Status Question 3
Answer: C

EDUCATIONAL OBJECTIVE: Identify possible drug or alcohol abuse in an older person with cognitive impairment.

Alcohol or drug use should be considered in any older person who presents with a history of fairly acute onset of irritability, distractability, and memory problems. Toxicity from multiple medications often produces the same symptoms. In this 89-year-old woman, the findings of an elevated serum alanine aminotransferase concentration and mean corpuscular volume, although not specific, suggest alcohol abuse.

Chronic dementia, such as Alzheimer's disease and multi-infarct dementia, does not present with an acute onset. Subdural hematoma can present in this way but usually includes focal neurologic findings. Although other acute disorders such as stroke or delirium from an underlying medical disorder should also be considered, alcohol abuse is a prime diagnosis in this patient and the most likely of the options presented.

Bibliography

1. **Widner S, Zeichner A.** Alcohol abuse in the elderly: review of epidemiology, research and treatment. Clin Gerontol. 1991;11:3-18.
2. **Willenbring ML.** Organic mental disorders associated with heavy drinking and alcohol dependence. Clin Geriatr Med. 1988;4:869-87.

Altered Mental Status Question 4
Answer: D

EDUCATIONAL OBJECTIVE: Assess postoperative delirium.

Postoperative delirium is common in elderly surgical patients. Its incidence varies from 10% to 40%, and it is three times more common in patients older than 75 years than in younger patients. Delirium ranges from mild disorientation to frank psychosis. It can be the sole early manifestation of such serious medical conditions as hypoxia, coronary ischemia, cerebrovascular accident, or infection, but more often it is a nonspecific response to such physiologic stressors as surgery, pain, and sleep deprivation, or is an adverse effect of common medications (for example, narcotics, sedatives, H_2-blockers, nonsteroidal anti-inflammatory drugs, and antiemetics). Although patients with dementia frequently develop delirium during a hospital stay, its occurrence does not necessarily indicate underlying organic brain disease. The next best step in the management of this patient is to discontinue morphine.

Should he not respond to withdrawal of morphine, alcohol withdrawal syndrome, a commonly overlooked cause of delirium in elderly patients, should be considered. In this patient, the mild hypertension, postoperative anxiety, and onset of his symptoms are consistent with the natural course of alcohol withdrawal. Nonetheless, cardiac, cerebral, infectious, and hypoxic events must be excluded as indicated by laboratory values.

Bibliography

1. **Pousada L, Leipzig RM.** Rapid bedside assessment of postoperative confusion in older patients. Geriatrics. 1990;45:59-64.

Altered Mental Status Question 5
Answer: B

EDUCATIONAL OBJECTIVE: Select the most appropriate imaging study to evaluate patients with dementia.

Several clinical criteria have been established to diagnose those patients who most likely have treatable causes of dementia. These criteria include the following: 1) onset before the age of 60 years; 2) duration of cognitive complaints less than 6 months; 3) focal signs, focal symptoms, papilledema; 4) new-onset seizures; 5) ataxic or apraxic gait. Patients who meet one or more of these criteria should undergo neuroimaging. This patient meets two of the criteria (<60 years old and duration of cognitive complaints <6 months), and the most appropriate neuroimaging study for this patient is routine magnetic resonance imaging.

More sophisticated imaging techniques that allow for quantification of cerebral blood flow or regional metabolism are not recommended in this routine clinical setting. Therefore, initial evaluation with xenon computed tomography (CT), single-photon emission CT, or positron emission tomography is not appropriate for this patient. Although a routine CT scan would also be appropriate, CT angiography is not indicated for the evaluation of patients with dementia, especially in the absence of clinical features suggestive of cerebrovascular disease.

Bibliography

1. Practice parameters for diagnosis and evaluation of dementia. Report of the Quality Standards Subcommittee of the American Academy of Neurology. Neurology. 1994;44:2203-6.

Altered Mental Status Question 6
Answer: D

EDUCATIONAL OBJECTIVE: Recognize findings that increase the likelihood of seizure recurrence.

Treating the patient who has had a single unprovoked seizure requires assessing the recurrence risk while weighing the risks and benefits of antiepileptic drug therapy. The overall risk of seizure recurrence averages approximately 30%, but estimates range from less than 10% to greater than 70%. Factors that have been associated with a low risk of seizure recurrence include precipitating factors that can be eliminated (for example, alcohol withdrawal is a common cause of generalized motor seizures occurring early in the work week). Normal findings on neurologic examination and a normal electroencephalogram (EEG) are associated with a low risk of seizure recurrence. Cocaine use alone is not a sufficient explanation for a generalized motor seizure. A single uncomplicated febrile seizure is not a risk factor for developing epilepsy in adulthood.

The risk of seizure recurrence within 12 months of a single unprovoked seizure in a patient with normal findings on electroencephalography (EEG) is 15% but increases to 41% in a patient with an abnormal EEG. The greatest risk factor for seizure recurrence during the first year following an unprovoked generalized motor seizure is an abnormal EEG; however, the absence of a recurrent seizure in the first year following a single unprovoked seizure does not eliminate the risk of further seizures: The overall risk rises from 26% in the first year to 40% by the third year.

Bibliography

1. **Hauser WA.** Seizure recurrence after a first unprovoked seizure. N Engl J Med. 1982;307:522-8.
2. **Shinnar S, Berg AT, Moshe SL, Petix M, Maytal J, Kang H, et al.** Risk of seizure recurrence following a first unprovoked seizure in childhood: a prospective study. Pediatrics. 1990;85:1076-85.

Altered Mental Status Question 7
Answer: E

EDUCATIONAL OBJECTIVE: Treat a patient with syncopal myoclonus.

Patients presenting with reported myoclonus or a generalized seizure clearly precipitated by syncope do not need additional testing or treatment. Patients with abnormalities on neurologic examination, particularly localizing signs, or a history of seizures not precipitated by syncope require electroencephalography, imaging studies, and appropriate antiepileptic drugs.

Multifocal myoclonus has been observed in most patients who experience syncope. Syncopal convulsions have been reported in a much smaller proportion of patients who experience syncope. These convulsions are generally characterized by tonic stiffening, but patients may exhibit tonic-clonic seizures.

Venipuncture is the most common procedure done by health care providers and is a leading cause of syncope. In a study of 4050 venipunctures done over a 3-year period, 3.4% of patients experienced serious complications, defined as cellulitis, phlebitis, diaphoresis, hypotension, near syncope, syncope, or seizure activity. Diaphoresis with hypotension occurred in 2.6% of patients, and syncope occurred in approximately 1% of the patients.

Syncope was precipitated in a group of 59 healthy volunteers by hyperventilation, orthostasis, and Valsalva's maneuver, and involuntary movements were studied during the syncopal spells via videotape. Ninety percent of the study subjects experienced multifocal arrhythmic jerks in proximal and distal muscles with common superimposition of generalized myoclonus. Additional involuntary movements seen in nearly 80% of the subjects included head turning and oral automatisms.

Bibliography

1. **Galena HJ.** Complications occurring from diagnostic venipuncture. J Fam Pract. 1992;34:582-4.
2. **Lempert T, Bauer M, Schmidt D.** Syncope: a videometric analysis of 56 episodes of transient cerebral hypoxia. Ann Neurol. 1994;36:233-7.

Altered Mental Status Questions 8-11
Answers: 8(B); 9(E); 10(D); 11(A)

EDUCATIONAL OBJECTIVE: Recognize the clinical features of the common causes of dementia.

The 62-year-old man has had a gradual worsening of cognitive functioning involving language, memory, and judgment over a period of at least 3 years. His occupational skills may have been impaired early in the course of his disease, and he is now no longer independent in all of his daily activities. Therefore, he meets the definition of dementia. With a gradual onset of impairment in multiple cognitive domains, especially involving cortical functions of language and praxis, he most likely has Alzheimer's disease.

Perhaps vascular dementia is the most difficult diagnosis to distinguish from Alzheimer's disease. Dementia due to cerebrovascular disease often presents in a step-wise fashion as patients accumulate cerebral infarctions, but gradual deterioration is not uncommon. The 76-year-old man initially developed signs of aphasia and mild cognitive impairment, followed nearly 2 years later by another stroke resulting in right-sided motor findings.

The 82-year-old woman has normal-pressure hydrocephalus, which is characterized by the clinical triad of dementia, urinary incontinence, and gait disorder. Dementia usually precedes the onset of urinary incontinence by 1 to 2 years. The typical gait disorder of patients with normal-pressure hydrocephalus is characterized by a marked inability in initiation of gait ("magnetic feet" or gait apraxia) with parkinsonian features of short shuffling steps and stooped posture. Imaging studies of the brain often show enlargement of the ventricles out of proportion to the degree of cortical atrophy.

Parkinsonian signs of bradykinesia, increased muscle tone, and gait disorder are more commonly seen in those patients with Alzheimer's disease who present before the age of 65. Patients with idiopathic Parkinson's disease, such as the 64-year-old woman, also have increased muscle tone and postural instability, but their findings are often asymmetric and usually include a resting tremor. Furthermore, although up to 30% of patients with Parkinson's disease develop dementia, cognitive impairment is rarely the presenting symptom and typically reflects a more subcortical pattern, characterized by psychomotor retardation, poor retrieval, and relatively preserved language function.

Creutzfeldt-Jakob disease is a rare, transmissible form of dementia characterized by rapidly progressive cognitive deterioration, seizures, and myoclonus. Electroencephalography often reveals periodic sharp discharges, but the diagnosis is confirmed by pathologic changes of diffuse cortical and cerebellar neuronal loss and microvacuolarization. Death usually occurs within 6 to 12 months of symptom onset.

Bibliography

1. **Corey-Bloom J, Thal LJ, Galasko D, Folstein M, Drachman D, Raskind M, et al.** Diagnosis and evaluation of dementia. Neurology. 1995;45:211-8.

2. Practice parameters for diagnosis and evaluation of dementia. Report of the Quality Standards Subcommittee of the American Academy of Neurology. Neurology. 1994;44:2203-6.

Altered Mental Status Questions 12-15
Answers: 12(D); 13(C); 14(A); 15(B)

EDUCATIONAL OBJECTIVE: Identify acute stroke syndromes that may result in cognitive or behavioral disturbances.

The 76-year-old man has an infarction in the nondominant parietal lobe. Infarctions in the nondominant parietal lobe (inferior lobule) may result in agitation, inattentiveness, delusional thinking and, rarely, visual hallucinations. Autonomic hyperactivity is also common. Contralateral visual neglect, hemiparesis, agraphesthesia, and astereognosis may be mild or absent. These lesions occur in the territory of the middle cerebral artery, but agitation may also result from infarctions in the anterior and posterior cerebral artery distributions to the nondominant hemisphere.

Lesions of the head of the caudate nucleus, as seen in the 75-year-old man, often result in neurobehavioral abnormalities characterized by confusion and abulia. Patients may suddenly become apathetic and have a marked slowness in their thoughts and movements. Occasionally, patients may become restless and agitated, with decreased attention to tasks. Motor symptoms are usually mild and transient and are attributable to extension of the infarction to involve the adjacent anterior limb of the internal capsule and putamen. The head of the caudate is supplied by small, penetrating lenticulostriate arteries and the recurrent arteries of Huebner.

The 74-year-old woman has the sudden onset of mutism, an inability to write, and weakness of the upper extremity, which all suggest an infarction in the frontal lobe (usually the left). Structures often involved include the inferior frontal lobe (Broca's area), insular cortex, and operculum. Speech may eventually become slow and effortful, with relatively preserved comprehension. Weakness preferentially affects the upper extremity and face, although the leg can be involved as well. The upper division of the middle cerebral artery supplies this territory.

The 66-year-old woman has clinical manifestations of thalamic infarctions. These manifestations depend upon the specific thalamic nuclei involved. Lesions in the territory of the paramedian thalamic arteries often produce a characteristic triad of depressed consciousness, neuropsychologic disturbances, and impaired vertical gaze. Impairment of consciousness may be severe, ranging from hypersomnolence to frank coma, and most likely results from involvement of intralaminar nuclei and the rostral midbrain reticular formation. As the impairment of consciousness improves, symptoms of amnesia, disorientation, and abulia may emerge. Up-gaze palsy is most common, but combined up-gaze and down-gaze palsies may also occur.

Bibliography

1. **Bogousslavsky J, Regli F, Uske A.** Thalamic infarcts: clinical syndromes, etiology, and prognosis. Neurology. 1988;38:837-48.

2. **Mohr JP, Pessin MS, Finkelstein S, Funkenstein HH, Duncan GW, Davis KR.** Broca aphasia: pathologic and clinical. Neurology. 1978;28:311-24.

3. **Caplan LR, Schmahmann JD, Kase CS, Feldmann E, Baquis G, Greenberg JP, et al.** Caudate infarcts. Arch Neurol. 1990;47:133-43.

4. **Mesulam MM, Waxman SG, Geschwind N, Sabin TD.** Acute confusional states with right middle cerebral artery infarctions. J Neurol Neurosurg Psychiatry. 1976;39:84-9.

Altered Mental Status Questions 16-19
Answers: 16(C); 17(B); 18(A); 19(D)

EDUCATIONAL OBJECTIVE: Distinguish important causes of confusion in older outpatients

Both short-term confusion (acute confusional state) and long-term confusion (chronic cognitive impairment) are common in older persons. Studies indicate that internists fail to recognize moderate to severely impaired persons. Most patients and families strongly desire a clear diagnosis when confusion is detected in order to rule out other causes of memory or behavior problems, to allow family members to get information about dementia, to decide about possible drug treatments, and to plan for the future (for example, advance directives and finances). In addition, internists need to evaluate confused patients for reversible components to the confusion or "excess disability." Evaluation of the clinical characteristics of the patient and the types of cognitive deficits, rather than laboratory or radiologic testing, is often the most useful approach for determining the most likely cause of the confusion.

The most common causes of chronic cognitive impairment are Alzheimer's dementia and vascular (multi-infarct) dementia. The predominant and earliest changes in Alzheimer's dementia are short-term and long-term memory problems and fluent aphasia. The language disorder is characterized by empty speech (for example, "he did that with the thing"), poor verbal and reading comprehension, and anomia. Over time, the speech becomes less fluent and mutism develops in late stages. Personality changes are also common: the patient may be described as a "shell" of his former self, as if the personality has drained away. Affected patients often appear bewildered or anxious, and persecutory delusions, centering on memory deficits, are common.

The findings in the 75-year-old man with memory loss are consistent with Alzheimer's dementia. Patients with mild Alzheimer's dementia may be candidates for treatment with donepezil, a once-daily medication with a low incidence of side effects. Randomized controlled trials have shown decreased functional decline over time in patients with early Alzheimer's dementia treated with donepezil, 5 to 10 mg/d.

In contrast, the deficits seen in vascular or multi-infarct dementia reflect the areas of vascular compromise. Patients may lose function insidiously or in a step-wise fashion. If strokes occur in the nondominant hemisphere, problems with visuospatial function, often evidenced by getting lost or wandering, as well as poor insight and safety awareness may occur. Problems in visuospatial functioning and safety awareness also occur in Alzheimer's disease, but memory and language deficits are present and usually dominate the picture. Vascular dementia occurs at a younger average age than Alzheimer's dementia, the incidence of which continues to rise with age.

The presenting symptoms of the 70-year-old man with driving accidents point to nondominant hemisphere dysfunction and do not include memory or aphasia problems. The absence of an early history of problems with memory or language makes Alzheimer's dementia unlikely. In the absence of a prominent memory deficit, delirium and pseudodementia (due to depression) are also less likely. Low-dose aspirin therapy should be prescribed for all patients with vascular dementia, based on dementia research as well as the greatly increased likelihood that these patients have concomitant coronary artery disease.

Multiple studies have established that benzodiazepines are independently associated with confusion, as well as with falls in older persons. Physicians should prescribe these drugs with great caution in elderly patients and maintain a low threshold for suspecting toxicity. A diagnosis of chronic cognitive impairment should not be made until the patient is evaluated after discontinuing benzodiazepine therapy. Therefore, without additional symptoms indicative of major depression, the 75-year-old woman taking lorazepam has delirium, or acute confusion, until proven otherwise.

Parkinson's disease–associated dementia is characterized by memory retrieval problems (patients can answer multiple-choice questions, whereas patients with Alzheimer's dementia, never having stored the information, cannot) and difficulty with such functions as planning, organizing, sequencing, and abstracting. Patients also have bradyphrenia, with slow response to questions. Apraxia, agnosia, and aphasia, which are features of Alzheimer's dementia, are not seen in this syndrome. Patients with Alzheimer's dementia also have difficulty with executive functions, but memory and language disturbances predominate.

Therefore, the 70-year-old woman with memory problems and difficulty planning and executing tasks most likely has Parkinson's disease–associated dementia, if she also has the motor features of Parkinson's disease. Parkinson's disease–associated dementia cannot be diagnosed in the absence of the milder findings of Parkinson's disease. The cognitive problems in this form of dementia do not respond to antiparkinsonian medications. These medications should be used only to treat the motor components of the disease.

Bibliography

1. **Connell CM, Gallant MP.** Spouse caregivers' attitudes toward obtaining a diagnosis of a dementing illness. J Am Geriatr Soc. 1996;44:1003-9.
2. **Callahan CM, Hendrie HC, Tierney WM.** Documentation and evaluation of cognitive impairment in elderly primary care patients. Ann Intern Med. 1995;122:422-9.
3. **Fleming KC, Adams AC, Petersen RC.** Dementia: diagnosis and evaluation. Mayo Clin Proc. 1995;70:1093-7.

Altered Mental Status Question 20
Answer: E

EDUCATIONAL OBJECTIVE: Select the most appropriate treatment option for a patient with a transient ischemic attack.

This 73-year-old man had a transient ischemic attack involving the left carotid artery territory while receiving aspirin therapy. The patient's symptoms are site-appropriate for an 80% left internal carotid artery stenosis. The preferred treatment for stroke prevention is left carotid endarterectomy.

Antiplatelet therapy is not as effective as carotid endarterectomy for stroke prevention if surgery can be accomplished with less than or equal to 5% morbidity and mortality. Warfarin has not been shown to be effective for stroke prevention in this clinical situation. Because the patient's neurologic deficit is rapidly improving, he is not a candidate for thrombolytic therapy.

The patient was initially treated with heparin. There is no rigorous evidence that this is effective in preventing an acute stroke. However, many physicians will use anticoagulation therapy until a long-term treatment plan is defined.

Bibliography

1. MRC European Carotid Surgery Trial: interim results for symptomatic patients with severe (70-99%) or with mild (0-29%) carotid stenosis. European Carotid Surgery Trialists' Collaborative Group. Lancet. 1991;337:1235-43.
2. Endarterectomy for moderate symptomatic carotid stenosis: interim results from the MRC European Carotid Surgery Trial. European Carotid Surgery Trial. Lancet. 1996;347:1591-3.
3. Beneficial effect of carotid endarterectomy in symptomatic patients with high-grade stenosis. North American Symptomatic Carotid Endarterectomy Trial Collaborators. N Engl J Med. 1991;325:445-53.

Altered Mental Status Question 21
Answer: D

EDUCATIONAL OBJECTIVE: Distinguish among various stroke syndromes.

This patient has findings consistent with the dysarthria–clumsy hand syndrome. This condition represents a lacunar infarction secondary to small artery occlusion in the contralateral pons. Hypertension and diabetes mellitus predispose patients to lacunar stroke. Patients are dysarthric as well as mildly hemiparetic and mildly to moderately ataxic ipsilateral to the weakness. The combination of symptoms is characteristic of this syndrome and does not suggest any other diagnosis. Control of risk factors is important; physicians often also prescribe aspirin, although evidence for its efficacy in this setting is slim.

Patients with a posterior-inferior cerebellar infarction can present with a cerebellar syndrome or lateral medullary syndrome. Weakness is not a component in either instance. This patient does not have a visual field deficit or hemisensory loss that might be expected with a middle cerebral artery occlusion. Clumsiness can occur following a right hemisphere infarction, not only from weakness but also from sensory loss of primary modalities as well as cortical sensory loss (parietal ataxia).

A cerebellar hemorrhage can cause an abnormal stance and gait, as well as ataxia, abnormal brain stem signs, and weakness. However, the latter two problems usually occur in a progressively deteriorating patient with impaired cognition. A thalamic lacunar stroke usually causes discrete impairments such as contralateral sensory loss or memory impairment (from an infarction in the dorsal medial nucleus).

Bibliography

1. **Glass JD, Levey AI, Rothstein JD.** The dysarthria-clumsy hand syndrome: a distinct clinical entity related to pontine infarction. Ann Neurol. 1990;27:487-94.

ANEMIA

Anemia Question 1
Answer: D

EDUCATIONAL OBJECTIVE: Manage a patient with a low vitamin B_{12} level but no hematologic evidence of deficiency.

Although serum vitamin B_{12} levels are often low in elderly patients (approximately 10% prevalence) and many of these patients have no clinical evidence of deficiency, it is important to remember that megaloblastic anemia is often absent in true deficiency. Blood counts are often normal in patients with pernicious anemia. Many such patients have neurologic dysfunction that can be mild or severe.

It is not clear whether this patient's forgetfulness is pathologic (the Mini-Mental State Examination is not sensitive enough) and possibly attributable to vitamin B_{12} deficiency or not. Similarly, the mild impairment of vibratory sense can be an early sign of vitamin B_{12} deficiency, evidence of mild diabetic neuropathy, or just the idiopathic diminution of vibratory sense seen in many otherwise healthy elderly people. However, the physician must always prove that the vitamin B_{12} deficiency is not present when the serum vitamin B_{12} level is low, especially when there is any suspicion of neurologic dysfunction. The possibility of deficiency is further strengthened by the mildly abnormal methylmalonic acid level. A Schilling test to assess vitamin B_{12} absorption and parenteral therapy to determine if neurologic symptoms reverse are both indicated.

Therefore, reassuring the patient that her low vitamin B_{12} level is insignificant or asking her to include red meat in her diet and re-evaluating her in 6 months is incorrect (moreover, the lack of red meat intake cannot explain the low vitamin B_{12} level because she eats chicken and fish, which are adequate sources of vitamin B_{12}). Prescribing 10 µg of vitamin B_{12} is inappropriate because it fails to address whether the patient has malabsorption of vitamin B_{12} and is inadequate if malabsorption exists. Most vitamin B_{12} deficiencies have a gastroenterologic cause. Unlike the Schilling test, endoscopy and gastric analyses for acid output address only one of the potential causes of vitamin B_{12} deficiency; moreover, they are invasive and premature and would probably be inconclusive.

Bibliography

1. **Metz J, Bell AH, Flicker L, Bottiglieri T, Ibrahim J, Seal E, et al.** The significance of subnormal serum vitamin B_{12} concentration in older people: a case control study. J Am Geriatr Soc. 1996;44:1355-61.
2. **Carmel R.** Cobalamin, the stomach, and aging. Am J Clin Nutr. 1997;66:750-9.
3. **Healton EB, Savage DG, Brust JC, Garrett TJ, Lindenbaum J.** Neurologic aspects of cobalamin deficiency. Medicine. 1991;70:229-45.

Anemia Question 2
Answer: D

EDUCATIONAL OBJECTIVE: Differentiate between cobalamin and folate deficiencies.

This woman clearly has megaloblastic anemia. The question posed is whether it is due to vitamin B_{12} or folate deficiency. The only direct, nonlaboratory clue would be the presence of neurologic dysfunction, which points to a vitamin B_{12} deficiency. However, like many patients with vitamin B_{12} deficiency, this patient has no neurologic dysfunction. Thus, only indirect clues from the history that suggest underlying diseases or disorders associated with one of these deficiencies are available in this patient.

This patient has a history of poor dietary intake for the past 6 months. Although her intake of meat and fish (the main dietary sources of vitamin B_{12}) was particularly poor, the history of intake largely limited to toast, tea, and infrequent fruit is also poor for folate. However, body stores of folate can be depleted by poor intake in a few months, whereas vitamin B_{12} depletion requires several years of poor intake. Thus, clinically significant vitamin B_{12} depletion is unlikely to have occurred in this woman so soon. Moreover, the suggestion of alcohol abuse in her history reinforces a focus on folate deficiency rather than vitamin B_{12} deficiency.

Because the history points to folate deficiency as the probable cause of this woman's megaloblastic anemia, low folate and high homocysteine levels would be expected. Homocysteine methylation to methionine depends on methyl tetrahydrofolate (but also requires methylcobalamin, and thus, homocysteine levels increase in vitamin B_{12} deficiency, too). Methylmalonic acid elevation, however, is a more specific marker for vitamin B_{12} deficiency and does not occur in folate deficiency. Thus, methylmalonic acid elevation would not be expected in this patient. Incidentally, either homocysteine or methylmalonic acid elevation in the blood may be spurious in even mild renal insufficiency.

Bibliography

1. **Green R.** Metabolite assays in cobalamin and folate deficiency. Baillieres Clin Haematol. 1995;8:533-66.

2. **Chanarin I.** The Megaloblastic Anaemias. 2nd ed. Oxford: Blackwell Scientific Publications; 1979:48-58.

3. **Lindenbaum J.** Drug-induced folate deficiency and the hematologic effects of alcohol. In: Lindenbaum J, ed. Contemporary Issues in Clinical Nutrition. Vol 5. Nutrition in Hematology. New York: Churchill Livingstone; 1983:33-58.

Anemia Question 3
Answer: C

EDUCATIONAL OBJECTIVE: Recognize the differential diagnosis of fragmentation hemolytic anemia associated with thrombocytopenia.

This patient's presentation is typical of thrombotic thrombocytopenic purpura with all of the cardinal features of the disease (hemolytic anemia, thrombocytopenia, renal abnormalities, fever, and a neurologic defect). All five features are usually present only 30% to 40% of the time. The sine qua non of the diagnosis is fragmentation hemolytic anemia associated with severe thrombocytopenia. This patient clearly had hemolytic anemia, as substantiated by a markedly elevated reticulocyte count, indirect serum bilirubinemia, and elevated lactate dehydrogenase. The most important test to be done in a patient who has hemolytic anemia is a review of erythrocyte morphology on the peripheral blood smear. In this patient, there were obvious fragmented erythrocytes, characteristic of fragmentation hemolytic anemia. Although the patient had proteinuria and hematuria, the patient's renal function was within normal limits, as it is in most of these patients. Although mild renal failure and/or prerenal azotemia may be seen in a significant number of these patients, progressive or irreversible renal failure in only occurs about 5% to 10% of the patients. The lactate dehydrogenase level of 3500 U/L is typical because of the severe hemolytic process.

Although acute leukemia is frequently characterized by severe anemia and thrombocytopenia, there usually is a markedly depressed reticulocyte count and a low serum bilirubin level, as seen in patients with erythroid hypoplasia. In addition, patients with acute leukemia usually do not have increased numbers of normal neutrophils in the peripheral blood, as was noted in this particular patient.

Although bacterial endocarditis may present with fever and focal neurologic findings (presumably from emboli from the affected valve), these patients rarely have fragmentation hemolysis and thrombocytopenia. In addition, there was no evidence that this patient had a valvular disorder nor was she an injection drug user.

Although hemolytic-uremic syndrome is characterized by fragmentation hemolysis along with thrombocytopenia, patients with this disorder present with either frank uremia or oliguria and progressive renal failure. There are many different causes of the hemolytic-uremic syndrome in adults, including those due to *Escherichia coli* and *Shigella,* malignant hypertension, cyclosporine, and cytotoxic anticancer drugs.

Although occasionally patients with systemic lupus erythematosus may present with the findings seen in this patient, it is very rare that this occurs at presentation. However, when a diagnosis of thrombotic thrombocytopenic purpura is made in a young woman, serologic tests should be obtained in order to rule out lupus.

Bibliography

1. **Moake JL.** Thrombotic thrombocytopenic purpura and the hemolytic-uremic syndrome. In: Hoffman R, Benz EJ Jr, Shattil SJ, Furie B, Cohen HJ, Silberstein LE, eds. Hematology: Basic Principles and Practice. 2nd ed. New York: Churchill Livingstone; 1995:1879-88.

2. **Ruggenenti P, Remuzzi G.** Thrombotic thrombocytopenic purpura and related disorders. Hematol Oncol Clin North Am. 1990;4:219-41.

3. **Thompson CE, Damon LE, Ries CA, Linker CA.** Thrombotic microangiopathies in the 1980s: clinical features, response to treatment, and the impact of the human immunodeficiency virus epidemic. Blood. 1992;80:1890-5.

Anemia Question 4
Answer: E

EDUCATIONAL OBJECTIVE: Select an appropriate strategy regarding transfusion for a patient with severe anemia.

This patient has megaloblastic anemia. The history does not allow clear differentiation between vitamin B_{12} and folate deficiency, although the vitamin B_{12} deficiency seems more likely. The management decision concerns how best to correct severe but reversible anemia in the elderly patient. The correct choice is to withhold transfusion, monitor the patient's status, and administer the necessary vitamin after the results have been received. Alternatively, the patient could be given both vitamins while waiting for the laboratory results. Incidentally, emergency institution of vitamin therapy is rarely necessary. Had immediate correction of anemia been necessary because of critical symptoms such as congestive heart failure or angina, transfusion would have been necessary because any hemoglobin response to vitamins would not begin for several days

This patient has a treatable cause of anemia, shows no signs of cardiac or pulmonary instability, has no evidence of neurologic compromise (such as altered consciousness or dizziness), and has no history of coronary or other coexisting disorders that might be seriously aggravated by anemia. Therefore, immediate transfusion in order to quickly raise the blood count is not indicated. It is clear from his history that his anemia is chronic and has progressed slowly over many weeks, if not months. Chronic anemia is usually well compensated by physiologic processes that improve oxygen delivery to the tissues, such as increased levels of 2,3-diphosphoglycerate, which shift the oxygen dissociation curve.

This patient's hemoglobin level was most likely well below 8 g/dL for many weeks before he sought medical attention and below 10 g/dL for even longer, and his symptoms were not alarming during that time. Thus, there is no urgent need to restore the blood count immediately to either of those hemoglobin levels (both arbitrary numbers in any case). Transfusion, despite its relative safety, still poses risks of infection that must be weighed against its benefits. If transfusion were to be chosen, however, the best approach would be to transfuse until relief of whatever critical symptoms prompted the decision to transfuse rather than to aim for a preselected numerical value.

Erythropoietin therapy would be ineffective in this patient. Endogenous levels of erythropoietin are already high in patients with megaloblastic anemia.

Bibliography

1. **Rossi EC.** Red cell transfusion therapy in chronic anemia. Hematol Oncol Clin North Am. 1994;8:1045-52.

2. Practice strategies for elective red blood cell transfusion. American College of Physicians. Ann Intern Med. 1992;116:403-6.

3. **Carmel R, Shulman IA.** Blood transfusion in medically treatable chronic anemia: pernicious anemia as a model for transfusion overuse. Arch Pathol Lab Med. 1989;113:995-7.

Anemia Question 5
Answer: D

EDUCATIONAL OBJECTIVE: Differentiate between iron deficiency and thalassemia.

Iron deficiency should be considered in any anemic woman of reproductive age, especially when the anemia is microcytic. However, thalassemia minor is both common and easily confused with iron deficiency, and iron therapy is not warranted and sometimes harmful. This patient's presentation illustrates a common dilemma. Her mild microcytic anemia indicates that there is a hematologic disorder, and recurrent iron deficiency and α-thalassemia are the most common causes. An additional option not listed but worth remembering, especially in a woman with mild microcytosis unresponsive to iron therapy, is hyperthyroidism.

In this patient, thalassemia minor is the most likely diagnosis because of the reasons given below that rule out other causes. This likelihood is enhanced by the relatively prominent microcytosis in relation to the patient's minimal anemia and the normal erythrocyte distribution width, both features more characteristic of thalassemia than iron deficiency (although the erythrocyte distribution width distinction between the two is not as consistent as originally thought).

The normal hemoglobin A_2 and hemoglobin F levels rule out β-thalassemia, in which suppression of β-globin chain synthesis diminishes the proportion of hemoglobin A in relation to one or both (depending on the specific molecular lesion) of those two minor hemoglobins. In α-thalassemia, on the other hand, the diminished availability of α-globin chains affects the production of all classes of globin equally, so that proportions thus remain unchanged. Definitive proof of β-thalassemia, probably the most common hemoglobinopathy in the world, would require further testing by β-globin gene analysis.

Recurrent iron deficiency, especially if attributed in an adult to the unlikely mechanism of poor dietary intake, can be ruled out in this patient because of the normal iron and ferritin levels. These results, especially the ferritin level, would not be masked by iron therapy discontinued some time ago. If her iron deficiency is severe enough to cause anemia, the ferritin level would be low (unless there was a coexisting reason for falsely elevated serum ferritin level, such as acute liver disease or inflammatory disease).

Anemia of chronic disease can be discounted because there is no suggestion of infection, inflammation, or cancer, and because a mean corpuscular volume of 72 fL is too low for anemia of chronic disease (in which the erythrocyte indices are most often normal and, even when low, the mean corpuscular volume rarely falls below 75 fL). Most importantly, the normal serum iron-binding capacity contradicts a diagnosis of anemia of chronic disease.

Finally, her previous physician's failure to follow up, recognize a lack of response, stop the unnecessary iron therapy, and re-evaluate the patient was a more serious error in this patient's earlier management than the automatic dispensing of iron treatment and the original assumption that her microcytic anemia was due to iron deficiency.

Bibliography

1. **Mach-Pascual S, Darbellay R, Pilotto PA, Beris P.** Investigation of microcytosis: a comprehensive approach. Eur J Haematol. 1996;57:54-61.

2. **Lafferty JD, Crowther MA, Ali MA, Levine M.** The evaluation of various mathematical RBC indices and their efficacy in discriminating between thalassemic and non-thalassemic microcytosis. Am J Clin Pathol. 1996;106:201-5.

3. **Higgs DR.** β-Thalassemia. Baillieres Clin Haematol. 1993;6:117-50.

4. **Lipschitz DA.** The anemia of chronic disease. J Am Geriatr Soc. 1990;38:1258-64.

5. **Nightingale S, Vitek PJ, Himsworth RL.** The haematology of hyperthyroidism. Q J Med. 1978;47:35-47.

Anemia Question 6
Answer: C

EDUCATIONAL OBJECTIVE: Recognize myelodysplasia as a long-term complication of immunosuppressive therapy for aplastic anemia.

Myelodysplasia, as well as acute myelocytic leukemia (AML) and paroxysmal nocturnal hemoglobinuria, occurs in up to 15% to 20% of patients who have been treated for aplastic anemia with immunosuppressive therapy and usually occurs between 2 and 10 years after therapy. Findings in some patients may evolve from a positive Ham test, which indicates a clonal disorder, to myelodysplasia and AML. Patients may present with either pancytopenia or an isolated cytopenia. Analysis of bone marrow specimen shows dysplastic morphology of the hematopoietic precursors and often an increase in blast cells.

Immunosuppressive therapy is an effective treatment for patients with aplastic anemia who cannot undergo bone marrow transplantation because of age, lack of donor, or medical condition. Although recurrence of aplastic anemia can occur in up to 25% of

patients following a response, this usually occurs within 1 to 2 years after therapy, often after discontinuation of the immunosuppressive medications. Some patients will respond again to immunosuppressive treatment.

This patient developed pancytopenia 7 years after successful treatment, making it unlikely that this is a recurrence of aplastic anemia. Although the patient's leukocyte count differential shows a predominance of lymphocytes, the absolute number is not elevated and does not support a diagnosis of chronic lymphocytic leukemia. Even though the mean corpuscular volume is high, the neutrophil and erythrocyte morphologies do not show any evidence of vitamin B_{12} deficiency. An elevated erythrocyte mean corpuscular volume can also be seen in patients who have myelodysplasia. Although disseminated infections such as miliary tuberculosis are a rare cause of pancytopenia, the patient did not show any evidence of clinical infection.

Bibliography

1. **Young NS, Maciejewski J.** The pathophysiology of acquired aplastic anemia. N Engl J Med. 1997; 336:1365-72.

2. **de Planque MM, Bacigalupo A, Wursch A, Hows JM, Devergie A, Frickhofen N, et al.** Long-term follow-up of severe aplastic anaemia patients treated with antithymocyte globulin. Severe Aplastic Anemia Working Party of the European Cooperative Group for Bone Marrow Transplantation (EBMT). Br J Haematol. 1989;73:121-6.

3. **Socie G, Henry-Amar M, Bacigalupo A, Hows J, Tichelli A, Ljungman P, et al.** Malignant tumors occurring after treatment of aplastic anemia. European Bone Marrow Transplantation-Severe Aplastic Anaemia Working Party. N Engl J Med. 1993;329:1152-7.

4. **Doney K, Leisenring W, Storb R, Appelbaum FR.** Primary treatment of acquired aplastic anemia: outcomes with bone marrow transplantation and immunosuppressive therapy. Seattle Bone Marrow Transplant Team. Ann Intern Med. 1997;126:107-15.

Anemia Question 7
Answer: D

EDUCATIONAL OBJECTIVE: Identify the complications of pernicious anemia.

Even though a Schilling test was not done, the positive anti-intrinsic factor antibody and the elevated serum gastrin level point to pernicious anemia as the cause of the vitamin B_{12} deficiency. The disease, moreover, is more common than originally thought in black women in their 40s.

Fourteen months after a complete hematologic response to standard vitamin B_{12} therapy was documented, a mild anemia reappeared. Although the anemia was not overtly macrocytic, the mean corpuscular volume had risen 7 fL since her 6-month follow-up visit.

Development of mild anemia with a rising mean corpuscular volume suggests either hypothyroidism or folate deficiency. However, hypothyroidism is a common complication of pernicious anemia (about 10% of cases) and its onset is typically insidious, whereas folate deficiency is not a noted complication. Most importantly, there was no change in dietary intake, which is the most common cause of folate deficiency, whereas the symptoms of constipation and menorrhagia suggest hypothyroidism.

This recurrence of anemia cannot be due to relapsed vitamin B_{12} deficiency because regular adequate treatment had been given. Even though the patient administered 0.5-mL injections instead of the prescribed 1-mL injections, smaller doses are effective, and she still received the required minimum of 1 to 2 μg/d. Ordering a Schilling test will not explain the anemia at this point, because even if the presumptive diagnosis of pernicious anemia (that is, lack of intrinsic factor) based on the gastrin and anti-intrinsic factor antibody results had been wrong, the diagnosis of vitamin B_{12} deficiency was not. Parenteral vitamin B_{12} would have been adequate treatment regardless of the underlying cause of the vitamin B_{12} deficiency.

Gastric cancer should always be considered as a potential complication of pernicious anemia, whether blood is detected in the stool or not. However, any accompanying anemia that results (usually iron deficiency or anemia of chronic disease) would not involve a rising mean corpuscular volume.

Bibliography

1. **Carmel R, Spencer CA.** Clinical and subclinical thyroid disorders associated with pernicious anemia. Observations on abnormal thyroid-stimulating hormone levels and on a possible association of blood group O with hyperthyroidism. Arch Intern Med. 1982;142:1465-9.

2. **Horton L, Coburn RJ, England JM, Himsworth RL.** The haematology of hypothyroidism. Q J Med. 1976;45:101-23.

3. **Carmel R.** Pernicious anemia and other megaloblastic anemias. In: Rakel RE, ed. Conn's Current Therapy 1995. Philadelphia: WB Saunders; 1995:311-4.

4. **Sjöblom SM, Sipponen P, Jarvinen H.** Gastroscopic follow-up of pernicious anaemia patients. Gut. 1993;34:28-32.

5. **Fairbanks VF, Wahner HW, Phyliky RL.** Tests for pernicious anemia: the "Schilling test." Mayo Clin Proc. 1983;58:541-4.

Anemia Questions 8-11
Answers: 8(E); 9(C); 10(A); 11(D)

EDUCATIONAL OBJECTIVE: Recognize the clinical significance of infectious agents transmitted by blood transfusion.

Recent estimates indicate that about 1/493,000 donated units (range 1/202,000 to 1/2,778,000) are infected with HIV. Each donated unit of whole blood is made into an average of about 1.8 products, such as packed erythrocytes, fresh frozen plasma, platelet concentrates, and cryoprecipitate. In March 1996, the HIV p24 antigen test was added to the battery of tests already done on all donated units, but this has detected only 1 unit infected with HIV in which other tests were negative among the first 2 million units tested.

Perhaps 50% of blood donors are seropositive for cytomegalovirus (CMV), although most seropositive donors do not transmit the virus. CMV usually causes no illness in immunocompetent patients but may cause serious and even fatal illness in immunosuppressed patients, such as recipients of allogeneic bone marrow transplants, premature infants, and patients with HIV infection. Fetuses are particularly susceptible, and intrauterine transfusions or transfusion of CMV-seronegative pregnant women is of particular concern. CMV transmission can be prevented by using blood from seronegative donors. Recent data suggest that filtration of cellular blood products to produce leukocyte-reduced products may also be effective in minimizing transmission.

The hepatitis C virus (HCV) usually causes asymptomatic infection; however, about 20% of infected persons have microscopic evidence of cirrhosis and a few will develop liver failure, usually after an incubation period of decades. The development of hepatocellular carcinoma is also associated with HCV infection, with a relative risk compared with persons without anti-HCV of about 6 to 8.

Bacterial contamination of blood products may occur as a result of asymptomatic bacteremia in the donor or, less often, by contamination of the product with skin flora. Usually such contaminated units cause no discernible effect, but heavily contaminated units cause immediate life-threatening reactions. About three fatal cases are reported annually in the United States.

Bibliography

1. **Schreiber GB, Busch MP, Kleinman SH, Korelitz JJ.** The risk of transfusion-transmitted viral infections. N Engl J Med. 1996;334:1685-90.

2. **Williams AE, Sullivan MT.** Transfusion-transmitted retro-virus infection. Hematol Oncol Clin North Am. 1995;9:115-36.

3. **Dodd RY.** Transfusion-transmitted hepatitis virus infection. Hematol Oncol Clin North Am. 1995;9:137-54.

4. **Bowden RA.** Transfusion-transmitted cytomegalovirus infection. Hematol Oncol Clin North Am. 1995;9:155-66.

5. **Krishnan LA, Brecher ME.** Transfusion-transmitted bacterial infection. Hematol Oncol Clin North Am. 1995;9:167-85.

Anemia Questions 12-16
Answers: 12(C); 13(A); 14(B); 15(E); 16(D)

EDUCATIONAL OBJECTIVE: Identify the mechanism of acute transfusion reactions.

By far the most common type of acute reaction to blood products is a febrile, nonhemolytic transfusion reaction. It is characterized by a fever (which may be accompanied by chills) that occurs during or within a couple of hours of a transfusion. It is caused by antibodies to donor leukocyte antigens, and accordingly, the use of leukocyte-reduced blood products is indicated to prevent subsequent reactions, particularly after a patient has had two or more episodes. These antigen-antibody reactions are thought to result in the stimulation and release of endogenous pyrogens (cytokines such as interleukin-1, interleukin-6, and tumor necrosis factor) by the donor leukocytes. It is critical to exclude a hemolytic reaction that often has fever as its presenting manifestation and that may result in much more serious morbidity. Cytokines may also accumulate in the cellular blood components during storage and, when infused, cause the typical symptoms characteristic of these reactions.

Hemolytic reactions are caused by erythrocyte incompatibility, that is, antibodies to antigens on the transfused erythrocytes. Severe, acute reactions have a mortality rate of about 5% to 10% and are usually caused by ABO blood group antibodies resulting from transfusion of blood of the wrong type (for example, type A blood to a type O patient). Inaccurate identification of the patient or of the unit of blood is the most common cause of these events. Extreme caution should be exercised to prevent such errors, which have been estimated to occur in about 1 in 12,000 transfusions. Manifestations of a severe hemolytic reaction may include fever, chills, signs of intravascular hemolysis (hemoglobinemia and hemoglobinuria), and systemic signs and symptoms, such as back or flank pain, dyspnea, nausea, and a sense of uneasiness or anxiety. The most severe reactions progress to renal failure, disseminated intravascular coagulation, multisystem organ failure, and death.

Less severe hemolytic reactions result from other erythrocyte alloantibodies that develop as a result of previous transfusions or pregnancies and are not detectable at the time of transfusion, but recur rapidly as part of an anamnestic reaction following transfusion. Such reactions most often become evident 1 day to 1 week following the transfusion and are called delayed hemolytic transfusion reactions. Manifestations include fever, signs of extravascular hemolysis, and an unexpected drop in hemoglobin without evidence of hemorrhaging.

Mild urticarial reactions complicate 1% to 3% of plasma infusions and have been attributed to the presence of recipient antibodies to foreign plasma proteins. For many of these reactions, however, the pathophysiologic mechanisms and mediators by which plasma products effect the allergic reaction are poorly understood.

Transfusion-associated circulatory overload causing pulmonary congestion is probably underdiagnosed and may occur as often as in 1 in 708 patients. Among reports to the Food and Drug Administration of transfusion-associated deaths, the third most common cause was acute pulmonary problems, including circulatory overload and transfusion-related acute lung injury.

Anaphylactic shock as a result of transfusion may result from preformed anti-IgA in the circulation of recipients. However, such antibodies probably account for only a few of these reactions, and most anaphylactic and anaphylactoid transfusion reactions have no detectable cause.

When symptoms occur following transfusion, the transfusion should be discontinued, the intravenous line should be kept open with saline, a clerical check should be done to confirm that the patient received the correct unit, and the reaction should be reported to the hospital blood transfusion service. Hospital policies vary, but most laboratories will request blood and urine specimens for visual inspection to exclude hemoglobinemia and hemoglobinuria. All paperwork will be checked to exclude clerical errors, the ABO and Rh typing will be repeated on donor and recipient specimens, and a direct antiglobulin test will be done on the post-transfusion specimen to determine if the patient's erythrocytes are coated with IgG and/or C3d. The results of this emergency work-up should be obtained before proceeding.

Bibliography

1. **Jeter EK, Spivey MA.** Noninfectious complications of blood transfusion. Hematol Oncol Clin North Am. 1995;9:187-204.

2. **Jenner PW, Holland PV.** Diagnosis and management of transfusion reactions. In: Petz LD, Swisher SN, Kleinman S, Spence RK, Strauss RG, eds. Clinical Practice of Transfusion Medicine. 3rd ed. New York: Churchill Livingstone; 1996:905-29.
3. **Popovsky MA, ed.** Transfusion Reactions. Bethesda, Maryland: AABB Press; 1996.

Anemia Questions 17-20
Answers: 17(B); 18(D); 19(A); 20(C)

Educational Objective: Recognize characteristic complete blood counts and blood-related chemistry test patterns in macrocytic anemias.

Of the two choices with pancytopenia, both Options B and C have suppressed reticulocyte counts as expected in patients with aplastic anemia. However, the elevated indirect bilirubin and lactate dehydrogenase levels in Option C suggest increased cell destruction as seen in either hemolysis or ineffective hematopoiesis (increased death of precursor cells in the bone marrow). In aplastic anemia, neither of these processes takes place because precursor cells are scant. Bilirubin levels are, if anything, decreased and lactate dehydrogenase levels are normal in patients with aplastic anemia.

Options D and E show reticulocytosis and elevated indirect bilirubin and lactate dehydrogenase levels and suggest hemolytic anemia. The mean corpuscular volume is usually normal in patients with hemolytic anemia but is sometimes high-normal or even high. Occasionally, the reticulocytosis may not be prominent in autoimmune hemolytic anemia, usually because reticulocytes are susceptible to immune destruction, too. However, even in such an event the hyperbilirubinemia and lactate dehydrogenase elevation that reflect increased erythrocyte destruction would still be seen. Option D best fits autoimmune hemolytic anemia because the microcytosis in Option E suggests chronic intravascular hemolytic anemia and coexisting iron deficiency. The thrombocytopenia in Option E, also unusual in autoimmune hemolysis, further suggests either a fragmentation hemolytic syndrome with platelet consumption or paroxysmal nocturnal hemoglobinuria.

Acute alcohol abuse often directly produces macrocytosis of erythrocytes, unrelated to any folate deficiency. Indeed, a high mean corpuscular volume in a nonanemic patient may be valuable as a diagnostic marker for recent alcohol abuse. Similarly, acute alcohol abuse often produces transient thrombocytopenia.

No intervention other than supportive care is needed. Option A illustrates both of these direct effects of alcohol without necessarily invoking features of chronic alcohol abuse, such as folate deficiency (Option C) or liver disease.

Option C illustrates a marked macrocytic anemia with low leukocyte and platelet counts. The indirect hyperbilirubinemia and high lactate dehydrogenase level in a patient with a low reticulocyte count suggest the characteristic ineffective hematopoiesis of megaloblastic anemia. These abnormal chemistry markers of ineffective hematopoiesis invariably occur when the megaloblastic anemia is severe, as it is here. Bacteria contaminating the small bowel can consume vitamin B_{12} and are often overlooked as a cause of vitamin B_{12} deficiency.

Bibliography
1. **Carmel R.** Megaloblastic anemia. In: Kelley WN, ed. Textbook of Internal Medicine. 3rd ed. Philadelphia: JB Lippincott; 1997:1446-54.
2. **Savage D, Lindenbaum J.** Anemia in alcoholics. Medicine. 1986;65:322-38.
3. **Renwick JH, Asker RL.** The time course of response of erythrocyte volume to ethanol and to its withdrawal. Clin Lab Haematol. 1982;4:325-6.
4. **Cowan DH.** Effect of alcoholism on hemostasis. Semin Hematol. 1980;17:137-47.

Anemia Question 21
Answer: C

Educational Objective: Identify the most likely cause of anemia in patients with renal insufficiency.

The most common cause of anemia in patients with renal insufficiency is erythropoietin deficiency. Because, as in this 43-year-old man, anemia is usually apparent when the glomerular filtration rate (GFR) falls below 30 to 40 mL/min (except in those with polycystic kidney disease), the diagnosis is usually not verified with a serum erythropoietin concentration, which is expensive. Therapy with exogenous erythropoietin is recommended once the hematocrit falls below 30%, but this agent worsens hypertension in at least 30% of patients.

Iron deficiency anemia is less likely in this patient with a mean corpuscular volume of 88 fL, but it should be excluded with a serum iron level and examination of the stool for occult blood before erythropoietin therapy is started to be sure iron stores are adequate to support increased erythropoiesis. Although hemodilution may be present in this patient with extracellular fluid expansion, it does not play a major role in chronic anemia. Decreased erythrocyte survival may occur in patients with uremia, but it does not contribute importantly to anemia except in patients with active hemolysis.

Bibliography

1. **Muirhead N, Bargman J, Burgess E, Jindal KK, Levin A, Nolin L, et al.** Evidence-based recommendations for the clinical use of recombinant human erythropoietin. Am J Kidney Dis. 1995;26(suppl 1):S1-24.

2. **Nissenson AR, Nimer SD, Wolcott DL.** Recombinant human erythropoietin and renal anemia: molecular biology, clinical efficacy, and nervous system effects. Ann Intern Med. 1991;114:402-16.

3. **Eschbach JW.** The anemia of chronic renal failure: pathophysiology and effects of recombinant erythropoietin. Kidney Int. 1989;35:134-48.

Anemia Questions 22-26
Answers: 22(C); 23(A); 24(B); 25(E); 26(D)

EDUCATIONAL OBJECTIVE: Recall distinctive features of the anemia of chronic renal failure and the type of anemia present to determine the cause of chronic renal failure.

Laboratory characteristics of the anemia of chronic renal failure (CRF) include normochromic normocytic indices (as in the 52-year-old woman), normal or high serum iron concentration, normal or slightly low iron-binding capacity, normal or high serum ferritin levels, decreased reticulocyte index, decreased radioactive isotope of chromium, erythrocyte survival, normal platelet count, increased bleeding time, and decreased hemoglobin-oxygen affinity. CRF is mainly caused by a lack of erythropoietin produced by the kidney and is potentially corrected by administering recombinant erythropoietin provided adequate iron stores are available and there is no inflammatory or neoplastic disease, osteitis fibrosa cystica, or aluminum-related bone disease that could diminish the effectiveness of exogenous erythropoietin administration. The prevailing erythropoietin levels, although normal to elevated, are relatively low for the prevailing oxygen tension. The diagnosis of the anemia of chronic renal disease should be made only when the influence of secondary causes (for example, iron and/or folate deficiency) has been appropriately ruled out.

The 45-year-old man has microcytic hypochromic anemia with iron deficiency (due to pulmonary hemorrhage), seen in Goodpasture's syndrome (rapidly progressive necrotizing glomerulonephritis with linear deposit of IgG antibody along glomerular basement membrane associated with fleeting pulmonary infiltrates and/or hemoptysis). Positive hemosiderin-laden macrophages may be seen on stains of pulmonary secretions.

The 64-year-old man has lead nephropathy. This usually manifests with the triad of hypertension, chronic renal failure, and gout ("saturnine" gout). It may lead to iron deficiency anemia due to lead toxicity, which is often seen in patients who use illicit whiskey. Basophilic stippling of erythrocytes on peripheral smear is another feature of this anemia.

In patients with chronic renal failure due to adult polycystic kidney disease, such as the 38-year-old man, the hematocrit level may be normal (or even slightly above normal) owing to increased productions of erythropoietin by the cystic kidneys.

In patients with malignant hypertension, such as the 40-year-old woman, microangiopathic hemolytic anemia occurs in about one third to one half of the patients. Fibrinoid necrosis in the small blood vessels (including the renal vasculature bed) triggers the hemolysis, which manifests as schistocytes (fragmented erythrocytes) on peripheral smear inspection. An element of thrombocytopenia may also occur. Increased lactate dehydrogenase and serum bilirubin levels are other biochemical markers of the syndrome. Control of blood pressure corrects the anemia and reverses the process.

Bibliography

1. **Eschbach JW.** The anemia of chronic renal failure: pathophysiology and the effects of recombination erythropoietin. Kidney Int. 1989;35:134-48.

2. **Eschbach JW, Adamson JW.** Anemia in renal disease. In: Schrier RW, Gottschalk CW, eds. Diseases of the Kidney. 5th ed. Boston, MA: Little, Brown, and Co; 1993:2743-58.

BACK PAIN

Back Pain Question 1
Answer: D

EDUCATIONAL OBJECTIVE: Diagnose and treat acute low back pain.

This patient is presenting with an episode of acute low back pain combined with a history of previous, milder episodes. Back pain is among the most common reasons for physician-office visits and is the most common cause of disability in patients under 45 years of age. The approach to the patient with acute low back pain must take into consideration the fact that 90% of patients with acute low back pain spontaneously recover and return to normal activity within 1 month. In the absence of signs of potentially dangerous underlying conditions (for example, cancer, infection, fracture) special diagnostic studies are not necessary. A careful history and focused physical examination are sufficient to assess patients with pain of less than 4 weeks' duration.

This patient's pain has all the characteristics of acute low back strain without serious disk herniation or neurologic compromise. The pain radiation down his right leg to the knee is a nonspecific finding. The reproduction of his back pain with a straight–leg maneuver does not indicate nerve root compression. A true-positive straight–leg-raise test produces pain below the knee at less than 70 degrees of elevation and generally indicates nerve root compression at L5 or S1. Crossover pain is an even stronger indication of nerve root compression but only if it produces pain below the knee. Walking on toes tests motor function at S1, and walking on heels primarily tests motor function at L4–L5. The ankle jerk tests S1 and knee jerk tests L4 primarily. His physical examination findings, which do not indicate nerve root compromise, his benign pattern of pain that is relieved by lying down, and the absence of constitutional symptoms are all consistent with acute strain.

The best course of action is to provide the patient with sufficient education so that he understands the basic pathophysiology of his acute low back pain and advise him to increase activity as tolerated so long as his pain gradually subsides. He should be advised that the natural history of this disorder is that, without activity modification, he can expect future episodes to occur.

Low-impact aerobics, abdominal strengthening exercises, and proper lifting techniques are all helpful in preventing future episodes. There is no known value to further bed rest after the first 2 to 3 days. Diagnostic studies (magnetic resonance imaging or radiography of the lumbosacral spine) are only indicated if signs of neurologic compromise are present or if the pain fails to resolve within 4 weeks. A lumbosacral spine radiograph would likely show evidence of degenerative disc disease, but this radiographic finding would have no bearing on his initial management. Imaging should be considered only if he fails to respond to conservative management. Surgical consultation would obviously be premature at this time.

Bibliography

1. Agency for Health Care Policy and Research. Clinical Practice Guideline. Acute Low Back Problems in Adults: Assessment and Treatment. U. S. Department of Health and Human Services. 1994; AHCPR Publication No. 95-0643:1-26.
2. **Malkmivaara A, Hakkinen U, Aro T, Heinrichs ML, Koskenniemi L, Kuosma E, et al.** The treatment of acute low back pain—bed rest, exercises, or ordinary activity? N Engl J Med. 1995;332:351-5.

Back Pain Question 2
Answer: D

EDUCATIONAL OBJECTIVE: Recognize acute spinal fracture in a patient with long-standing ankylosing spondylitis.

Spinal fracture, particularly involving an ankylosed lower cervical spine, is an uncommon but very dangerous complication of long-standing ankylosing spondylitis. Minor trauma is the most common precipitating event generally following falls or motor vehicle accidents. On occasion, fractures occur with no history of trauma.

This patient's paresthesias suggest an unstable spine and the need for urgent evaluation. Severe neurologic sequelae, including quadriplegia, are common, so suspicion of a possible fracture should be treated with neck and spinal immobilization until definitive tests have ruled out a fracture. Radiographic evaluation may be difficult because of osteopenia, so the absence of a fracture or displacement on cervical spine radiography cannot be considered sufficient to rule out fracture. Bone scanning, tomography, computed tomography, and magnetic resonance imaging may be necessary. If a fracture is shown and there are no neurologic deficits present, the patient may be treated conservatively with immobilization. Healing may be delayed up to 3 months.

Apical pulmonary fibrosis and myxomatous degeneration of the aortic root are both associated with long-standing ankylosing spondylitis. The history does not suggest acute aortic insufficiency, which cannot explain the paresthesias and neck pain. Aortic dissection should always be considered in a patient with hypertension and acute back pain. The intact pulses and paresthesias in the arms do not support this diagnosis. Pneumothorax can occur as a complication of bullous emphysema, but the physical findings, particularly the paresthesias, cannot be explained by intrathoracic pathology alone. The patient clearly has back muscle spasm, but it would be wrong to attribute his symptoms to muscle strain alone.

Bibliography

1. **Murray GC, Persellin RH.** Cervical fracture complicating ankylosing spondylitis: a report of eight cases and review of the literature. Am J Med. 1981;70:1033-41.

2. **Hunter T, Dubo HI.** Spinal fracture complicating ankylosing spondylitis. A long-term follow-up study. Arthritis Rheum. 1983;26:751-9.

Back Pain Question 3
Answer: B

EDUCATIONAL OBJECTIVE: Recognize the clinical manifestations of malignancy of the spine.

Most low back pain is caused by structural spine or disc disease. It is aggravated by use and relieved significantly when the spine is unloaded. A change in the pattern of back pain, especially in an older person such as this 75-year-old man, is a red flag and should be worked up thoroughly. The normal laboratory studies and relatively low erythrocyte sedimentation rate do not suggest a paraproteinemia-associated pain; a plain radiograph is the best screening test for this problem.

Metastatic deposits in the epidural space or in the spine itself can be seen on plain radiographs if the malignancy is osteolytic, such as in prostate, breast, thyroid, and kidney cancer. However, a plain radiograph does not exclude metastases, and a bone scan

or magnetic resonance imaging would be needed. Metabolic bone disease, such as osteoporosis, has a structural pain pattern: pain in the upright position; pain relieved in the supine position. A compression fracture or a herniated disc would have rapid onset and be relieved by unloading the spine. Lumbar spinal stenosis causes back, buttock, and leg pain that is usually bilateral and aggravated by spine extension and walking and relieved by spine flexion or sitting.

Back Pain Question 4
Answer: B

EDUCATIONAL OBJECTIVE: Recognize the clinical manifestations of lumbar spinal stenosis.

This 79-year-old man has a history typical of lumbar spinal stenosis, which has been called pseudoclaudication. The claudication pattern of peripheral vascular disease may be distinguished from spinal stenosis in that symptom relief in peripheral vascular disease comes promptly after the patient stops walking, and the pulses are diminished. In patients with spinal stenosis, the resolution of symptoms takes several minutes. Degenerative lumbar spinal stenosis arises from compression of the exiting nerve roots from elements of the spine that include the disc, osteophytes, and hypertrophy of the ligaments. Pseudoclaudication is at one end of a spectrum of manifestations that can include myelopathy with bowel and bladder involvement. Rarely, paraspinal tumor deposits or infection may cause the syndrome.

The physical findings most useful in the diagnosis are a wide-based gait, abnormal results on Romberg's test, thigh pain after 30 seconds of lumbar extension, and neuromuscular deficits, but patients may have few or no physical findings. The keys to diagnosis are a history suggestive of the disease and confirmatory magnetic resonance imaging. Myeloma would be unlikely with the low erythrocyte sedimentation rate; the plain radiograph shows normal bone.

Bibliography

1. **Katz JN, Dalgas M, Stucki G, Katz NP, Bayley J, Fossel AH, et al.** Degenerative lumbar spinal stenosis. Diagnostic value the history and physical examination. Arthritis Rheum. 1995;38:1236-41.

CANCER

Cancer Question 1
Answer: E

EDUCATIONAL OBJECTIVE: Identify risk factors for melanoma.

Constitutional risk factors for malignant melanoma include light skin and hair color as well as a propensity to burn rather than tan with sun exposure. The incidence of melanoma has been increasing 4% to 6% per year. This is thought to be related to increased sun exposure. Suspicious lesions should not be observed.

Our main defense against the rapid increase in the incidence of melanoma is removing suspicious lesions. Survival in patients with melanoma is directly related to the thickness of individual lesions. Although surgery for melanoma is best with lesions less than 0.75 mm in thickness, lesions in the area of 0.75 to 1.5 mm in thickness are frequently totally cured by surgical excision. Although melanomas may enlarge rapidly, this is not something that is noted on a regular basis. Asymmetry, irregular Borders, Color variation, and Diameters greater than 6 mm (ABCD criteria) are the hallmarks of melanoma.

Bibliography
1. **Johnson TM, Smith JW 2d, Nelson BR, Chang A.** Current therapy for cutaneous melanoma. J Am Acad Dermatol. 1995;32:689-707.

Cancer Question 2
Answer: B

EDUCATIONAL OBJECTIVE: Identify the most important prognostic indicator of survival for patients with malignant melanoma.

Malignant melanoma is currently the eighth most common cancer in the United States. Its frequency is increasing rapidly, although the case fatality rate has declined. It is believed that early diagnosis is primarily responsible for this improved survival rate. Currently, survival in patients with melanoma is routinely predicted almost exclusively on the basis of tumor thickness. Patients who have melanomas with greater than 1.5 mm of invasion have significantly decreased survival.

In one study, 488 patients were followed prospectively for a median of 13.5 years, and four variables were found to be independent predictors of survival. Tumor thickness is still associated with the most predictive strength (odds ratio, 50.8). Survival is improved in women compared with men (odds ratio, 2.0), in patients less than 60 years of age compared with those older than 60 years of age (odds ratio, 3.0), and in extremity melanomas compared with truncal melanomas (odds ratio, 4.4).

Bibliography
1. **Schuchter L, Schultz DJ, Synnestvedt M, Trock BJ, Guerry D, Elder DE, et al.** A prognostic model for predicting 10-year survival in patients with primary melanoma. The Pigmented Lesion Group. Ann Intern Med. 1996;125:369-75.

Cancer Question 3
Answer: B

EDUCATIONAL OBJECTIVE: Recognize appropriate surveillance for the breast cancer survivor.

Breast cancer survivors are at risk for metastatic disease, recurrent disease within the conserved breast, or a new breast primary tumor. Potentially curative therapy exists for recurrent disease within the conserved breast or a new breast primary tumor. Therefore, breast self-examination, regular breast examination by a health care provider, and annual mammography are recommended for women with a history of early-stage breast cancer.

In contrast, therapy for metastatic breast cancer is largely palliative. Two large randomized trials have failed to show a survival advantage for routine laboratory screening in the follow-up of women with early-stage breast cancer. In both studies, the majority of distant recurrences were detected by the patient between office visits, even in patients who underwent blood studies as often as every 3 months. Therefore, laboratory testing is warranted only for evaluation of new symptoms or abnormalities on physical examination. The tumor markers, carcinoembryonic antigen and CA-2729, are frequently used to monitor efficacy of therapy for metastatic breast cancer, but routine measurement of these markers in survivors of early-stage breast cancer has not been shown to improve outcome.

Bibliography

1. American Society of Clinical Oncology. Recommended breast cancer surveillance guidelines. J Clin Oncol. 1997;15:2149-56.

2. American Society of Clinical Oncology. Clinical practice guidelines for the use of tumor markers in breast and colorectal cancer. J Clin Oncol. 1996;14:2834-77.

3. **Del Turco MR, Palli D, Cariddi A, Ciatto S, Pacini P, Distante V et al.** Intensive diagnostic follow-up after treatment of primary breast cancer. A randomized trial. National Research Council Project on Breast Cancer Follow-up. JAMA. 1994;271:1593-7.

4. The GIVIO Investigators. Impact of follow-up testing on survival and health-related quality of life in breast cancer patients. A multicenter randomized controlled trial. JAMA. 1994;271:1587-92.

Cancer Question 4
Answer: B

EDUCATIONAL OBJECTIVE: Recognize the hereditary nonpolyposis colon cancer syndrome.

This young adult man has a family history of colon cancer at a young age in his mother and brother, and an aunt had ovarian cancer. This pedigree is highly suggestive of the familial genetic syndrome known as hereditary nonpolyposis colon cancer (HNPCC). Families with HNPCC often include persons with multiple primary cancers, which in women include endometrial or ovarian cancer in addition to colorectal tumors. The median age at which adenocarcinomas of the large bowel appear is less than 50 years, and these neoplasms occur with an unusually high frequency in the proximal large bowel.

HNPCC has been associated with germline mutations of several genes, particularly in chromosomes 2 and 3, with these mutations leading to errors in DNA replication, resulting in DNA instability and abnormal cell growth and tumor development. It has been recommended that members of such families undergo biennial colonoscopy beginning at 25 years of age, and such an examination would be indicated at this time for this 30-year-old man with such a strong family history. The HNPCC syndrome has not been associated with breast cancer.

HNPCC should be distinguished from familial adenomatous polyposis (also known as polyposis coli), which is an autosomal dominant disorder characterized by the appearance of thousands of adenomatous polyps, each typically smaller than 1 cm in diameter, throughout the entire large bowel. This familial condition is associated with a deletion in chromosome 5, which apparently leads to an abnormal proliferative pattern in the colonic mucosa. Patients with polyposis coli are born with normal-appearing colonic mucosa, but polyps develop during the second and third decades of life. If surgical treatment is not performed, colorectal cancer is almost certain to develop before 40 years of age. Consequently, prophylactic colectomy has been advocated to prevent malignant transformation.

Bibliography

1. **Lynch HT, Smyrk T.** Hereditary nonpolyposis colorectal cancer (Lynch syndrome). An updated review. Cancer. 1996;78:1149-67.

2. **Rustgi AK.** Hereditary gastrointestinal polyposis and nonpolyposis syndromes. N Engl J Med. 1994;331:1694-702.

Cancer Question 5
Answer: B

EDUCATIONAL OBJECTIVE: Recognize current concepts of diagnosis and management of early-stage prostate cancer.

Screening for prostate cancer is controversial, and the level of information based on opinion outweighs that based on evidence. The normal range for prostate-specific antigen (PSA) rises with age above 60 years, and this is important to avoid the reporting of a falsely "elevated" PSA that leads inappropriately to further investigation. To date, randomized clinical trials have not been completed to resolve the question regarding the role of population screening for prostate cancer. There is, therefore, no firm evidence to confirm the useful role of PSA screening in saving lives, as compared with data that support the role of screening for breast or cervix cancer.

Large surveys have shown that neither transrectal ultrasonography nor digital rectal examination is sufficiently sensitive or specific for use as population screens; some studies have suggested that the combination of digital rectal examination, transrectal ultrasonography, and PSA measurement will identify early-stage prostate cancer more effectively than the use of each technique alone. However, such screening has not been proven to save lives in large community-based trials. There have been no well-conducted randomized clinical trials that compare surgery and radiotherapy for early-stage prostate cancer in otherwise healthy patients. In equivalently staged cases in comparable clinical populations, there is no evidence of a major difference in survival at 5 or 10 years for men with early-stage prostate cancer treated by radical radiotherapy or radical prostatectomy.

Bibliography

1. **Coley CM, Barry MJ, Fleming C, Mulley AG.** Early detection of prostate cancer. Part I: Prior probability and effectiveness of tests. Ann Intern Med. 1997;126:394-406, Part II: Estimating the risks, benefits, and costs. Ann Intern Med. 1997;126:468-79.

2. **Morgan TO, Jacobsen SJ, McCarthy WF, Jacobson DJ, McLeod DG, Moul JW.** Age-specific reference ranges for serum prostate-specific antigen in black men. N Engl J Med. 1996;335:304-10.

3. **Fowler FW Jr, Barry MJ, Lu-Yao G, Wasson JH, Bin L.** Outcomes of external beam radiation therapy for prostate cancer: a study of Medicare beneficiaries in three surveillance, epidemiology and end results areas. J Clin Oncol. 1996;14:2258-65.

Cancer Question 6
Answer: C

EDUCATIONAL OBJECTIVE: Recognize the presentation and management of the superior vena cava syndrome.

The superior vena cava syndrome is usually not regarded as a medical emergency, and it is now viewed as more important initially to establish a tissue diagnosis, rather than to begin urgent treatment. This patient, with a significant history of cigarette smoking and ischemic heart disease, is at risk for lung cancer. The central location of the tumor, with dominant mediastinal lymphadenopathy and possible superior vena cava obstruction, is consistent with a diagnosis of small cell anaplastic lung cancer. However, it is also possible that this is a non–small cell lung cancer or even a lymphoma, malignant germ cell tumor, or malignant thymoma. A tissue diagnosis is required before beginning treatment.

Bronchoscopy has a high yield, and is usually safe in a patient with superior vena cava obstruction, in contrast to mediastinoscopy, which may be associated with excessive hemorrhage due to the obstructed venous return. Urgent initiation of radiotherapy is not necessary and may interfere with obtaining an adequate histologic sample for diagnosis. Similarly, urgent chemotherapy is usually not appropriate; the use of

etoposide and carboplatin would not be optimal chemotherapy for several of these tumors. Although high-dose corticosteroid therapy is often used for patients with superior vena cava obstruction, it is not clear that it offers a clinical benefit, and such therapy may obscure the diagnosis, particularly in a patient with lymphoma.

Bibliography

1. **Johnson DH, Eisert DR.** Treatment of small cell lung cancer. In: Roth JA, Ruckdeschel JC, Weisenburger TH, eds. Thoracic Oncology. 2nd ed. Philadelphia: WB Saunders Co; 1995:201-24.

2. **Carbone DC.** The biology of lung cancer. Semin Oncol. 1997;24:388-401.

Cancer Questions 7-8
Answers: 7(D); 8(C)

EDUCATIONAL OBJECTIVE: Provide appropriate analgesia, and recognize spinal cord compression.

One of the most common errors in pain management is the avoidance of using narcotic analgesics when they are appropriate. The requirement for narcotics may be reduced by the use of coanalgesics, for example, nonsteroidal anti-inflammatory drugs (NSAIDs) reduce production of prostaglandins and inflammation associated with bone metastases. A careful history must be taken to ensure that there are not other complications of progressive malignancy in addition to the problem of pain. In prostate cancer, the use of luteinizing hormone-releasing hormone agonists alone as urgent treatment runs the risk of a transient tumor flare reaction, due to the agonist effect of this agent; it should be used under coverage of a peripheral antagonist, which has been started several days earlier. Urgent radiotherapy is often appropriate for bone pain, but it takes several days to some weeks to have an effect; thus, urgent analgesia should take precedence. The use of a morphine infusion can be helpful for a patient with severe pain, but it can mask many other medical problems and should not be implemented before a careful history and examination; in addition, in the case of bone pain, coanalgesics will reduce the requirement for morphine. The use of sedatives and tranquilizers may be helpful to control pain, but usually they do not provide a substitute for adequate analgesia.

In this case, the symptoms in an elderly patient with prostate cancer and bone metastases may reflect an emerging spinal cord compression. The initiation of physical therapy to strengthen lower limb function before making a diagnosis could cause the patient to become paraplegic. The various choices that are offered would constitute reasonable care once a diagnosis had been achieved and the possibility of spinal cord compression has been excluded. In general, laxatives should be used before constipation has become established as a major problem. In addition, increased use of laxatives and enemas will not be useful in the patient with an emerging spinal cord compression, which is a medical emergency. Unnecessary delay in definitive treatment of spinal cord compression may allow paraparesis to progress to irreversible paraplegia. Either mitoxantrone or strontium may help alleviate the pain from bony metastases, but both modalities take up to 6 to 8 weeks to have such an effect.

Bibliography

1. **Jacox A, Carr DB, Payne R.** New clinical-practice guidelines for the management of pain in patients with cancer. N Engl J Med. 1994;330:651-5.
2. **Levy MH.** Pharmacologic treatment of cancer pain. N Engl J Med. 1996;335:1124-32.

Cancer Question 9
Answer: B

EDUCATIONAL OBJECTIVE: Manage stage IIIA non–small cell lung cancer.

The clinical presentation in this case is most consistent with a stage IIIA non–small cell lung cancer in view of the smoking history and the presence of the spiculated mass and enlarged mediastinal nodes on CT scan. The presence of vocal cord paresis is consistent with involvement of the recurrent laryngeal nerve, which is often associated with stage IIIA non–small cell lung cancer.

Lung cancer is now the most common cause of cancer deaths in women, having eclipsed breast cancer. Mammography is not a specifically appropriate test in this clinical scenario, despite the family history of breast cancer, as there is no clinical evidence of breast cancer; although breast cancer can masquerade as lung cancer, it is usually associated with diffuse endobronchial involvement or with extensive interstitial changes. The clinical history makes this unlikely. Bronchoscopy and mediastinoscopy will allow a tissue diagnosis to be obtained and will facilitate accurate mediastinal staging. CT scans may yield false-positive results, identifying lymph nodes that are enlarged on a reactive basis.

If this is stage IIIA non–small cell lung cancer, randomized trials have shown that the best results are obtained by use of combined modality treatment, incorporating chemotherapy plus radiotherapy or chemotherapy plus surgery. Fine-needle biopsy, although reasonable, will provide less information than bronchoscopy and mediastinoscopy, specifically with respect to the involvement of mediastinal nodes. Upper respiratory infection is a common cause of hemoptysis in a young woman, but it does not explain the persistent hoarseness, vocal cord paresis, and spiculated mass on radiograph. A common error is unnecessary delay in diagnosis due to antibiotic prescribing; in this clinical context, antibiotic therapy would be inappropriate. In the past, with a clinical suspicion of lung cancer in a young patient, thoracotomy and mediastinal node dissection were implemented after basic staging, allowing both diagnosis and treatment to be effected quickly. However, it has now been demonstrated in several randomized trials that combined-modality treatment gives superior results. The role of adjuvant chemotherapy after tumor resection has not yet been proven.

Bibliography

1. **Pritchard RS, Anthony SP.** Chemotherapy plus radiotherapy compared with radiotherapy alone in the treatment of locally advanced, unresectable, non-small-cell lung cancer. A meta-analysis. Ann Intern Med. 1996;125:723-9.
2. **Zang EA, Wynder EL.** Differences in lung cancer between men and women: examination of the evidence. J Natl Cancer Inst. 1996;88:183-92.
3. **Roth JA, Fossella F, Komacki R, Ryan MB, Putnam JB Jr, Lee JS, et al.** A randomized trial comparing perioperative chemotherapy and surgery with surgery alone in resectable stage IIIA non-small-cell lung cancer. 1994;86:673-80.

Cancer Question 10
Answer: B

EDUCATIONAL OBJECTIVE: Recognize that advanced ovarian cancer presenting as malignant ascites is potentially curable.

Most patients with ovarian cancer present with such nonspecific symptoms as abdominal distention or discomfort. Therefore, ovarian cancer is usually diagnosed at more advanced stages, such as stage III, in which disease is confined to the abdominal cavity, or stage IV, in which disease is disseminated beyond the abdomen. Nonetheless, combination chemotherapy with platinum-based and paclitaxel-based chemotherapy and aggressive debulking surgery can result in long-term survival in a significant number of patients with stage III ovarian cancer. In addition intraperitoneal chemotherapy may sometimes be indicated if residual intra-abdominal disease is small. Careful gynecologic evaluation is critical for this patient.

The presence of malignant ascites in patients with breast, colon, or gastric carcinoma would give a diagnosis of advanced stage IV disease. In each case, palliative chemotherapy is available, but the likelihood of long-term control of the disease is quite small.

Bibliography

1. **McGuire WP, Hoskins WJ, Brady MF, Kucera PR, Partridge EE, et al.** Cyclophosphamide and cisplatin compared with paclitaxel and cisplatin in patients with stage III and IV ovarian cancer. N Engl J Med. 1996;334:1-6.

2. **Alberts DS, Liu PY, Hannigan EV, O'Toole R, Williams SD, Young JA, et al.** Intraperitoneal cisplatin plus intravenous cyclophosphamide versus intravenous cisplatin plus intravenous cyclophosphamide for stage III ovarian cancer. N Engl J Med. 1996;335:1950-55.

3. **Van der Burg ME, van Lent M, Buyse M, Kobierska A, Colombo N, Favalli G, et al.** The effect of debulking surgery after induction chemotherapy on the prognosis in advanced epithelial ovarian cancer. Gynecological Cancer Cooperative Group of the European Organization for Research and Treatment of Cancer. N Engl J Med. 1995;332:629-34.

Cancer Question 11
Answer: D

EDUCATIONAL OBJECTIVE: Recognize proper follow-up for a patient surgically treated for Dukes' A colon cancer.

This woman has Dukes' stage A colon cancer. Radiation therapy is not effective in colon cancer and should not be given. The adjuvant therapy trials have not yet shown a benefit for early-stage colon cancer. Therapy with 5-fluorouracil (5-FU) and leucovorin has shown some advantage in advanced or metastatic colon cancer.

Sulindac, a nonsteroidal anti-inflammatory drug, has been shown to reduce polyp size and number, but it is unclear whether this therapy will be useful as a preventive measure for colon cancer or whether it will be beneficial as an adjuvant to surgery for early colon cancer. The best choice is to observe the patient. Most experts would recommend annual colonoscopy, although this is controversial.

Bibliography

1. **Moertel CG.** Surgical adjuvant treatment of colorectal carcinoma in adjuvant therapy. In: Salmon SE, ed. Cancer, Vol VII. Philadelphia: JB Lippincott Co; 1993.

2. **Wolmark N, Rockette H, Fisher B.** Adjuvant therapy for carcinoma of the colon: review of NSABP clinical trials. In: Salmon SE, ed. Cancer, Vol. VII. Philadelphia: JB Lippincott Co; 1993:300-6.

Cancer Question 12
Answer: D

EDUCATIONAL OBJECTIVE: Choose the appropriate diagnostic evaluation for a patient with potentially resectable non–small cell lung cancer.

This patient has squamous cell carcinoma in the right middle lobe bronchus. She is relatively healthy otherwise. Computed tomography (CT) can be useful in the evaluation of patients with lung cancer; however, one must be very cautious in interpreting whether mediastinal lymph nodes are involved with regional spread of carcinoma.

Many nodes smaller than 2 cm in diameter are hyperplastic but contain no malignancy. Nodes larger than 2 cm are more likely to contain metastatic tumor; however, even a small percentage of these are hyperplastic, enlarged, benign nodes. Therefore, the most appropriate action would be to evaluate the mediastinal nodes by mediastinoscopy. Should they be free of obvious metastases, then the patient would be a good candidate for resection for potential cure. If, however, the nodes are positive, it would be very unlikely that surgery would offer any advantage as a single modality of therapy, and other forms of treatment would be indicated. The other options would not provide critical information necessary for her management and would not therefore be the appropriate next approach in this patient.

Bibliography

1. **Line BR, Armstrong MR, Hendick WJ, Killam DA.** Radiographic studies of lung cancer. In: Roth JA, Ruckdeschel JC, Weisenburg TH, eds. Thoracic Oncology. Philadelphia: WB Saunders Company; 1989:108-32.

Cancer Question 13
Answer: D

EDUCATIONAL OBJECTIVE: Recognize Paget's disease of the nipple.

Paget's disease of the nipple is an often-misdiagnosed unusual form of breast cancer presentation, occurring in 1% to 3% of cases. An eczematoid eruption on the nipple is the diagnostic initial biopsy hallmark. In fact, an eczematoid eruption on the nipple should be considered Paget's disease until proven otherwise. A negative mammogram cannot exclude Paget's disease, which is proven by biopsy of a clinically suspicious lesion.

Although a 2-week trial of topical therapy was described, an immediate referral for mammography and biopsy would have been appropriate. The external lesion is a manifestation of intraductal malignancy involving ducts near the nipple. There may or may not be an accompanying mass, and there may or may not be an invasive component.

Bibliography
1. **Osteen RT.** Paget disease of the nipple. In: Harris JR, Hellman S, Henderson IC, Kinne DW, eds. Breast Disease. 2nd ed. Philadelphia: JB Lippincott Co; 1991:797-803.

Cancer Question 14
Answer: D

EDUCATIONAL OBJECTIVE: Recognize that screening for malignancy in ulcerative colitis should be performed only when the disease is quiescent.

Microscopic evaluation for early dysplasia in ulcerative colitis is difficult to interpret. Inflammation may alter the interpretation so that patients with otherwise benign colonic mucosa may have biopsies that suggest severe dysplasia and may lead to a colectomy when it would not have been otherwise indicated.

Surveillance should not therefore be undertaken during periods of colitis activity. Patients due for screening who have active colitis should have their colitis treated and should not be screened until the colitis is in remission.

Bibliography
1. **Bernstein CN, Weinstein WM, Levine DS, Shanahan F.** Physicians' perceptions of dysplasia and approaches to surveillance colonoscopy in ulcerative colitis. Am J Gastroenterol. 1995;90:2106-14.

2. **Lashner BA, Hanauer SB, Silverstein MD.** Optimal timing of colonoscopy to screen for cancer in ulcerative colitis. Ann Intern Med. 1988;108:274-8.

Cancer Questions 15-18
Answers: 15(C); 16(A); 17(D); 18(B)

EDUCATIONAL OBJECTIVE: Distinguish appropriate local therapy options for women with various forms of early-stage breast cancer.

Women who have received radiotherapy during adolescence (for example, for treatment of Hodgkin's disease or in the past for treatment of thymic enlargement or acne) are at higher risk for breast cancer. High-dose radiotherapy such as that required for treatment of Hodgkin's disease precludes later breast-conservation therapy because the dose of radiation recommended for breast-conserving therapy superimposed on that administered during mantle radiotherapy exceeds the tolerance of normal tissue. Thus, the 39-year-old woman would require modified radical mastectomy. She could undergo immediate or delayed reconstruction if she wished.

A fibroadenoma is a benign finding that requires no further intervention. Lobular carcinoma in situ is often an incidental finding, as in the 42-year-old woman. Women with this lesion have about a 1% per year chance of developing invasive breast cancer in either breast. Thus, most women are followed conservatively with regular physical examination and annual mammography. Women who are extremely anxious or who have such major risk factors for breast cancer as a strong family history may opt for bilateral simple mastectomies. This surgery removes the breast including the nipple; removal of axillary lymph nodes is not warranted. Women considering such surgery should be counseled that it is not completely protective against breast cancer.

Women with small mammographically detected invasive breast cancers, such as the 65-year-old woman, are excellent candidates for breast-conserving therapy. Such therapy should include excision to negative margins, axillary dissection to guide selection of adjuvant chemotherapy, and breast radiotherapy. Numerous randomized clinical trials have documented that survival is identical to that seen with modified radical mastectomy. Breast conservation generally is preferred by patients given that option.

Increased use of screening mammography has led to more frequent diagnosis of ductal carcinoma in situ, as in the 47-year-old woman. Such lesions should be excised with negative pathologic margins. A randomized trial has shown that the addition of radiotherapy decreases recurrence rate within the breast by about one half compared with excision alone. There is no role for axillary node dissection, as the incidence of lymph node metastasis is 2% to 3%. Simple mastectomy is indicated for patients who have diffuse disease.

Bibliography

1. National Institutes of Health Consensus Development Panel. Consensus statement: treatment of early-stage breast cancer. Monogr Natl Cancer Inst. 1992;11:1-5.

2. **Fisher B, Costantino J, Redmond CK, Fisher ER, Margolese R, Dimitrov N, et al.** Lumpectomy compared with lumpectomy and radiation therapy for treatment of intraductal breast cancer. N Engl J Med. 1993:328:1581-6.

3. **Fonseca R, Hartmann LC, Petersen IA, Donahue JH, Crotty TB, Gisvold JJ.** Ductal carcinoma in situ of the breast. Ann Intern Med. 1997;127:1013-22.

Cancer Questions 19-22
Answers: 19(C); 20(D); 21(E); 22(B)

EDUCATIONAL OBJECTIVE: Distinguish the risk factors associated with various gastrointestinal tract malignancies.

An increasingly common form of gastric lymphoma known as a mucosa-associated lymphoid tissue (MALT) tumor has been shown to arise following chronic infection with *Helicobacter pylori*. MALT tumors are low-grade, clonal B-cell malignancies that often remain restricted to the mucosa but may occasionally become invasive and life-threatening. Several reports have shown that eradication of *Helicobacter pylori* has resulted in regression and even disappearance of the MALT tumor.

Squamous cell carcinomas of the anus have been linked etiologically to the same forms of human papillomavirus that have been associated with the development of squamous cell carcinomas of the cervix and penis. Human papillomavirus is a causative agent for the genital warts (condylomata acuminata), which are precursors of anal cancer. Additionally, it has been proposed that one explanation for the increased incidence of anal carcinoma in patients with HIV infection is the impaired ability of the immunosuppressed host to eradicate human papillomavirus, thereby leading to a higher likelihood of infection and carcinogenesis.

Hepatocellular carcinoma develops in essentially any condition that leads to cirrhosis. Approximately 60% to 80% of patients in the United States with hepatocellular carcinoma have a cirrhotic liver, and more than 10% of persons with a cirrhotic liver eventually develop hepatocellular carcinoma. The risk appears to be highest in patients whose liver disease is caused by inherited hemochromatosis or by hepatitis B or hepatitis C virus infection. Chronic infection with a hepatitis C virus progresses to cirrhosis in 20% to 30% of cases. Hepatocellular carcinoma has been observed to occur in approximately 10% of patients who develop hepatitis C viral infection after a blood transfusion. It is uncertain whether the risk of developing hepatocellular carcinoma can be reduced by the treatment of hepatitis C virus infection with interferon alfa.

Although little is known about the causes of pancreatic cancer, cigarette smoking represents the most consistently observed risk factor for the disease. The tumor is two to three times more common in heavy smokers than in nonsmokers.

Schistosoma haematobium, endemic in the Middle East, is associated with the development of squamous cell carcinoma of the urinary bladder.

Bibliography

1. **Mayer RJ.** Gastrointestinal cancer. In: Dale DC, Federman DD eds. Scientific American Medicine. New York, Scientific American, 1996: Oncology VIII, 1-22.

Chest Pain

Chest Pain Question 1
Answer: C

EDUCATIONAL OBJECTIVE: Recognize and treat post-infarction unstable angina pectoris.

The recurrence of angina during the early morning hours within the first few weeks following myocardial infarction places the patient at high risk for re-infarction and/or cardiac death. Accordingly, an aggressive treatment approach is warranted. The absence of indicators of myocardial ischemia on his exercise stress test several months ago would imply that his current instability is mediated by a recently disrupted plaque within a single coronary artery. Coronary angiography with a view toward percutaneous transluminal coronary angioplasty, possibly to include adjunctive use of a specific platelet glycoprotein IIB/IIIA receptor antagonist (abciximab), would offer the best chance for prompt stabilization. This strategy is a class I recommendation of the American Heart Association/American College of Cardiology Task Force for the Management of the Post–Myocardial Infarction Patient.

Neither low-level nor symptom-limited exercise stress testing is appropriate in the setting of early postinfarction angina. Ambulatory electrocardiographic monitoring is similarly unnecessary to establish the high-risk nature of the situation. Such monitoring may not provide information regarding prognostic risk beyond that which can be obtained from exercise stress testing in patients without markers of spontaneous ischemia.

Bibliography

1. **Ryan TJ, Antman EM, Brooks NH, Califf RM, Hillis LD, Hiratzka LF, et al.** 1999 update: ACC/AHA guidelines for the management of patients with acute myocardial infarction. A report of the American College of Cardiology/American Heart Association Task Force on Practice Guidelines (Committee on Management of Acute Myocardial Infarction). J Am Coll Cardiol. 1999;34:890-911.

2. **Gill FB, Cairns JA, Roberts RS, Constantini L, Sealey BJ, Fallen EF, et al.** Prognostic importance of myocardial ischemia detected by ambulatory monitoring early after myocardial infarction. N Engl J Med. 1996;334:65-70.

3. The CAPTURE Investigators. Randomized placebo-controlled trial of abciximab before and during coronary intervention in refractory unstable angina: the CAPTURE study. Lancet. 1997;349:1429-35.

Chest Pain Question 2
Answer: C

EDUCATIONAL OBJECTIVE: Assist the patient in developing an informed choice about coronary revascularization.

The rate of restenosis following percutaneous transluminal coronary angioplasty (PTCA) is approximately 40% and not reduced by directional or rotablation atherectomy. During the first year following PTCA, 50% of patients with multivessel disease have an ischemic event or require further revascularization procedures. In randomized trials comparing coronary artery bypass graft (CABG) with PTCA, at 1 year there is comparable angina control and no mortality difference. PTCA patients require repeat procedures and more medication, and CABG patients have a higher rate of myocardial infarction. The Bypass Angioplasty Revascularization Investigation (BARI) trial, a comparison of PTCA and CABG in patients with multivessel coronary artery disease eligible for either procedure, showed a comparable 5-year survival rate (87%) and rate of Q-wave myocardial infarction (20%). In diabetic patients taking insulin or oral hypoglycemic agents, the 5-year survival rate with CABG was approximately 80%, whereas that with PTCA was significantly less at 65%. Because the number of enrollees was small and selected from a much larger cohort, the recommendations for CABG over PTCA in diabetic patients should be tempered.

Coronary stenting has been shown to reduce short-term restenosis to 20% to 25% and has good long-term patency. In long-term studies of stent patients, diabetes is an independent predictor of need for repeat revascularization. Whether stenting with or without intravascular ultrasonography will improve the outcome in diabetic patients to the level of CABG is not yet known.

Bibliography

1. **Elliot JM, Berdan LG, Holmes DR, Isner JM, King SB, Keeler GP, et al.** One year follow-up in the Coronary Angioplasty Versus Excisional Atherectomy Trial (CAVEAT I). Circulation. 1995; 91:2158-66.

2. **Hamm CW, Reimers J, Ischinger T, Rupprecht HJ, Berger J, Bleifield W, et al.** A randomized study of coronary angio-

plasty compared with bypass surgery in patients with symptomatic multi-vessel coronary disease. A German Angioplasty Bypass Surgery Investigation. N Engl J Med. 1994;331:1037-43.

3. Comparison of coronary bypass surgery with angioplasty in patients with multivessel disease. The Bypass Angioplasty Revascularization Investigation (BARI) Investigators. N Engl J Med. 1996;335:217-25.

4. **Laham RJ, Carrozza JP, Berger C, Cohen DJ, Kuntz RE, Bain DS, et al.** Long-term (4- to 6-year) outcome of Palmaz-Schatz stenting: paucity of late clinical stent related problems. J Am Coll Cardiol. 1996;28:820-6.

Chest Pain Question 3
Answer: D

EDUCATIONAL OBJECTIVE: Assess risk and initiate appropriate medical therapy for newly recognized angina pectoris.

The clinical presentation is consistent with new-onset angina, which, although it may fall broadly under the category of unstable angina pectoris, entails a low short-term risk of death or myocardial infarction. Given the high pretest likelihood of coronary artery disease on the basis of the history alone, as well as the clear need for antihypertensive therapy, it would first be most appropriate to institute medical treatment in the form of aspirin and β-blockade before an assessment of its efficacy with symptom-limited exercise stress testing. Given the consistent exertional nature of this man's symptoms at a moderate workload, the presence of untreated hypertension, and the lack of signs suggestive of left ventricular dysfunction, the initial evaluation and management can proceed on an outpatient basis. Admission to a chest pain observation unit is not necessary in the absence of acute symptoms or more compelling electrocardiographic changes.

The presence of left ventricular hypertrophy on the resting electrocardiogram may confound the results of routine stress electrocardiographic testing. In particular, the ST-segment response is nonspecific, and concomitant radionuclide or echocardiographic imaging (as dictated by local expertise and available technology) is warranted. In general, pharmacologic stress testing (with dobutamine, dipyridamole, or adenosine) with either radionuclide or echocardiographic imaging should be reserved for patients who cannot exercise. At the very least, this patient would benefit from a simulation of the conditions present during his individual exercise stress test sessions.

Coronary angiography is the recommended first step in the evaluation of patients with new-onset angina

when high-risk indicators (such as recent myocardial infarction or congestive heart failure) are present.

Exercise stress testing to further stratify risk in this patient can be done as soon as his medical program is optimized. The impact of medical therapy on his exercise test parameters must be taken into consideration when assessing the results of such testing. One would expect, for example, a blunted heart rate response as a result of β-blockade. Even in more unstable patients, exercise testing can be done safely after 2 to 3 days of optimal medical management. Exercise test indicators of high risk include provocation of ischemia at a low workload (less than 6 metabolic equivalents [METs]), exercise-induced ventricular tachycardia, exercise-induced decrease in systolic blood pressure, and 2-mm ST-segment depressions in multiple electrocardiographic leads that persist through several minutes of recovery. Patients with these indicators should be referred for coronary angiography. A low-risk test would be characterized by the ability to achieve a higher workload (for example, stage 3 or 4 of the Bruce protocol) with mild or no angina (or its equivalent) and less than 2-mm ST-segment depression. Such patients can be continued on medical therapy and reassessed at periodic intervals. An exercise prescription can be provided on the basis of the test results.

The assessment of risk using treadmill exercise testing in patients with unstable angina pectoris who have received optimal medical therapy has thus far relied heavily on the extrapolation of observations made in large populations of patients with stable coronary artery disease. Because the pathophysiology of unstable angina differs in some respects from that of stable angina pectoris, these extrapolations may inherently underestimate risk in the former group of patients.

Bibliography

1. **Braunwald E, Jones RH, Mark DB, Brown J, Brown L, Cheitlin MD, et al.** Diagnosing and managing unstable angina. Agency for Health Care Policy and Research. Circulation. 1994;90:613-22.

2. **Mark DB, Shaw L, Harrell FE Jr, Hlatky MA, Lee KL, Bengtson JR, et al.** Prognostic value of a treadmill exercise score in outpatients with suspected coronary artery disease. N Engl J Med. 1991;325:849-53.

3. **Moss AJ, Goldstein RE, Hall WJ, Bigger JT Jr, Fleiss JL, Greenberg H, et al.** Detection and significance of myocardial ischemia in stable patients after recovery from an acute coronary event. Multicenter Myocardial Ischemia Research Group. JAMA. 1993;269:2379-85.

4. **Nyman I, Larsson H, Areskog NH, Wallentin L.** The predictive value of silent ischemia at an exercise test before discharge after an episode of unstable coronary artery disease. RISC Study Group. Am Heart J. 1992;123:324-31.

Chest Pain Question 4
Answer: D

EDUCATIONAL OBJECTIVE: Recognize the role of atrioventricular sequential pacing in the treatment of medically refractory hypertrophic disease.

The vast majority of patients with documented hypertrophic cardiomyopathy have mild to moderate symptoms that can be managed with medical therapy, which may include high doses of β-adrenergic antagonists, calcium channel blockers, and negative inotropic agents such as disopyramide. Optimal medical therapy may include one or more of these drugs alone or in combination. Dyspnea and exertional chest pain are the most common symptoms of hypertrophic disease. Angina due to subendocardial myocardial ischemia typically occurs despite the presence of normal coronary arteries. Relief of left ventricular outflow obstruction may not only improve anginal symptoms but also result in resolution of reversible myocardial perfusion abnormalities that are frequently evident on thallium-201 imaging. Dyspnea is multifactorial in origin and may result from dynamic outflow tract obstruction, variable degrees of mitral regurgitation, and marked diastolic dysfunction. This patient has advanced hypertrophic disease, as evidenced by his young age at diagnosis, the extent of septal and free wall hypertrophy, the presence of biventricular involvement, and a marked resting and provokable left ventricular outflow tract gradient.

The most appropriate treatment option for this patient is dual-chamber atrioventricular sequential (DDD) pacing, which has been reported to decrease left ventricular outflow gradient by at least 50% and to produce substantial symptomatic and functional benefits. Right ventricular pacing alters the sequence of left ventricular activation and may result in paradoxical septal motion. This effect appears to widen the outflow tract itself and decrease the extent of systolic anterior motion of the mitral valve. Dual-chamber pacing has been shown to be more effective than ventricular pacing alone. When used, the atrioventricular conduction interval must be kept shorter than the normal physiologic delay to ensure ventricular capture at all times, particularly during exercise. Programmed atrioventricular intervals typically have been between 50 and 100 msec but must be individualized to ensure maximum hemodynamic benefit. To date, there have been no studies directly comparing DDD pacing to septal myotomy-myectomy. Based upon its low risk and morbidity, many centers are now recommending DDD pacing for medical treatment failure before consideration of septal myectomy. Long-term outcomes following DDD pacing require careful evaluation.

Additional medical therapy is unlikely to improve this patient's limiting symptoms sufficiently to permit him to return to work. He is unlikely to respond to low-dose β-blockers, and he has previously been unable to tolerate high-dose therapy due to intolerable side effects. Amiodarone has not been shown to improve symptoms and its ability to lower the risk of sudden cardiac death remains unproved.

Surgical septal myotomy-myectomy (the Morrow procedure) is a reasonable treatment option and had been the treatment of choice for more than 25 years for patients with medically refractory symptoms and documented left ventricular outflow obstruction. Myectomy thins the ventricular septum and widens the outflow tract, thereby abolishing systolic anterior motion of the mitral valve; this not only relieves left ventricular outflow obstruction but also decreases the amount of mitral regurgitation. The surgical mortality rate is below 5% at most centers, and the 10-year survival rate exceeds 85%; peak outflow gradient under basal conditions is relieved or abolished in approximately 95% of patients. Approximately 70% of patients have marked objective improvement in symptoms and functional capacity shown by treadmill testing. Most patients continue to receive medical therapy following surgery but at substantially reduced doses. Anecdotal reports suggest that myotomy-myectomy may also lower the risk of sudden cardiac death in patients with marked outflow tract obstruction. Neither pacing nor septal myectomy is effective in relieving symptoms of patients with marked ventricular hypertrophy who lack evidence for resting or provokable outflow tract obstruction.

Bibliography

1. **Wigle ED, Rakowski H, Kimball BP, Williams WG.** Hypertrophic cardiomyopathy. Clinical spectrum and treatment. Circulation. 1995;92:1680-92.

2. **Maron BJ.** Hypertrophic cardiomyopathy. Curr Probl Cardiol. 1993;1:639-704.

3. **Cannon RO 3rd, Dilsizian V, O'Gara PT, Udelson JE, Tucker E, Panza JA, et al.** Impact of surgical relief of outflow obstruction on thallium perfusion abnormalities in hypertrophic cardiomyopathy. Circulation. 1992; 85:1039-45.

4. **Cohn LH, Trehan H, Collins JJ Jr.** Long-term follow-up of patients undergoing myotomy-myectomy for obstructive hypertrophic cardiomyopathy. Am J Cardiol. 1992; 70:657-60.

5. **Cannon RO 3rd, Tripodi D, Dilsizian V, Panza JA, Fananapazir L.** Results of permanent dual-chamber pacing in symptomatic nonobstructive hypertrophic cardiomyopathy. Am J Cardiol. 1994;73:571-6.

Chest Pain Question 5
Answer: C

EDUCATIONAL OBJECTIVE: Recognize the importance of pericardial findings in patients with connective tissue abnormalities.

This young woman has evidence of acute pericarditis and several features (body habitus, straight back, and pectus excavatum) that suggest an underlying connective tissue abnormality. The history of forceful shaking would provide a possible mechanism for rapid deceleration injury similar to that experienced by patients who have been in motor vehicle accidents.

The aorta is most commonly injured near the area of its fixation to the posterior chest wall in the region of the ligamentum arteriosum or near its annular attachment to the base of the left ventricle. Patients with weakening of the aortic media from cystic medial necrosis are particularly prone to transsection or dissection of the aorta under conditions of such trauma. Pericardial findings always imply some involvement of the ascending aorta, either as the primary site of aortic pathology or as a site of secondary involvement from retrograde extension. The increased dimension of the cardiac silhouette on chest radiograph does not provide distinguishing information because this finding may simply relate to her pectus deformity with straight back. Once the potential connection between pericarditis and an underlying connective tissue abnormality is made, an echocardiogram, with transesophageal imaging if necessary, should be obtained immediately.

One would expect the erythrocyte sedimentation rate to be elevated in this clinical setting, yet its confirmation would not be of diagnostic value. The likelihood of coronary artery disease of any type is low, and the electrocardiographic changes described are classic for pericarditis; a creatine kinase determination would be unnecessary. Likewise, the case history does not suggest systemic lupus erythematosus as a cause of the pericarditis, and an antinuclear antibody titer, which would not be available for 1 to 2 days, would not be useful. The D-dimer test, which has been used as a screening test for pulmonary thromboembolism, is not specific, and an elevated D-dimer has been associated with recent surgery, myocardial infarction, sepsis, or other systemic illness.

In this patient, transesophageal echocardiography study confirmed the presence of a type A dissection, and the entry point was determined to be at the level of the ligamentum arteriosum beyond the origin of the left subclavian artery. She underwent prompt resection and replacement of the ascending aorta and returned for additional surgery on the descending thoracic aorta 3 months later.

Bibliography

1. **Saner HE, Gobel FL, Nicoloff DM, Edwards JE.** Aortic dissection presenting as pericarditis. Chest. 1987;91:71-4.
2. **Goldhaber SZ, Simons GR, Elliott CG, Haire WD, Toltzis R, Blacklow SC, et al.** Quantitative plasma D-dimer levels among patients undergoing pulmonary angiography for suspected pulmonary embolism. JAMA. 1993;270:2819-22.
3. **Hirsch DR, Lee TH, Morrison RB, Carlson W, Goldhaber SZ.** Shortened hospitalization by means of adjusted-dose subcutaneous heparin for deep venous thrombosis. Am Heart J. 1996;131:276-80.

Chest Pain Question 6
Answer: B

EDUCATIONAL OBJECTIVE: Manage coronary artery disease with exertional angina in an elderly woman.

This patient has a decrease in anginal threshold over several months. The laboratory evaluation excludes anemia and thyroid disorders for explaining the worsening angina. The approach to managing angina pectoris is more often one of style than outcome-based, but there is a cost-effective strategy. Although there is no evidence that nitrates reduce mortality or event rates in patients with coronary artery disease (CAD) with angina, long-acting nitrates are effective and inexpensive antianginal agents when added to β-blocking agents. There are several nitrate options. The new mononitrates are easily administered and prevent nitrate tolerance. Topical nitrates and isosorbide dinitrate with an 8- to10-hour nitrate-free period are good alternatives. Because the indication is relief of angina, cost and compliance are important variables when choosing a nitrate preparation. The heart rate of 56/min is consistent with effective β-blockade, and no increment is necessary or possible. Calcium channel blocking drugs such as verapamil are complementary to β-blockers but should be used as the third agent after nitrates or in cases of nitrate intolerance. The short-acting calcium channel blockers (particularly nifedipine) have been associated with an increase in mortality when used in patients with hypertension and unstable angina. This should not discourage use of sustained-release nifedipine in conjunction with β-blockers. When β-blockers cannot be used, it may be possible to use diltiazem, verapamil, or amlodipine alone in patients who have angina associated with effort or emotion. Considering the low heart rate in this patient, diltiazem and verapamil should not be added to β-blockade. Substituting diltiazem or verapamil for the β-blocker would sacrifice the benefits of reduction in sudden death reported in both hypertensive patients and patients with CAD following myocardial infarction. The addition of amlodipine to β-blockade rather than nitrates is an expensive alternative with no known outcome advantage. Elderly women with CAD and a low-density lipoprotein cholesterol greater than 125 mg/dL have been shown to benefit from a hydroxymethylglutaryl–coenzyme A (HMG-CoA) reductase inhibitor. Although these drugs may reduce coronary events, improve endothelial function, and reduce silent ischemia, the benefits on reducing symptomatic angina are minimal.

Bibliography

1. **Carbajal EV, Deedwania PC.** Contemporary approaches in medical management of patients with stable coronary artery disease. Med Clin North Am. 1995:79:1063-84.

2. **Mangione N, Glasser SP.** Phenomenon of nitrate tolerance. Am Heart J. 1994:128:137-46.

3. **Kendall MJ, Lynch KP, Hjalmarson A, Kjekshus J.** Betablockers and sudden cardiac death. Ann Intern Med. 1995;123:358-67.

4. **Furberg CD, Psaty BM, Meyer JV.** Nifedipine. Dose-related increase in mortality in patients with coronary heart disease Circulation. 1995;92:1326-31

Chest Pain Question 7
Answer: A

EDUCATIONAL OBJECTIVE: Recognize and treat the syndrome of chest pain with normal coronary arteries.

Angina-like chest pain with no evidence of coronary artery disease on coronary arteriography has been recognized for several years and is known as microvascular angina or syndrome X. Classic coronary risk factors may or may not be present. The pain has many potential mechanisms. The two most commonly considered mechanisms are ischemia due to abnormal endothelial function in the microvasculature and unusual myocardial pain reception (increased nociception). This patient's presentation is classic. The atypical presentation, duration, and fatigue, with a sense of seriousness (and even panic), are commonly described. The work-up usually includes a stress electrocardiogram with imaging (nuclear or echocardiographic), which is often followed by coronary arteriography. The left ventricular end-diastolic pressure is characteristically mildly increased (> 12 to 15 mm Hg).

Estrogen deficiency is associated with reversible impairment of endothelial function, and one report suggested a benefit of estrogen in women with syndrome X. In postmenopausal women with atypical chest pain and a low coronary risk profile, a trial of estrogens may eliminate the need for expensive studies and coronary arteriography. In this patient, vasospastic angina is unlikely based on the exertional component, duration, and inconsistency, and no features are suggestive of dyspepsia or reflux. β-blockade and calcium channel blockers can be tried for syndrome X but are often ineffective; nitroglycerin relief is inconsistent. Refractory patients can be tried on the antidepressant imipramine. Anxiolytics may be used to decrease associated panic attacks but have little impact on the chest pain. There is no role for nonsteroidal anti-inflammatory drugs in syndrome X.

Bibliography

1. **Kaski JC, Elliott PM.** Angina pectoris and normal coronary arteriograms: clinical presentation and hemodynamic characteristics. Am J Cardiol. 1995;76:35D-42D.

2. **Rosano GM, Collins P, Kaski JC, Lindsay DC, Sarrel PM, Poole-Wilson PA.** Syndrome X in women is associated with estrogen deficiency. Eur Heart J. 1995;16:610-4.

3. **Rosano GM, Peters NS, Lefroy D, Lindsay DC, Sarrel PM, Collins P, et al.** 17-beta-Estradiol therapy lessens angina in post-menopausal women with syndrome X. J Am Coll Cardiol. 1996;28:1500-5.

4. **Cannon RO 3rd, Quyyumi AA, Mincemoyer R, Stine AM, Gracely RH, Smith WB, et al.** Imipramine in patients with chest pain despite normal coronary angiograms. N Engl J Med. 1994;330:1411-7.

Chest Pain Question 8
Answer: D

EDUCATIONAL OBJECTIVE: Recognize aortic dissection as an important complication of treated temporal arteritis.

Aortic dissection may be the most serious long-term complication in patients who have had temporal arteritis. The fact that it is so common indicates that the vasculitis in temporal arteritis involves more than the cranial arteries. Presumably these patients develop a vasculitis in the aorta, resulting in weakness that later leads to dissection.

Given the patient's symptoms, the other diagnoses deserve serious consideration, but they are less likely. Myocardial infarction would be expected to show changes on electrocardiogram, as would acute pericarditis. In addition, pericarditis is rarely this acute. Esophageal disease, either rupture or esophagitis, can mimic other syndromes. However, acute esophagitis rarely produces pain of this magnitude. Esophageal rupture usually follows prolonged vomiting or esophageal occlusion by a bone or some other object, and although there is acute pain, it typically begins at a low to moderate intensity and progressively worsens over the next several hours.

Bibliography

1. **Evans JM, O'Fallon WM, Hunder GG.** Increased incidence of aortic aneurysm and dissection in giant cell (temporal) arteritis. A population-based study. Ann Intern Med. 1995;122:502-7.

CONGESTIVE HEART FAILURE

Congestive Heart Failure Question 1
Answer: D

EDUCATIONAL OBJECTIVE: Construct a differential diagnosis for acute left ventricular dysfunction in an HIV-positive patient.

The patient has zidovudine-induced cardiotoxicity. A growing number of antiretroviral agents have been associated with the development of a dilated cardiomyopathy. Onset may occur within a few weeks or many months. Although HIV cardiomyopathy is a possibility in this patient, the presence of cardiac and skeletal muscle involvement suggests an idiosyncratic reaction to zidovudine. Case reports have implicated interferon-α, zidovudine, dideoxycytidine (ddC), and dideoxyinosine (ddI). The importance of recognizing drug-induced left ventricular dysfunction cannot be overemphasized, because it is often totally reversible if the offending agent is withdrawn.

Most patients with chronic HIV infection are serologically positive for both cytomegalovirus and toxoplasmosis. However, direct cardiac involvement with either infectious agent is quite rare unless systemic infection is present. The clear-cut, short-duration atrial fibrillation combined with the modest increase in ventricular response rate make tachycardia-induced cardiomyopathy an unlikely possibility.

Echocardiographic studies have documented dilated cardiomyopathy in 11% to 22% of HIV-infected adults. It is more common in patients with markedly depressed CD4 counts. Ventricular function may fluctuate considerably in asymptomatic or minimally symptomatic patients. Myocarditis is a frequent pathologic finding at autopsy. Some patients with unexplained left ventricular dysfunction may undergo biopsy, and corticosteroids are occasionally administered to those with biopsy-verified myocarditis. Controlled trials have not examined the safety or efficacy of this approach.

Bibliography

1. **Herskowitz A, Willoughby SA, Baughman KL, Schulman SP, Bartlett JD.** Cardiomyopathy associated with antiretroviral therapy in patients with HIV infection: a report of six cases. Ann Inter Med. 1992;116:311-3.

2. **DeCastro S, d'Amati G, Gallo P, Cartoni D, Santopadre P, Vullo V, et al.** Frequency of development of acute global left ventricular dysfunction in human immunodeficiency virus infection. J Am Coll Cardiol. 1994;24:1018-24.

3. **Herskowitz A, Vlahov D, Willoughby S, Chaisson RE, Schulman P, Neumann DA, et al.** Prevalence and incidence of left ventricular dysfunction in patients with human immunodeficiency virus infection. Am J Cardiol. 1993;71:955-8.

4. **Blanchard DG, Hagenhoff C, Chow LC, McCann HA, Dittrich HC.** Reversibility of cardiac abnormalities in human immunodeficiency virus (HIV)-infected individuals: a serial echocardiographic study. J Am Coll Cardiol. 1991;17:1270-6.

5. **Herskowitz A, Wu TC, Willoughby SB, Vlahou D, Ansaria A, Beschorner WE, et al.** Myocarditis and cardiotropic viral infection associated with severe left ventricular dysfunction in late-stage infection with human immunodeficiency virus. J Am Coll Cardiol. 1994;24:1025-32.

Congestive Heart Failure Question 2
Answer: C

EDUCATIONAL OBJECTIVE: Identify critical aortic stenosis as a cause for acute pulmonary edema despite the presence of a soft systolic murmur.

The clinical picture in this patient is most consistent with critical aortic stenosis. Progressive stenotic valvular heart disease should always be considered in the differential diagnosis of acute left-sided heart failure. A bicuspid valve is the most likely etiology, given the long-standing murmur and age of the patient at the time of symptomatic presentation. The degree of stenosis may progress rapidly in mildly symptomatic elderly patients with calcific disease.

Echocardiography is the initial diagnostic study needed to confirm the clinical suspicion of critical aortic stenosis. The presence of a very soft systolic murmur does not exclude the possibility of critical stenosis, because the intensity of the murmur is related not only to the valve area but also to the rapidity of forward blood flow across the valve. Although risky in this critically ill patient, preoperative coronary angiography to exclude the presence of severe epicardial coronary artery disease is desirable. Many centers would proceed directly to surgery based upon echocardiographic confirmation of severe aortic stenosis in younger patients with a lower probability of "silent" coronary artery disease. Despite severely depressed left ventricular function, as judged by the presence of a third heart sound, left ventricular ejection fraction can be expected to return to normal following aortic valve replacement, if coronary artery disease is not a concomitant finding.

The long-standing nature of the heart murmur and the left ventricular hypertrophy on electrocardiography point to a diagnosis of valvular rather than ischemic heart disease. There is no history or electrocardiographic findings to suggest a recent myocardial infarction. The location, intensity, and character of the murmur are not suggestive of acute mitral regurgitation or a ventricular septal defect. Furthermore, the left ventricle on examination lacks the hyperdynamic features that accompany acute volume overload lesions such as mitral regurgitation or a ventricular septal defect.

Bibliography

1. **Beppu S, Suzuki S, Matsuda H, Ohmori F, Nagata S, Miyatake S.** Rapidity of progression of aortic stenosis in patients with congenital bicuspid aortic valves. Am J Cardiol. 1993;71:322-7.

2. **Pellikka PA, Nishimura RA, Bailey KR, Tajik AJ.** The natural history of adults with asymptomatic, hemodynamically significant aortic stenosis. J Am Coll Cardiol. 1990;15:1012-7.

3. **Rediker DE, Boucher CA, Block PC, Akins CA, Buckley MJ, Fifer MA.** Degree of reversibility of left ventricular systolic dysfunction after aortic valve replacement for isolated aortic valve stenosis. Am J Cardiol. 1987;60:112-8.

4. **Shah PM, Graham BM.** Management of aortic stenosis: is cardiac catheterization necessary? Am J Cardiol. 1991;67:1031-2.

Congestive Heart Failure Question 3
Answer: D

EDUCATIONAL OBJECTIVE: Identify high-risk patients with acute coronary syndromes who require an aggressive diagnostic strategy.

Despite the absence of both chest pain and a diagnostic increase in serum cardiac markers, there are several clues in the patient's history and laboratory data to suggest the presence of high-grade and potentially life-threatening coronary artery disease. The assessment of myocardial viability in the presence of this degree of left ventricular dysfunction should be done after delineation of the coronary anatomy. In general, presentation with unstable angina pectoris, or its symptomatic equivalent, and pulmonary edema should prompt early catheterization unless the patient's comorbidities indicate otherwise. The absence of both significant left ventricular dilatation and widespread pathologic Q waves on the electrocardiogram would intuitively suggest that the associated degree of left ventricular dysfunction may indeed be a transient reflection of a recent ischemic insult rather than the expression of a fixed and chronic process.

Repeat echocardiography under conditions of rest would be of little incremental value. The performance of any provocative imaging study, with either echocardiographic or radionuclide techniques, places this marginally compensated patient at high risk for an adverse outcome.

The term *viability* implies that left ventricular function will improve following revascularization. *Hibernation* refers to a state of chronic, low-flow ischemia resulting in myocardial contractile dysfunction. Myocardial stunning, on the other hand, is a more transient phenomenon of postischemic contractile dysfunction despite reflow. It may be more appropriate to re-evaluate left ventricular function weeks, rather than days, after a myocardial infarction.

Several noninvasive techniques have been applied to the study of viability. Thallium perfusion imaging and dobutamine echocardiography appear to be equally sensitive. Positron emission tomography (PET) is perhaps the most sensitive technique, but its use is limited by its high cost.

In this particular patient, the right heart pressures were normal at rest and a coronary angiogram showed high-grade left main and proximal three-vessel coronary artery disease, with distal vessels suitable for surgical revascularization. The ejection fraction was estimated at 40% by echocardiography on postoperative day 4.

Bibliography

1. **Braunwald E, Jones RH, Mark DB, Brown J, Brown L, Cheitlin MD, et al.** Diagnosing and managing unstable angina. Agency for Health Care Policy and Research. Circulation. 1994;90:613-22.

2. **Brown KA.** Prognostic value of cardiac imaging in patients with known or suspected coronary artery disease: comparison of myocardial perfusion imaging, stress echocardiography, and positron emission tomography. Am J Cardiol. 1995;75:35D-41D.

3. **Dilsizian V, Bonow RO.** Current diagnostic techniques of assessing myocardial viability in patients with hibernating and stunned myocardium. Circulation. 1993;87:1-20.

4. **Picano E, Mathias W Jr, Pingitore A, Bigi R, Previtali M.** Safety and tolerability of dobutamine-atropine stress echocardiography: a prospective, multicentre study. Echo Dobutamine International Cooperative Study Group. Lancet. 1994;1190-2.

5. **Yusuf S, Zucker D, Peduzzi P, Fisher LD, Takaro T, Kennedy JW, et al.** Effect of coronary artery bypass graft surgery on survival: overview of 10-year results from randomized trials by the Coronary Artery Bypass Graft Surgery Trialists' Collaboration. Lancet. 1994;344:563-70.

Congestive Heart Failure Question 4
Answer: C

EDUCATIONAL OBJECTIVE: Recognize various forms of radiation-induced pericardial disease.

Various forms of pericardial disease may be caused by radiation therapy. Patients with constrictive pericarditis, such as this 42-year-old man, characteristically present with a progressive and insidious increase in abdominal girth, which is then followed by lower-extremity edema. Although exertional dyspnea and orthopnea are common, paroxysmal nocturnal dyspnea (PND) is not. Indeed, the presence of the latter historical fact may be useful in distinguishing between left heart failure (in which PND is common) and constrictive pericarditis (in which PND is rare). The reason for this distinction is that in patients with constrictive pericarditis, both left and right ventricular filling are usually limited. Thus, the increased right heart filling that leads to PND in patients who have left heart failure does not occur. Patients with constrictive pericarditis characteristically have remarkably high jugular venous pressures. Such patients, like others with similar degrees of jugular venous pressure, frequently do not have external jugular venous distention when examined. The key to recognizing the true venous pressure in such instances is to examine these patients while they are either sitting or standing to observe a pulsation at the level of their earlobes (or higher). Gentle compression over an area of 4 to 5 cm at the base of the neck will virtually eliminate, or significantly reduce, the magnitude of this pulsation, which can then be assumed to be venous in origin. Failure to correctly estimate significant jugular venous distention when it is present in patients who have right heart failure is probably the most frequent oversight in the cardiac examination.

The diastolic sound described in this patient is a pericardial knock. It is distinguished from an opening snap by its later occurrence after the S_2 (that is, opening snaps are usually heard about 0.06 to 0.10 seconds after S_2, whereas pericardial knocks are detected about 0.12 to 0.14 seconds after S_2). An S_3 is usually detected later than 0.16 seconds after S_2 and is lower in pitch than either an opening snap or pericardial knock.

Effusive pericarditis is the most frequent form of pericardial disease caused by radiation therapy. These effusions are most often asymptomatic when discovered during the initial 6 to 12 months after completion of radiation therapy and are usually detected when a routine chest radiograph is obtained and shows cardiomegaly. Not infrequently, however, such asymptomatic pericardial effusions may occur many years after mantle field radiotherapy, at which time they are discovered in a similar fashion. In these instances, the association with previous radiation therapy is a process of exclusion, and often other processes (including relapse of the patient's cancer) are considered before the true cause of the effusion is ascertained. Occasionally, patients with radiation-induced pericardial effusions will complain of exertional dyspnea. Pericardial friction rubs are infrequently detected in such individuals. Echocardiography virtually always confirms the presence of a pericardial effusion and is an appropriate study in these circumstances.

The characteristic presentation of occult constrictive pericarditis is that of unexplained exertional dyspnea and/or chest pain at any time following radiation therapy. Usually there is a period of several years between the completion of radiation therapy and the appearance of this entity. The physical examination is usually unremarkable. However, if the patient is examined in a well-hydrated state, unexplained elevation in mean venous pressure (> 9 cm H_2O) is frequently noted. Neither a pericardial friction rub nor pericardial knock is heard in patients who have occult constrictive pericarditis and in whom edema does not occur. The diagnosis is confirmed by showing a thickened pericardium on either CT scan or MRI; it is confirmed by a right heart catheterization and a fluid challenge of warmed normal saline. Occult constrictive pericarditis is treated conservatively; it seldom progresses to chronic constrictive pericarditis.

Idiopathic dilated cardiomyopathy is not a consideration in this patient because the heart was not dilated on examination. Additionally the absence of a systolic murmur or atrial or ventricular gallop also makes this diagnosis unlikely. Finally, dilated cardiomyopathy is a relatively unusual consequence of radiation therapy.

The exclusion of a restrictive cardiomyopathy is more difficult. The presence of the pericardial knock strongly favors the diagnosis of constrictive pericarditis. However, these two conditions—constrictive pericarditis and restrictive cardiomyopathy—can coexist in patients who have radiation-induced heart disease. When this is the case, the diagnosis of cardiomyopathy can be exceedingly difficult preoperatively. The finding of significant myocardial fibrosis on endomyocardial biopsy can be helpful diagnostically. Ultimately, however, the diagnosis of restrictive cardiomyopathy is made at the time of surgery for what is believed to be constrictive pericarditis. The treatment of restrictive cardiomyopathy is at best difficult, whereas constrictive pericarditis can often be treated with pericardiectomy if the visceral pericardium is uninvolved and/or can be completely resected if it is thickened. However, complete pericardiectomy in these patients can be extremely challenging, and the clinical results are often less than ideal. For this reason, conservative therapy with the aggressive use of diuretics is best; surgery should be reserved for refractory patients and be done by those who have experience with this disease.

Finally, it is uncertain if patients who have radiation-induced cardiac disease are candidates for heart transplantation. Concerns have been raised as to whether their immune status would allow them to receive the immunosuppressive therapy necessary following this surgical procedure as well as whether relapse of their malignancy might occur.

Bibliography

1. **Applefeld MM, Wiernik PH.** Cardiac disease after radiation therapy for Hodgkin's disease: Analysis of 48 patients. Am J Cardiol. 1983;51:1679-81.

2. **Bush CA, Stang JM, Wooley CF, Kilman JW.** Occult Constrictive Pericardial Disease. Circulation. 1977;56:924-30.

Congestive Heart Failure Question 5
Answer: E

EDUCATIONAL OBJECTIVE: Recognize diastolic heart failure.

This patient's clinical presentation is consistent with left-sided heart failure due to abnormal diastolic filling. Treatment of diastolic heart failure is frequently ineffective and is aimed at decreasing ventricular preload without unduly compromising forward cardiac stroke volume. Published consensus guidelines on heart failure management support the judicious use of diuretics and nitrates as the only treatments that have proven efficacy in treating diastolic heart failure. Addition of oral or transdermal nitrates will decrease preload and may improve this patient's congestive symptoms. This approach is preferable to a further increase in diuretics in this patient, who has newly established prerenal azotemia.

Angiotensin-converting enzyme (ACE) inhibitors may be useful over the long-term in promoting regression of hypertensive left ventricular hypertrophy, but these agents do not yield short-term symptomatic improvement. A β-blocker might have been useful for this patient, if significant tachycardia or hypertension had developed during exercise testing. Neither calcium channel antagonists nor β-adrenergic blockers have been shown to provide consistent symptomatic benefit in patients who do not have uncontrolled hypertension, excessive tachycardia, or hypertrophic cardiomyopathy. No treatment has been shown to improve prognosis in diastolic heart failure. Clinical trials that compare treatment modalities are needed in this population.

Hypertension, age, and diabetes mellitus predispose this woman to impairment in diastolic function. Abnormal left ventricular diastolic function in hypertensive patients may result from the effects of myocyte hypertrophy, increased myocardial connective tissue deposition, and alterations in myocardial relaxation. The noncompliant ventricle exhibits a greater sensitivity of left ventricular diastolic pressure to modest changes in left ventricular volume. Diastolic stiffness may also be altered in a dynamic fashion by changes in ventricular relaxation. Relaxation at the myocyte level is an active, energy-dependent process directed at transporting calcium ions from the cytoplasm back into the sarcoplasmic reticulum. Normal aging is associated with increased myocardial collagen deposition and decreased sarcoplasmic reticular function. Both abnormalities increase the susceptibility of the elderly patient to the development of symptomatic diastolic heart failure. The findings are consistent with diastolic dysfunction. Diastolic, rather than systolic, dysfunction may account for 30% to 40% of symptomatic heart failure in patients over 70 years of age. Although ischemic heart disease is often the primary cause or an accompanying feature, this patient's normal exercise technetium-sestamibi study has a high sensitivity for excluding this diagnostic possibility. The absence of right ventricular involvement argues somewhat against hypertrophic or restrictive cardiomyopathy.

Bibliography

1. **Bonow RO, Udelson JE.** Left ventricular diastolic dysfunction as a cause of congestive heart failure. Mechanisms and management. Ann Int Med. 1992;117:502-10.

2. **Kitzman DW, Higginbotham MB, Cobb FR, Sheikh KH, Sullivan MJ.** Exercise intolerance in patients with heart failure and preserved left ventricular systolic function: failure of the Frank-Starling mechanism. J Am Coll Cardiol. 1991;17:1065-72.

3. **Setaro JF, Soufer R, Remetz MS, Perlmutter RA, Zaret BL.** Long-term outcome in patients with congestive heart failure and intact systolic left ventricular performance. Am J Cardiol. 1992; 69:1212-6.

4. **Fleg JL.** Normative aging changes in cardiovascular structure and function. Am J Geriatric Cardiol. 1996;1:7-15.

5. ACC/AHA Task Force Report: guidelines for the evaluation and management of heart failure. J Am Coll Cardiol. 1995; 26:1376-98.

Congestive Heart Failure Question 6
Answer: A

EDUCATIONAL OBJECTIVE: Recognize the proven risks and benefits of long-term β-blocker therapy in patients with chronic heart failure.

Although β-blockers have been used sporadically for the treatment of patients with chronic heart failure for the past two decades, controlled clinical trials evaluating their safety and efficacy have only recently been undertaken. Excessive sympathetic activation is evident in advanced heart failure and may contribute to disease progression through down-regulation of β-receptors, excessive tachycardia, promotion of subendocardial myocardial ischemia, and provocation of ventricular arrhythmias.

The patient's symptoms are likely to improve with metoprolol therapy. This patient shows signs and symptoms of progressive biventricular heart failure despite appropriate medical treatment with digoxin, diuretics, and an angiotensin-converting enzyme (ACE) inhibitor. Further increases in diuretics would be expected to result in worsening renal dysfunction, and the patient's relative hypotension limits the possibility of adding a second smooth muscle vasodilator, such as hydralazine or isosorbide dinitrate, to improve forward cardiac output. The principal role of currently available β-blockers in heart failure management is to provide symptomatic relief. Identification of the patient most likely to achieve long-term benefit from β-blocker therapy is not yet possible based on clinical or hemodynamic indicators. Although patients with significant resting sinus tachycardia were originally felt to be the most likely candidates to achieve benefit, no consistent relationship has been shown in clinical trials between resting heart rate and therapeutic response. Likewise, patients with either idiopathic dilated cardiomyopathy or ischemic cardiomyopathy may improve with β-blocker therapy.

Results of the Metoprolol in Dilated Cardiomyopathy (MDC) Trial have clarified outcomes of long-term metoprolol therapy in patients with idiopathic dilated cardiomyopathy. When initiated at a low dose, metoprolol is well tolerated in over 90% of patients. β-blocker treatment should not generally be instituted during the acute phase of decompensated heart failure, but rather following several weeks of clinical stability. A remarkably small percentage of patients (< 10%) do not tolerate long-term therapy if the dose is slowly up-titrated. Left ventricular ejection fraction and submaximal and maximal exercise performance usually fall during the first month of treatment, but both will improve during long-term therapy. Left ventricular ejection fraction rose by 8% and exercise duration by 15% during the MDC Trial. Despite clinically significant improvements in ejection fraction, exercise duration, and quality of life, no survival benefit has been shown for metoprolol in any controlled trial. The results of the MDC Trial with metoprolol have recently been confirmed for bucindolol in the CIBIS Trial. Carvedilol, a complex third-generation β-blocker that also possesses antioxidant properties, is the only β-blocker that has been convincingly shown to prolong survival in patients with heart failure. Additional studies are under way to determine this drug's long-term safety and efficacy. Carvedilol may soon replace other β-blockers as the agent of choice in heart failure management.

Initiation of a β-blocker in a patient with advanced left ventricular dysfunction is often risky and requires close monitoring by a physician experienced in the use of this treatment for patients with chronic heart failure.

Bibliography

1. **Waagstein F, Bristow MR, Swedberg K, Camerini F, Fowler MB, Silver MA, et al.** Beneficial effects of metoprolol in idiopathic dilated cardiomyopathy. Metoprolol in Dilated Cardiomyopathy (MDC) Trial Study Group. Lancet. 1993;342:1441-6.

2. **Eichhorn EJ, Heesch CM, Risser RC, Marcoux L, Hatfield B.** Predictors of systolic and diastolic improvement in patients with dilated cardiomyopathy treated with metoprolol. J Am Coll Cardiol. 1995;25:154-62.

3. **Kendall MJ, Lynch KP, Hjalmarson A, Kjekhus J.** Beta-blockers and sudden cardiac death. Ann Int Med. 1995;123:358-67.

4. CIBIS Investigators and Committees. A randomized trial of beta-blockade in heart failure. The Cardiac Insufficiency Bisoprolol Study (CIBIS). Circulation. 1994;90:1765-73.

5. **Packer M, Bristow MR, Cohn JN, Colucci WS, Fowler MB, Gilbert EM, et al.** Effect of carvedilol on morbidity and mortality in chronic heart failure. US Carvedilol Heart Failure Study Group. N Engl J Med. 1996;374:1349-55.

Congestive Heart Failure Question 7
Answer: E

EDUCATIONAL OBJECTIVE: Recognize rapid, uncontrolled, supraventricular tachycardia as a reversible form of dilated cardiomyopathy.

Rapid ventricular pacing is a well-established experimental model for producing a progressive dilated cardiomyopathy in animals. Ectopic atrial tachycardia is an infrequently recognized cause of reversible left ventricular dysfunction in infants and children. Sustained supraventricular tachycardia was first described as producing cardiomegaly in adults by Phillips and Levine in 1949; however this entity remains an infrequent but important and overlooked cause for deterioration of left ventricular function. Management involves either termination of the arrhythmia or controlling the ventricular response rate. Although pharmacologic agents that increase AV nodal refractoriness are generally effective, an occasional patient may require atrioventricular nodal ablation and permanent pacer insertion. In a series of patients with uncontrolled atrial fibrillation described by Grogan, all patients were unaware of their tachycardia. Following correction of the accelerated ventricular response rate, the mean left ventricular ejection fraction rose from 25% to 52%; improvement occurred over 1 to 12 months.

Hypertension may result in cardiomyopathy, but it must be severe and sustained for many years. Although alcohol is a common cause of cardiomyopathy, it would be unusual for it to produce a cardiomyopathy after a long period of abstinence. Ischemic heart disease always merits consideration in a middle-aged man, but the negative stress test, absence of anginal symptoms, and global left ventricular hypokinesis on echocardiography decrease the likelihood of this diagnosis. Idiopathic dilated cardiomyopathy is possible but is always a diagnosis of exclusion. Attention should always focus on potentially reversible forms of left ventricular dysfunction such as uncontrolled tachycardia.

Bibliography

1. **Grogan M, Smith HC, Gersh BJ, Wood DL.** Left ventricular dysfunction due to atrial fibrillation in patients initially believed to have idiopathic dilated cardiomyopathy. Am J Cardiol. 1992;69:1570-3.
2. **Tomita M, Spinale FG, Crawford FA, Zile MR.** Changes in left ventricular volume, mass, and function during the development and regression of supraventricular tachycardia-induced cardiomyopathy. Disparity between recovery of systolic versus diastolic function. Circulation. 1991;83:635-44.
3. **Rinaldi CA, Thompson DS.** Tachycardia-induced cardiomyopathy caused by atrial flutter responding to DC conversion. Hosp Med. 1999;60:305-6.

Congestive Heart Failure Question 8
Answer: D

EDUCATIONAL OBJECTIVE: Identify the potential benefits of structured aerobic exercise for patients with chronic heart failure.

Patients with chronic New York Heart Association (NYHA) class II, III, or IV heart failure symptoms have traditionally been advised to rest and avoid regular exercise because of concerns that their underlying cardiac condition would further deteriorate. Various studies have clearly shown that left ventricular ejection fraction is not related to peak exercise performance. Furthermore, exercise training in patients with ischemic heart disease (particularly in the postinfarction setting) has been convincingly shown to improve symptoms, functional capacity, and clinical outcome. In most patients who have had an infarction, limiting physical activity is not only unnecessary but undesirable because it leads to further deconditioning.

The appropriate advice for the patient is that aerobic exercise training is safe and may improve exercise capacity and decrease heart failure symptoms. Exercise training has only recently been studied in patients with heart failure. Six uncontrolled and three randomized, controlled studies have now examined the safety and utility of structured exercise training in this population. Training periods have ranged from as short as 4 weeks to as long as 18 months; all patients have had left ventricular ejection fractions below 40%. These studies indicate that moderate levels of aerobic training (such as bicycling, walking, or jogging) can decrease heart failure symptoms and improve both submaximal and maximal exercise capacity as measured by peak oxygen consumption or a change in treadmill time. Peripheral adaptations, including an increase in peak skeletal muscle blood flow and enhancement of skeletal oxidative metabolism, also occur. There is no evidence to suggest that properly prescribed aerobic exercise increases the risk of sudden cardiac death or accelerates disease progression provided that exercise does not induce high-grade ventricular arrhythmias or produce a substantial degree of myocardial ischemia. A randomized controlled trial of exercise in patients with heart failure (Keteyian, 1996) showed that exercise training improved exercise tolerance, as measured by increases in peak Vo_2, exercise duration, and power output. This improved exercise tolerance was caused in part by an increase in peak heart rate.

Bibliography

1. **McKelvie RS, Teo KK, McCartney N, Humen D, Montague T, Yusuf S.** Effects of exercise training in patients with congestive heart failure: a critical review. J Am Coll Cardiol. 1995;25:789-96.

2. **Coats AJS, Adamopoulos S, Radaelli A, McCance A, Meyer TE, Bernardi L, et al.** Controlled trial of physical training in chronic heart failure. Exercise performance, hemodynamics, ventilation, and autonomic function. Circulation. 1992;85:2119-31.

3. **Sullivan MJ, Higginbotham MB, Cobb FR.** Exercise training in patients with severe left ventricular dysfunction. Hemodynamic and metabolic effects. Circulation. 1988;78:506-15.

4. **Horning B, Maier V, Drexler H.** Physical training improves endothelial function in patients with chronic heart failure. Circulation. 1996;93:210-4.

5. **Hambrecht R, Niebauer J, Fiehn E, Kalberer B, Olfner B, Hauer K, et al.** Physical training in patients with stable chronic heart failure: effects on cardiorespiratory fitness and ultra- structural abnormalities of leg muscles. J Am Coll Cardiol. 1995;25:1239-49.

6. **Keteyian SJ, Levine AB, Brawner CA, Kataoka T, Roger FJ, Schairer JR, et al.** Exercise training in patients with heart failure. A randomized, controlled trial. Ann Intern Med. 1996:124:1051-7.

Congestive Heart Failure Question 9
Answer: B

EDUCATIONAL OBJECTIVE: Recognize acute severe aortic regurgitation.

Based on the presentation, this patient has acute infective endocarditis caused by a virulent organism, probably *Staphylococcus aureus*. Indications for surgery in patients with this disease include relapse of infection following an adequate course of antibiotic therapy; evidence of intra-cardiac infection (for example, heart block, myocardial abscess, heart failure, and rupture of a papillary muscle, chordae tendineae, or valve) despite therapy; and possibly the presence of large vegetations. In this case a mechanical complication—namely, acute severe aortic regurgitation—is the indication to proceed directly to surgery. This complication is suspected on the basis of history and physical examination and may be confirmed by echocardiography. The symptoms are those of heart failure manifested by dyspnea, tachypnea, and a reduced pulse oximetry.

The pathophysiology of acute severe aortic regurgitation is reflux of a significant amount of blood into a nondilated, noncompliant left ventricle. In turn, this causes a significant increase in left ventricular end-diastolic pressure such that the characteristic widened pulse pressure usually expected in chronic aortic regurgitation does not occur. Additionally, the elevated left ventricular end-diastolic pressure is also responsible for premature mitral valve closure, thus leading to an S_1 that is reduced in intensity. Another consequence of the elevated left ventricular end-diastolic pressure and increased heart rate is that the long diastolic murmur expected in severe aortic regurgitation is not noted. Acute severe aortic regurgitation is a true medical emergency and should be dealt with by prompt aortic valve replacement. A preoperative echocardiogram is indicated to confirm the diagnosis of aortic regurgitation, and mitral valve preclosure (consistent with acute severe aortic regurgitation) should be readily identified; but this study must be obtained expeditiously.

Bibliography

1. **Perloff JK.** Acute aortic regurgitation: Recognition and management. J Cardiovasc Med. 1983;8:209.

2. **Benotti JR, Dalen JE.** Aortic valvular regurgitation: Natural history and medical treatment. In: Cohn LH, DiSesa VJ. Aortic Regurgitation: Medical and Surgical Management. New York: Marcel Dekker; 1986:1-54.

3. **Carabello BA, Crawford FA Jr.** Valvular heart disease. N Engl J Med. 1997;337:32-41.

Chronic Obstructive
Pulmonary Disease

Chronic Obstructive Pulmonary Disease
Question 1
Answer: D

EDUCATIONAL OBJECTIVE: Evaluate and manage a patient with severe pulmonary hypertension.

Pulmonary angiography remains the definitive test to diagnose chronic large vessel thromboemboli. Two or more segmental defects on perfusion lung scan suggest large vessel chronic thromboembolic pulmonary hypertension. However, defects on the perfusion lung scan are not specific and may be seen with chronic obstructive pulmonary disease as well as large vessel chronic thromboemboli. In the latter disease, defects on the perfusion lung scan often are not as striking as the abnormalities that are identified on a pulmonary angiogram. Computed tomography with intravenous contrast is not sensitive for this diagnosis, but it may aid in identifying the proximal extent of such thrombi. Computed tomography also may complement pulmonary angiography by analyzing pulmonary arteries distal to angiographic cutoff lesions and by detecting and characterizing pulmonary infarctions.

Although this patient has mild airflow obstruction and hypoxemia, it does not explain his extreme dyspnea, severe pulmonary hypertension, and right ventricular failure. Pulmonary hypertension accompanying chronic airflow obstruction is not usually severe. Therefore, titration of oxygen therapy, while generally appropriate, does not adequately address this patient's problem. It overlooks clues to surgically treatable disease. Similarly, nifedipine to reduce pulmonary artery pressure and aerosolized bronchodilators to relieve airflow obstruction may provide some benefit, but they would not lead to the correct diagnosis and more definitive treatment (thromboendarterectomy).

Bibliography

1. **Moser KM, Auger WR, Fedullo PF, Jamieson SW.** Chronic thromboembolic pulmonary hypertension: clinical picture and surgical treatment. Eur Respir J. 1992;5:334-42.

2. **Moser KM, Auger WR, Fedullo PF.** Chronic major-vessel thromboembolic pulmonary hypertension. Circulation. 1990;81:1735-43.

3. **Rich S, Levitsky S, Brundage BH.** Pulmonary hypertension from chronic thromboembolism. Ann Intern Med. 1988;108:425-34.

4. **Tardivon AA, Musset D, Maitre S, Brenot F, Dartevelle P, Simonneau G, et al.** Role of CT in chronic pulmonary embolism: comparison with angiography. J Comput Assist Tomogr. 1993;17:345-51.

Chronic Obstructive Pulmonary Disease
Question 2
Answer: B

EDUCATIONAL OBJECTIVE: Manage a patient with chronic obstructive pulmonary disease who requires surgery for gallstones.

This patient requires upper abdominal surgery. The risk for postoperative pulmonary complications is substantial, particularly if abnormalities of pulmonary function are present. Although routine preoperative screening of pulmonary function is not necessary for all patients who are scheduled to undergo high-risk procedures, this patient should undergo such testing because her history (> 75 pack-years of cigarette smoking) and her physical examination (decreased intensity of breath sounds) suggest moderate or severe chronic obstructive pulmonary disease. A forced expiratory volume in 1 sec (FEV_1) less than 1 L or an increased $Paco_2$ suggests a high likelihood for postoperative complications, and either finding should lead to preoperative interventions (for example, smoking cessation or bronchodilation) and careful postoperative follow-up in order to manage pulmonary complications.

Laparoscopic cholecystectomy does not clearly reduce the risk for perioperative pulmonary complications; the procedure should not be undertaken without first documenting the presence and severity of chronic airflow obstruction. Preoperative measurements of total lung capacity and single-breath $DLco$ do not predict postoperative pulmonary complications.

Bibliography

1. **Zibrak JD, O'Donnell CR.** Indications for preoperative pulmonary function testing. Clin Chest Med. 1993;14:227-36.

2. **American Thoracic Society.** Standards for the diagnosis and care of patients with chronic obstructive pulmonary disease. Am J Respir Crit Care Med. 1995;152:S77-S121.

Chronic Obstructive Pulmonary Disease
Questions 3-6
Answers: 3(C); 4(E); 5(D); 6(A)

EDUCATIONAL OBJECTIVE: Recognize the appropriate evaluation and indications for long-term oxygen therapy in patients with chronic airflow obstruction.

Prescribing physicians must understand the efficacy and indications for long-term oxygen therapy. Audit studies have found that nearly 40% of community patients receiving such therapy do not meet accepted criteria for its utilization.

The 62-year-old man recovering from an acute exacerbation of chronic obstructive pulmonary disease requires reassessment of his need for long-term oxygen therapy after 1 to 3 months of clinical stability and optimal medical management. Although he was symptomatically at his personal baseline at the time of hospital discharge, his arterial Pao_2 may gradually improve over 1 to 3 months to concentrations that no longer require long-term oxygen therapy. In multicenter, controlled trials, 30% to 45% of hypoxemic patients thought to be clinically stable improved enough over 1 to 3 months of outpatient observation and treatment so that oxygen therapy could be discontinued.

The 66-year-old man should continue long-term oxygen therapy indefinitely despite the recent room air arterial blood gas study showing Pao_2 of 58 mm Hg. He was initially hypoxemic at a time of apparent clinical stability, and hypoxemia was reconfirmed after 3 months of adequate medical management. There is evidence that up to 25% of patients receiving long-term oxygen therapy for months to years for stable, chronic, hypoxemic chronic obstructive pulmonary disease may show an improvement in Pao_2 and decrease in alveolar-arterial oxygen gradient and no longer meet criteria for long-term oxygen. This may result from a reduction in hypoxic pulmonary vasoconstriction, although the exact mechanism of this improvement in Pao_2 is unknown. Removal of long-term oxygen therapy from these patients may promptly increase pulmonary hypertension and again impair gas exchange. They should continue to receive long-term oxygen therapy.

The 67-year-old woman with symptomatic chronic obstructive pulmonary disease should have measurement of arterial oxygenation during exercise, most conveniently with pulse oximetry. Because she has a resting room air Pao_2 of 58 mm Hg and no clinical evidence of cor pulmonale or erythrocytosis (hematocrit above 55%), she does not qualify for continuous long-term oxygen therapy. For patients with Pao_2 greater than 55 mm Hg at rest but exercise arterial oxygen desaturation ($Sao_2 > 88\%$), oxygen therapy during exercise may decrease dyspnea and increase exercise tolerance and peak exercise level; long-term benefits of supplemental oxygen in this setting have not been studied. Exercise testing with pulse oximetry should be done at a level of exertion equal to or greater than the patient's usual daily activities such as during walking or with upper extremity exercises, if dyspnea is prominent at those times. If arterial oxygen desaturation is detected, oxygen therapy with exercise is initiated and titrated to maintain an Sao_2 greater than 90% utilizing the patient's personal oxygen delivery device. Exercise arterial oxygen desaturation with resting Pao_2 greater than 55 mm Hg does not justify continuous long-term oxygen therapy. Oxygen therapy is not indicated to relieve dyspnea in patients who have neither resting nor exercise arterial hypoxemia.

The 68-year-old woman with chronic productive cough, progressive exertional dyspnea, and severe airflow obstruction requires a room air arterial blood gas study despite her normal Sao_2 measured in the office by pulse oximetry. Because she is a heavy smoker she may have a substantial elevation of carboxyhemoglobin. Pulse oximetry may significantly overestimate the level of oxyhemoglobin and arterial oxygen saturation in the presence of high levels of carboxyhemoglobin, and so this patient may possibly still have significant arterial hypoxemia. Additionally, because her airflow obstruction is severe, she may also have significant elevation of $Paco_2$ that will not be detected by pulse oximetry. Measurement of room air arterial blood gases rather than pulse oximetry alone is recommended to confirm the need for initiation of long-term oxygen therapy, to assess the level of $Paco_2$ in severe airflow obstruction, and to accurately determine the adequacy of arterial oxygenation in patients with moderate or severe airflow obstruction who continue to smoke.

Screening overnight oximetry is indicated only if there is evidence of cor pulmonale or erythrocytosis despite adequate daytime oxygenation, or if there is a clinical suspicion of sleep-disordered breathing.

Bibliography

1. **American Thoracic Society.** Standards for the diagnosis and care of patients with chronic obstructive pulmonary disease. Am J Respir Crit Care Med. 1995;152:S77-S121.

2. **Bongard F, Sue D.** Pulse oximetry and capnography in intensive and transitional care units. West J Med. 1992;156:57-64.

3. **O'Donohue WJ Jr.** Home oxygen therapy. Med Clin North Am. 1996;80:611-22.

4. **O'Donohue WJ Jr.** Effect of oxygen therapy on increasing arterial oxygen tension in hypoxemic patients with stable chronic obstructive pulmonary disease while breathing ambient air. Chest. 1991;100:968-72.

5. **Timms RM, Kvale PA, Anthonisen NR, Boylen CT, Cugell DW, Petty TL, Williams GW.** Selection of patients with chronic obstructive pulmonary disease for long-term oxygen therapy. JAMA. 1981;245:2414-5.

Chronic Obstructive Pulmonary Disease
Questions 7-10
Answers: 7(A); 8(C); 9(B); 10(D)

EDUCATIONAL OBJECTIVE: Identify flow-volume loops for various airway obstructive disorders.

Graphic displays of lung volume and airflow (flow-volume loops) provide characteristic patterns for certain respiratory disorders. They are particularly useful for recognition of upper airway obstruction.

The 34-year-old woman presents a characteristic history for upper airway obstruction following prolonged tracheal intubation. Tracheal stenosis, an uncommon but serious complication of tracheal intubation, commonly occurs at the site where the balloon cuff of the tracheal tube presses against the tracheal wall. Although tracheal stenosis may occur after only 1 or 2 days of tracheal intubation, it occurs more commonly after longer periods of tracheal intubation, as in this patient. Flow-volume loop A shows a plateau during both forced inspiration and expiration. This pattern is characteristic of a fixed upper airway obstruction such as tracheal stenosis.

The 70-year-old woman has severe fixed obstructive lung disease as evidenced by the history (> 75 pack-years of cigarette smoking and severe exertional dyspnea) and the physical examination (diminished intensity of breath sounds on chest auscultation). Flow-volume loop C shows very low flow with no change following aerosolized bronchodilator, a characteristic pattern for severe fixed airflow obstruction.

This pattern contrasts with the pattern observed in the 40-year-old man with asthma. Flow-volume loop B shows a moderate reduction in airflow with a marked improvement following inhalation of aerosolized bronchodilator.

The pattern is distinctly different from the normal flow-volume pattern D seen in the otherwise healthy 65-year-old man who has exertional dyspnea.

Bibliography

1. **Crapo RO.** Pulmonary-function testing. N Engl J Med. 1994;331:25-30.

2. **Stauffer JL, Olson DE, Petty TL.** Complications and consequences of endotracheal intubation and tracheotomy. Am J Med. 1981;70:65-76.

3. **Kryger M, Bode F, Antic R, Anthonisen N.** Diagnosis of obstruction of the upper and central airways. Am J Med. 1976;61:85-93.

Chronic Obstructive Pulmonary Disease
Question 11
Answer: C

EDUCATIONAL OBJECTIVE: Distinguish emphysema from asthma.

An increase in lung volume, particularly the total lung capacity and residual volume, often occurs in patients with chronic obstructive pulmonary disease, both with asthma and emphysema. Similarly, emphysema may have a reversible component and as in asthma the FEV_1 will improve with administration of a bronchodilator. With severe compromise of the airway caliber, small changes induced by methacholine can cause dramatic reduction in airflow, and therefore patients with severe emphysema typically have a positive methacholine bronchial challenge. Asthma may develop either in the presence or absence of allergic sensitization and therefore allergy skin testing will not help differentiate these conditions.

Typically, asthma is associated with an elevation of DLco for reasons that are not entirely clear but may relate to increased blood flow through the lungs. Emphysema with its destruction of the lungs can cause dramatic reduction of the diffusing capacity, and therefore measuring the DLco would be useful in distinguishing these two conditions.

Bibliography

1. **Meslier N, Racineux JL, Six P, Lockhart A.** Diagnostic value of reversibility of chronic airway obstruction to separate asthma from chronic bronchitis: a statistical approach. Eur Respir J. 1989;2:497-505.

2. **Snider GL.** Distinguishing among asthma, chronic bronchitis, and emphysema. Chest. 1985;87:35S-9S.

3. **Clausen JL.** The diagnosis of emphysema, chronic bronchitis, and asthma. Clin Chest Med. 1990;11:405-16.

4. **Martinez FJ.** Diagnosing chronic obstructive pulmonary disease. The importance of differentiating asthma, emphysema, and chronic bronchitis. Postgrad Med. 1998;103:112-7, 121-2, 125.

Chronic Obstructive Pulmonary Disease
Questions 12-15
Answers: 12(C); 13(A); 14(B); 15(D)

EDUCATIONAL OBJECTIVE: Distinguish potential adverse events associated with various antimicrobial agents.

Ciprofloxacin causes a reduction in the metabolism of theophylline, increasing the serum levels by 30%. Signs and symptoms of theophylline toxicity include nausea, vomiting, palpitations, flushing, and headache. Cimetidine will not hinder the absorption of ciprofloxacin. Care must be taken that ciprofloxacin is not given at the same time as aluminum- and magnesium-containing antacids, because absorption will be markedly decreased.

The most common bacterial pathogens associated with an exacerbation of chronic bronchitis include *Streptococcus pneumoniae, Haemophilus influenzae,* and *Moraxella catarrhalis.* Cephalexin would be adequate to treat most *S. pneumoniae* but would not be active against *H. influenzae* and *M. catarrhalis.*

Clarithromycin, like erythromycin, impairs the activity of the cytochrome P-450 enzyme system which impairs catabolism of other medications and thus increases their serum concentration. Increased concentrations of astemizole and cisapride have been associated with prolonged QT intervals and ventricular arrhythmias. Other agents such as ketoconazole and itraconazole have similar effects on the cytochrome P-450 enzymes and should not be given to patients taking astemizole or cisapride. Spectrum of activity would be reasonable, although the activity against *H. influenzae* is marginal.

Norfloxacin, although having similar spectrum of activity as ciprofloxacin, achieves poor serum concentrations. Norfloxacin is only indicated for treatment of urinary tract infections and bacterial diarrhea. Because the serum concentrations are low, there is little effect on theophylline metabolism. There has been no association with ventricular arrhythmias.

Bibliography

1. **Tran HT.** Torsades de pointes induced by nonantiarrhythmic drugs. Conn Med. 1994;58:291-5.
2. **Fuhr U, Anders EM, Sorgel F, Staib AH.** Inhibitory potency of quinolone antibacterial agents against cytochrome P450IA2 activity in vivo and in vitro. Antimicrob Agents Chemother. 1992;36:942-8.

Chronic Obstructive Pulmonary Disease
Question 16
Answer: C

EDUCATIONAL OBJECTIVE: Manage dyspnea in a patient with end-stage lung disease.

This 69-year-old man has end-stage emphysema with persistent dyspnea despite aggressive therapy that is unrelated to an acute precipitating event. The use of opiates (such as codeine) to relieve dyspnea in patients with severe lung disease is well-documented. In short-term controlled trials, oral opiate therapy has improved exercise performance and dyspnea scores with mild or infrequent side effects. The subjective relief may be significant. The results of long-term studies have been somewhat inconsistent, but opiate therapy appears to have a role in the management of distressing dyspnea in selected patients with advanced but not necessarily terminal lung disease.

Although increased levels of anxiety are common in patients with lung disease, the use of anxiolytics to treat dyspnea has been disappointing. In clinical trials, benzodiazepines have failed to show beneficial effect for the relief of breathlessness and generally are not recommended.

In the absence of wheezing, bronchospasm or documented bronchodilator response on pulmonary function testing, the effectiveness of corticosteroid therapy, either as an inhaled or oral agent, in end-stage emphysema is not well-established. With proper technique and the use of a spacer device, metered-dose inhalers are as effective as hand-held nebulizers in delivering inhaled medications. However, patients should be directly observed to ensure that they use proper technique. This patient's oxyhemoglobin saturation is adequate on his current flow rate of supplemental oxygen. More severe hypercapnia may develop if the flow rate of oxygen were increased.

Bibliography

1. **Tobin MJ.** Dyspnea. Pathophysiologic basis, clinical presentation, and management. Arch Intern Med. 1990;150:1604-13.
2. **Silvestri GA, Mahler DA.** Evaluation of dyspnea in the elderly patient. Clin Chest Med. 1993;14:393-404.
3. **Light RW, Muro JR, Sato RI, Stansbury DW, Fischer CE, Brown SE.** Effects of oral morphine on breathlessness and exercise tolerance in patients with chronic obstructive pulmonary disease. Am Rev Respir Dis. 1989;139:126-33.

Cough

Cough Question 1
Answer: C

EDUCATIONAL OBJECTIVE: Distinguish various triggers and therapeutic approaches in treating perennial rhinitis with coexisting asthma.

Environmental control measures for indoor allergens and irritants are essential for optimal asthma control. Inhalant indoor allergens due to house dust mites, animal dander and saliva, and mold spores from plants need to be controlled or eliminated. These exposures can lead to a greater requirement for medication, decreased pulmonary function, and significant loss of work.

Airborne dust mite particles and cat saliva and molds are known to exacerbate allergic reactions and the development of asthma. High-efficiency particulate air (HEPA) cleaning devices are useful in reducing airborne cat dander, mold spores, and tobacco smoke but not dust mite. An association of atopic dermatitis with dust mite exposure has also been noted.

Bibliography

1. **Woodfolk JA, Hayden ML, Couture N, Platts-Mills TA.** Chemical treatment of carpets to reduce allergen: comparison of the effects of tannic acid and other treatments on proteins derived from dust mites and cats. J Allergy Clin Immunol. 1995;96:325-33.
2. **Reisman RE, Mauriello PM, Davis GB, Georgitis JW, DeMasi JM.** A double-blind study of the effectiveness of a high-efficiency particulate air (HEPA) filter in the treatment of patients with perennial allergic rhinitis and asthma. J Allergy Clin Immunol. 1990;85:1050-7.

Cough Questions 2-5
Answers: 2(E); 3(B); 4(D); 5(C)

EDUCATIONAL OBJECTIVE: Identify the most appropriate management in patients presenting with cough.

The 24-year-old man has symptoms consistent with a upper respiratory infection. Such infections are predominantly viral and neither antibiotic therapy nor diagnostic testing is typically indicated. Although an antihistamine–decongestant may alleviate the nasal symptoms, this patient's major residual complaint is a nagging cough. An antitussive preparation containing dextromethorphan may provide some relief until this common and self-limited illness resolves.

The nasal symptoms reported by the 32-year-old woman with a persistent cough for 3 months are important in that postnasal drip is the probable cause in one half to two thirds of patients with chronic cough. One study found that in the absence of such symptoms, an empiric trial of an antihistamine–decongestant was effective in a large proportion of patients with chronic cough and should be considered as the first step unless there is clear evidence on history or physical examination of other causes. Although the patient reports occasional dyspepsia, gastroesophageal reflux is a less common cause of cough than postnasal drip, and the diagnosis of gastroesophageal reflux as well as its long-term management are somewhat more difficult.

The 64-year-old man has an acute exacerbation of his chronic obstructive pulmonary disease, including a worsening cough that has now become productive of discolored sputum. Although antibiotic therapy for acute bronchitis in patients without underlying lung disease is controversial, there is evidence that antibiotic therapy is a useful adjunct in patients with chronic obstructive pulmonary disease who develop an acute respiratory illness with a worsening productive cough.

Asthma is the second most common cause of chronic cough after postnasal drip. The 42-year-old man reports no nasal symptoms, and therapy with antihistamines and decongestants has been ineffective. If the patient had clinical features suggestive of asthma (for example, episodic wheezing or worsening of cough after exertion), an empiric trial of treatment for asthma might be warranted. When there are no clinical features of asthma other than cough, a positive methacholine challenge test is highly suggestive of a cough related to reactive airways and merits a trial of a β-adrenergic agonist or other asthma therapy.

Bibliography

1. **Saint S, Bent S, Vittinghoff E, Grady D.** Antibiotics in chronic obstructive pulmonary disease exacerbations. A meta-analysis. JAMA. 1995;273:957-60.
2. **Irwin RS, Curley FJ, French CL.** Chronic cough. The spectrum and frequency of causes, key components of the diag-

nostic evaluation, and outcome of specific therapy. Am Rev Respir Dis. 1990; 141:640-7.

3. **Irwin RS, Curley FJ, Bennett FM.** Appropriate use of antitussives and protussives. A practical review. Drugs. 1993;46:80-91.

Cough Question 6
Answer: B

EDUCATIONAL OBJECTIVE: Manage a lung mass with suspicious mediastinal lymphadenopathy.

The right upper lobe lesion detected on chest radiograph is consistent with a primary bronchogenic carcinoma, particularly when considered with the patient's smoking history. It must now be determined whether surgical resection is appropriate, based both on staging and on predicted post-resection pulmonary function.

The patient's baseline FEV_1 of 1.7 L should be sufficient for lobectomy, which would be the standard procedure if surgery is performed. Quantitative perfusion scanning would be useful primarily if his pulmonary function were worse and if there were concern that his post-resection FEV_1 might not exceed 0.8 L.

The therapeutic approach to this patient (surgery versus nonsurgical or combined therapy) depends on whether the enlarged mediastinal lymph node is positive for carcinoma, which will alter the staging. Even though the lymph node is enlarged, the predictive value for finding carcinoma is not high enough to dictate further therapy without a tissue diagnosis from the lymph node. Surgical resection as the sole form of therapy (either lobectomy or wedge resection) would be inappropriate if the mediastinal node is positive for carcinoma. Alternatively, either radiation therapy or chemotherapy, used alone or combined with surgery, would not be appropriate if the lymph node is hyperplastic and not involved with malignancy.

Therefore, obtaining tissue from the lymph node is critical for staging and for the optimal therapeutic approach to the patient. A pretracheal, retrocaval lymph node is easily obtained by a standard suprasternal mediastinoscopy, in which the scope follows a course directly anterior to the trachea. Alternatively, a transtracheal needle aspiration of the node through a fiberoptic bronchoscope (Wang needle aspiration) would be helpful if the cytologic specimen were positive, but would not be useful if the results were negative.

Bronchoscopy alone, not given as a possible answer to this question, has a limited role here for diagnosis of the peripheral nodule, as the yield is only 40% to 50% for nodules between 2 and 4 cm in diameter. Mediastinoscopy would also still need to be done

unless transthoracic needle aspiration of the pretracheal lymph node performed during bronchoscopy was positive.

Bibliography

1. **Karsell PR, McDougall JC.** Diagnostic tests for lung cancer. Mayo Clin Proc. 1993;68:288-96.
2. **McLoud TC, Bourgouin PM, Greenberg RW, Kosiuk JP, Templeton PA, Shepard JA, et al.** Bronchogenic carcinoma: analysis of staging in the mediastinum with CT by correlative lymph node mapping and sampling. Radiology. 1992;182:319-23.
3. **Mountain CF.** Lung cancer staging classification. Clin Chest Med. 1993;14:43-53.
4. **Midthun DE, Swensen SJ, Jett JR.** Approach to the solitary pulmonary nodule. Mayo Clin Proc. 1993;68:378-85.

Cough Question 7
Answer: D

EDUCATIONAL OBJECTIVE: Recognize a potentially delayed presentation of cystic fibrosis, an inherited genetic illness.

The physician caring for the adolescent must consider a broad differential when confronted with a complex problem. Few disease entities are specific to adolescents and young adults. However, diseases usually diagnosed in children may present in adolescents, and diseases that usually begin in the third decade may present early.

Cystic fibrosis, once believed to present only in children, has now been diagnosed in the third and fourth decades. In this case of a male in late adolescence, the clues to diagnosis are the chronic cough, the small stature, and the disproportionately low weight. A positive family history for this inherited disorder would sway the clinician to order a quantitative pilocarpine iontophoresis sweat test to confirm the diagnosis.

The differential of chronic cough is broad. Postnasal drip is extremely common, but the clinician will usually find swollen nasal turbinates and posterior pharyngeal lymphoid hyperplasia. Sarcoidosis is usually asymptomatic and would not cause growth retardation but can present with many symptoms, especially lymphadenopathy and fatigue. Gastrointestinal reflux can present as chronic cough, though it would not change the growth parameters. Stress would be a diagnosis of exclusion, with historic factors linking increased cough with specific activities.

Bibliography

1. **Weinberger SE.** Medical progress: recent advances in pulmonary medicine. Part 1. N Engl J Med. 1993;328:1389-97.

DEPRESSION

Depression Question 1
Answer: C

EDUCATIONAL OBJECTIVE: Recognize that combined vision and hearing deficits can lead to substantial loss of functional ability in older persons.

Older persons such as this 72-year-old woman who has both vision and hearing loss are in double jeopardy, because neither the visual nor the auditory system can compensate for deficits in the other. Older persons with combined vision and hearing loss are at risk for falls and accidents. In addition, because they have difficulty in ambulation, driving an automobile, and hearing in crowded social situations, they often become more homebound. Lack of sensory stimulation and social activity can lead to depression.

It is possible that early Alzheimer's disease could account for most of this patient's findings, but the neurologic examination is normal and there is no history of forgetfulness or memory problems. Her problems playing bridge are more likely explained by hearing disability. Apathetic hyperthyroidism is possible, but the sensory disorder should be addressed before other less likely diagnoses are pursued. Finally, the presence of a few extrasystoles on electrocardiography is not sufficient to suggest sick sinus syndrome, and there is no adequate history of syncope in this patient.

Bibliography

1. **Johnson CA, Adams AJ, Lewis RA.** Evidence for a neural basis of age-related visual field loss in normal observers. Invest Ophthalmol Vis Sci. 1989;30:2056-64.
2. **Uhlmann RF, Teri L, Rees TS, Mozlowski KJ, Larson EB.** Impact of mild to moderate hearing loss on mental status testing. Comparability of standard and written Mini-Mental State Examinations. J Am Geriatr Soc. 1989;37:223-8.

Depression Question 2
Answer: B

EDUCATIONAL OBJECTIVE: Distinguish depression from physical disease.

Although the patient seems classically depressed, measurement of thyroid function and vitamin B_{12} is a basic screen for medical disorders presenting with depression. Electrolyte abnormalities, calcium disarray, and giant cell arteritis should also be sought by appropriate laboratory studies. Measurement of antinuclear antibodies is of little value without other evidence of lupus.

Imaging of the brain is not indicated at this point, given the normalcy of physical examination and the fact that the headache is typically associated with stress affecting the neck. A therapeutic trial of any agent would be premature before the chemical studies return.

Bibliography

1. **Katon W, Sullivan MD.** Depression in chronic medical illness. J Clin Psychiatry. 1990;51:S3-S14.

Depression Questions 3-5
Answers: 3(C); 4(A); 5(D)

EDUCATIONAL OBJECTIVE: Select the optimal therapy for patients with depression.

The 26-year-old woman has a situational depression related to the recent death of her mother. She has a supportive family and, at least at this point, does not meet the criteria for major depression. Her major manifestation is sleep disturbance, which can be treated with a sleeping medication. Close follow-up is important to watch for the development of major depression, but this is not the usual course of a grief reaction.

The 45-year-old man manifests important criteria for major depression and is at high risk for suicide—he is single, lives alone, has been drinking heavily, and has had thoughts of hurting himself. These are all criteria that should lead a primary care physician to refer the patient to a psychiatrist immediately.

The 30-year-old woman has somatic complaints as a replacement for depressive symptoms. There is no evidence of intrinsic heart disease. Her chest pain appears to be a situational reaction to losing her job. The primary care physician should offer the patient counseling, and should discuss with her the likely etiology of her chest complaints. She has no criteria for major depression and need not be treated with anti-depressants.

Antidepressants can be used by the internist to treat patients who have major depression. The physician must identify suicidal patients; these patients may need hospital admission. Severely depressed patients who need significant counseling should be referred to a psychiatrist; these patients probably should be started on antidepressant medication by the internist while awaiting psychiatric intervention.

Bibliography

1. **Perez-Stable EJ, Miranda J, Munoz RF, Ying YW.** Depression in medical outpatients. Underrecognition and misdiagnosis. Arch Intern Med. 1990;150:1083-8.

2. **Eisenberg L.** Treating depression and anxiety in primary care. Closing the gap between knowledge and practice. N Engl J Med. 1992;326:1080-4.

3. **Lin EH, Von Korff M, Wagner EH.** Identifying suicide potential in primary care. J Gen Intern Med. 1989;4:1-6.

4. **Rush AJ.** Problems associated with the diagnosis of depression. J Clin Psychiatry. 1990;51:15-25.

Depression Question 6
Answer: E

EDUCATIONAL OBJECTIVE: Recognize generalized anxiety disorder.

At least one out of five primary care patients has anxiety and depressive disorders, which frequently present as somatic rather than emotional complaints and may be treatable with either psychotropic medications or nonpharmacologic therapies.

This patient gives a typical history for generalized anxiety disorder, including the somatic complaints, excessive worry about multiple matters, irritability, and an almost obsessional preoccupation with these fears, despite the fact she realizes that the degree and the disabling nature of her worries are unreasonable.

Major depression (as well as other depressive disorders) shares a number of symptoms in common with anxiety disorders, and some affected patients meet criteria for both depression and anxiety. Fatigue, insomnia, irritability, and somatic complaints are equally likely in major depression, and the clinician would need to inquire about depressed mood, anhedonia, changes in appetite or weight, problems in concentration or memory, feelings of guilt, and thoughts of suicide.

In obsessive–compulsive disorder, the obsessions are usually about things most people would not dwell on, such as repeated thoughts about contamination, having things in a particular order, fears of hurting someone, or sexual imagery.

An adjustment disorder is characterized by anxiety (or depression) about a single stressful event rather than multiple worries, and the course is typically not chronic. Hypochondriasis is a preoccupying conviction that one has a serious disease that persists despite medical evaluation and reassurance to the contrary.

Bibliography

1. **Rickels K, Schweizer E.** The clinical course and long-term management of generalized anxiety disorder. J Clin Psychopharmacol. 1990;10:101S-110S.

2. **Black JL.** Obsessive compulsive disorder: a clinical update. Mayo Clin Proc. 1992;67:266-75.

Depression Question 7
Answer: C

EDUCATIONAL OBJECTIVE: Distinguish a normal grieving reaction from pathologic grief reactions.

The mild depression-like symptoms of normal grief, as seen in this 74-year-old widow, do not extend to extreme vegetative symptoms, anhedonia, active tendencies toward suicide, or a persistent severely depressed mood that would suggest superimposed major depression. The symptoms of normal grief often mimic a mild depression and may include some guilt. This does not convey a worse prognosis. Likewise, it may be normal for grieving persons to withdraw somewhat from their usual activities, especially in the initial weeks following the loss. The phase of acute grief includes somatic distress such as choking, sighing, and a sense of emptiness and normally persists for days after the loss. The patient in this case has progressed beyond that phase. She shows no sign of complicated grief characterized by denial, persistent yearning, searching, or disbelief in the loss.

Bibliography

1. **Prigerson HG, Frank E, Kasl SV, Reynolds CF 3rd, Anderson B, Zubenko GS, et al.** Complicated grief and bereavement-related depression as distinct disorders: preliminary empirical validation in elderly bereaved spouses. Am J Psychiatry. 1995;152:22-30.

Depression Question 8
Answer: D

EDUCATIONAL OBJECTIVE: Recognize depression after myocardial infarction.

Many patients experience a major depression and anxiety after myocardial infarction, with additional elements of post-traumatic stress disorder after bypass surgery. Equally significant is that the diagnosis may not be made. Depression is a key element in hindering return to work and has been shown to be an independent risk factor for mortality 18 months after a myocardial infarction. A critical point therefore is the need to recognize depression when it is concomitantly present with other major illness, as for example in myocardial infarction and stroke patients. To consider the depression as "understandable" in the context of devastating illness prevents its being treated, thereby adding unnecessary morbidity to the underlying disease.

Recent data show that depression is not associated with β-blocker therapy. The myocardial effects of the tricyclic antidepressants would not make them the agents of choice in this setting. A selective serotonin reuptake inhibitor such as paroxetine would be safer in that this class of agents appears to be free of proarrhythmic effects and orthostatic hypotension and appear to have no adverse effect on the pulse. A stimulant is not indicated nor is a benzodiazepine alone because the major problem of depression would not be addressed. The pharmacotherapy for depression is enhanced by concomitant psychotherapy.

Bibliography

1. Clinical Practice Guideline, Number 5. Depression in Primary Care: Volume 1. Detection and diagnosis. U.S. Department of Health and Human Services, Public Health Service, Agency for Health Care Policy and Research. April, 1993.
2. Clinical Practice Guideline, Number 5. Depression in Primary Care: Volume 2. Treatment of major depression. U.S. Department of Health and Human Services, Public Health Service, Agency for Health Care Policy and Research. April, 1993.
3. Crowe JM, Runions J, Ebbesen LS, Oldridge NB, Streiner DL. Anxiety and depression after acute myocardial infarction. Heart Lung. 1996;25:98-107.
4. Frasure-Smith N, Lesperance F, Talajic M. Depression and 18-month prognosis after myocardial infarction. Circulation. 1995; 91:999-1005.
5. Gerstman BB, Jolson HM, Bauer M, Cho P, Livingston JM, Platt R. The incidence of depression in new users of beta-blockers and selected antihypertensives. J Clin Epidemiol. 1996;49:809-15.
6. Roose SP, Glassman AH. Antidepressant choice in the patient with cardiac disease: Lessons from the cardiac arrhythmia suppression trial (CAST) studies. J Clin Psychiatry. 1994;55 (suppl A):83-87.

Depression Question 9
Answer: D

EDUCATIONAL OBJECTIVE: Distinguish chronic fatigue syndrome from major depression.

Chronic fatigue syndrome continues to be a controversial illness that shares symptoms not only with major depression but also with other medical and psychiatric disorders, particularly fibromyalgia and somatoform disorders. Although fatigue is required for the diagnosis of chronic fatigue syndrome, it is also one of the diagnostic criteria for major depression and is exceptionally common in fibromyalgia and somatoform disorders. Likewise, myalgias and other pain complaints, sleep disturbances, other somatic symptoms, and chronicity are common in all these conditions.

Half of patients who suffer their first episode of major depression will suffer another, and the recurrence rate is 80% after a second episode. In a patient with symptoms common to chronic fatigue syndrome and major depression, a history of depression, particularly if accompanied by symptoms more specific (although not unique) to a mood disorder, such as depressed mood, anhedonia, appetite changes, or feelings of guilt, make a partial recurrence of major depression more likely than a diagnosis of chronic fatigue syndrome.

Although various mild, nonspecific immunologic abnormalities can occur in some patients with chronic fatigue syndrome, there are no laboratory abnormalities diagnostic of the disorder. "Chronic mononucleosis" was a popular diagnosis in the early 1980s, but Epstein-Barr virus infection (often subclinical) has occurred in a majority of persons by the age of 30, and positive Epstein-Barr viral serology is common in asymptomatic persons. Also, elevated serologic titers to other viruses have been reported in patients with chronic fatigue syndrome, leading some experts to speculate this is an epiphenomenon secondary to immune dysregulation rather than a primary viral infection. Although no large clinical trials have been published, antidepressants have frequently been reported to be beneficial in some patients with chronic fatigue syndrome, so that a response to antidepressants cannot be used as a diagnostic test.

Bibliography

1. **Wessely S, Chalder T, Hirsch S, Pawlikowska T, Wallace P, Wright DJ.** Postinfectious fatigue: prospective cohort study in primary care. Lancet. 1995;345:1333-8.

2. **McKenzie R, Straus SE.** Chronic fatigue syndrome. Adv Intern Med. 1995;40:119-53

3. **Cathebras PJ, Robbins JM, Kirmayer LJ, Hayton BC.** Fatigue in primary care: prevalence, psychiatric comorbidity, illness behavior, and outcome. J Gen Intern Med. 1992;7:276-86.

4. **Bates DW, Buchwald D, Lee J, Kith P, Doolittle T, Rutherford C, et al.** Clinical laboratory test findings in patients with chronic fatigue syndrome. Arch Intern Med. 1995;155:97-103.

5. **Wilson A, Hickie I, Lloyd A, Wakefield D.** The treatment of chronic fatigue syndrome: science and speculation. Am J Med 1994;96:544-50.

Depression Questions 10-14
Answers: 10(D); 11(A); 12(C); 13(B); 14(E)

EDUCATIONAL OBJECTIVE: Differentiate various types of depression.

Major depression includes a depressed mood or anhedonia for at least 2 weeks. At least four additional symptoms must be present including weight loss or decreased appetite; insomnia or hypersomnia; psychomotor retardation or agitation; fatigue; inappropriate worthlessness or guilt; indecisiveness or inability to concentrate; and/or suicidal ideation or recurrent thoughts of death. This description best fits the second patient whose brother was diagnosed with leukemia. Seasonal affective disorder has similar features but has occurred at least twice in relation to a particular season, usually winter, like the third patient whose three episodes have all occurred in November.

Atypical depression is a subtype of major depression also characterized by overeating, oversleeping, weight gain, and sensitivity to personal rejection related to external events, as exemplified by the fourth patient who has gained weight, oversleeps, and is having problems at work. Dysthymia is more chronic than major depression, at least 2 years in duration, and milder. Affected patients have subjective depression plus at least two additional symptoms, like the fifth patient who admits to having felt depressed for years.

Depression not otherwise specified (NOS) consists of frequent episodes over a period of time, each one too brief for dysthymia, and each one too mild to be considered a major depression, like the first patient.

Bibliography

1. Task Force on DSM-IV. Diagnostic and Statistical Manual of Mental Disorders. Fourth edition. American Psychiatric Association. Washington, D.C. 1994. 317-392.

2. Depression guideline panel. Depression in primary care: volume one. Detection and diagnosis. volume two. Treatment of major depression. US Department of Health and Human Services. Public Health Service, Agency for Healthcare Policy and Research. Rockville, MD. Clinical Practice Guideline 5. April, 1993.

DIABETES MELLITUS

Diabetes Mellitus Question 1
Answer: A

EDUCATIONAL OBJECTIVE: Manage hypoglycemia in a patient with type 1 diabetes mellitus.

Hypoglycemia unawareness commonly develops after many years of type 1 diabetes mellitus. It is not usually directly caused by autonomic neuropathy. It tends to occur on intensive insulin regimens as a result of frequent episodes of even mild hypoglycemia. Catecholamine warning signs are delayed or lost because the brain, including the glucose-sensing centers in the hypothalamus, adapts to repetitive hypoglycemia. This occurs by increasing the rate of glucose transport into the brain and of consequent brain glucose utilization at low plasma glucose concentrations that would previously have triggered counterregulatory responses. In this way hypoglycemia is thought to beget hypoglycemia and a vicious circle ensues, sometimes culminating in multiple episodes of coma or convulsions. This cycle can sometimes be reversed by virtually eliminating any hypoglycemia for several months. This entails very frequent contact between the patient and the health care team and a modest increase in hemoglobin A_{1c} (HbA_{1c}) of 0.5% to 1.0%.

The intensive insulin regimen should not be stopped, and HbA_{1c} should not be allowed to increase to 9% because the patient already has evidence of early retinopathy and nephropathy, the progression of which can be greatly reduced by maintaining HbA_{1c} around 7%. Giving an α-adrenergic blocker will help control his hypertension but may not lessen any impairment in gluconeogenesis produced by metoprolol. The β-blocker would ordinarily be stopped and replaced with a calcium channel blocker or a diuretic agent for hypertension. However, β-blockers improve mortality during the first year after a myocardial infarction and for that reason could still be used in this patient. The constant presence of a sympathomimetic drug will not improve response to hypoglycemia and will worsen hypertension. The morning plasma cortisol of 20 µg/dL makes it unlikely that this patient's hypoglycemia is caused by autoimmune primary adrenal insufficiency. Because the latter does occur with increased frequency in patients with type 1 diabetes mellitus, a low nor-

mal or borderline low cortisol value or any history of skin darkening should have prompted a cosyntropin stimulation test.

Bibliography

1. **Boyle PJ, Kempers SF, O'Connor AM, Nagy RJ.** Brain glucose uptake and unawareness of hypoglycemia in patients with insulin-dependent diabetes mellitus. N Engl J Med. 1995;333:1726-31.
2. **Fanelli CG, Epifano L, Rambotti AM, Pampanelli S, De Vincenzo A, Modarelli F, et al.** Meticulous prevention of hypoglycemia normalizes the glycemic thresholds and magnitude of most neuroendocrine responses to, symptoms of, and cognitive function during hypoglycemia in intensively treated patients with short-term IDDM. Diabetes. 1993;42:1683-9.
3. **Gold AE, MacLeod KM, Frier BM.** Frequency of severe hypoglycemia in patients with type I diabetes with impaired awareness of hypoglycemia. Diabetes Care. 1994;17:697-703.
4. **Mokan M, Mitrakou A, Veneman T, Ryan C, Korytkowski M, Cryer P, Gerich J.** Hypoglycemia unawareness in IDDM. Diabetes Care. 1994;17:1397-403.
5. **Widom B, Simonson DC.** Intermittent hypoglycemia impairs glucose counterregulation. Diabetes. 1992;41:1597-602.

Diabetes Mellitus Question 2
Answer: B

EDUCATIONAL OBJECTIVE: Recognize potential consequences of bicarbonate therapy on potassium concentrations in diabetic ketoacidosis.

The sequence of events in this patient strongly suggests the rapid development of profound hypokalemia. She had a low-normal serum potassium concentration on admission to the hospital, and standard insulin doses stimulated the usual transfer of potassium intracellularly from the extracellular space. However, this was accelerated markedly by a rapid increase in arterial pH caused by bicarbonate therapy, which also promoted entry of potassium into the cells in exchange for hydrogen ions. This catastrophe could have been prevented by hourly monitoring of serum potassium and electrocardiography, with extra administration of potassium to maintain the serum concentration at least where it was on admission.

Hyperkalemia would be extremely unlikely in these circumstances and does not typically cause respiratory failure before cardiac arrest. This is not the clinical picture of cerebral edema, which is seldom seen in adults. Cerebral edema does not usually develop until 8 to 12 hours after treatment when the patient has shown biochemical improvement. Manifestations include headache, vomiting, a worsening of mental status after initial improvement, diabetes insipidus, and papilledema. There is no simple physiologic relationship between the plasma glucose concentrations on admission and the amounts of insulin required to reverse ketoacidosis. If anything, giving larger doses of insulin would have made matters worse by aggravating hypokalemia. Administration of bicarbonate will increase both serum bicarbonate and Pco_2 concentrations. The latter diffuses into the cerebrospinal fluid more readily than does bicarbonate, so there may be a transient decrease in cerebrospinal fluid pH. However, there are no proven clinical consequences of this phenomenon. Clinical signs of hypophosphatemia and phosphate depletion do not usually occur this rapidly. Because most patients with diabetic ketoacidosis have hypochloremia and a tendency to hyperphosphatemia on admission, potassium chloride is the most logical initial choice for potassium repletion in diabetic ketoacidosis.

Bibliography

1. **Hamblin PS, Topliss DJ, Chosich N, Lording DW, Stockigt JR.** Deaths associated with diabetic ketoacidosis and hyperosmolar coma, 1973-1988. Med J Aust. 1989;151:439-44.
2. **Podolsky S, Emerson K Jr.** Potassium depletion in diabetic ketoacidosis (KA) and in hyperosmolar nonketotic coma (HNC). Diabetes. 1973;22:299.
3. **Riley L Jr, Cooper M, Narins R.** Alkali therapy of diabetic ketoacidosis: biochemical physiologic and clinical perspectives. Diabetes Metab Rev. 1989;5:627-36.
4. **Soler NG, Bennet MA, Dixon K, Fitzgerald M, Malins J.** Potassium balance during treatment of diabetic ketoacidosis with special reference to the use of bicarbonate. Lancet. 1972;2:665-7.
5. **Walker M, Marshall SM, Alberti KG.** Clinical aspects of diabetic ketoacidosis. Diabetes Metab Rev. 1989;5:651-63.

Diabetes Mellitus Question 3
Answer: D

EDUCATIONAL OBJECTIVE: Manage secondary sulfonylurea failure in a patient with type 2 diabetes mellitus.

Approximately 50% of patients with type 2 diabetes mellitus who are initially well-controlled with sulfonylurea drugs show loss of response to this therapy in the succeeding 5 to 10 years. This is due to progression of the disease with declining beta-cell function. Nonetheless, many placebo-controlled studies have suggested that if insulin is added to glyburide (so-called combination therapy), glucose toxicity is diminished. The glyburide may then again contribute to lowering glycemic levels by stimulating some resurgence of endogenous insulin secretion. Giving the NPH insulin at bedtime selectively attacks fasting hyperglycemia and minimizes further weight gain as metabolic control is improved.

A near maximum benefit from glyburide alone is reached at 10 mg per day. Metformin is usually no more effective than the original sulfonylurea drug in patients with secondary failure to the latter. Although substituting NPH insulin in the morning is likely to improve the patient's glycemia, it is more likely to cause further weight gain in this already obese patient. Adding acarbose might improve hemoglobin A_{1c} (HbA_{1c}) modestly (0.5% to 1.0%) but would likely leave the patient's diabetic control still poor (HbA_{1c} about 9.0%).

Bibliography

1. **Chiasson JL, Josse RG, Hunt JA, Palmason C, Rodger N, Ross, SA, et al.** The efficacy of acarbose in the treatment of patients with non–insulin-dependent diabetes mellitus. Ann Intern Med. 1994;121:928-35.
2. **DeFronzo RA, Goodman AM, the Multicenter Metformin Study Group.** Efficacy of metformin in patients with non–insulin-dependent diabetes mellitus. N Engl J Med. 1995;333:541-9.
3. **Genuth S.** Management of the adult onset diabetic with sulfonylurea drug failure. Diabetes mellitus: perspective on therapy. Endocrinol Metab Clin North Am. 1992; 21:351-70.
4. **Stenman S, Melander A, Groop PH, Groop LC.** What is the benefit of increasing the sulfonylurea dose? Ann Intern Med. 1993;118:169-72.
5. **Yki-Jarvinen H, Kaupilla M, Kujansuu E, Lahti J, Marjanen T, Niskanen L, et al.** Comparison of insulin regimens in patients with non–insulin-dependent diabetes mellitus. N Engl J Med. 1992;327:1426-33.

Diabetes Mellitus Question 4
Answer: E

EDUCATIONAL OBJECTIVE: Manage complications in the treatment of diabetic ketoacidosis.

This patient's history of diabetic ketoacidosis symptoms for 48 hours before starting treatment and the low-normal serum potassium and phosphate concentrations on admission suggest severe depletion of these intracellular ions at the outset of treatment. The improvement in bicarbonate indicates significant reversal of ketoacidosis. The increased creatine kinase concentration and muscle pains suggest rhabdomyolysis caused by hypophosphatemia. Muscle weakness, even that of respiratory muscles, can occur. Option E is correct because it provides everything that is necessary: continuation of insulin at a lower but adequate rate to inhibit recurring ketosis; glucose at a rate sufficient to sustain central nervous system metabolism of glucose; a doubling of the rate of potassium input to 20 meq/h to bring serum potassium concentration back to normal (80 mmol of potassium phosphate equals 120 meq of potassium); and a significant amount of phosphate to treat rhabdomyolysis and the potential threat of renal failure.

The first option is incorrect because discontinuing insulin, while aborting threatened hypoglycemia, can lead to recurrent ketoacidosis and does not provide a sufficient increase in potassium or phosphate concentration. Option B is insufficient because it provides no phosphate and may not provide enough extra potassium for this rate of insulin infusion. Option C is harmful because this rate of insulin infusion is now excessive; this will perpetuate hypokalemia, hypophosphatemia, and a tendency for hypoglycemia. Furthermore, there is no increase in the input of needed potassium or phosphate. Option D will prevent hypoglycemia but does not correct the clinically significant phosphate deficit and may not improve the serum potassium concentration enough.

Bibliography

1. **Berger W, Keller U.** Treatment of diabetic ketoacidosis and non-ketotic hyperosmolar diabetic coma. Baillieres Clin Endocrinol Metab. 1992;6:1-22.

2. **Fleckman AM.** Diabetic ketoacidosis. Endocrinol Metab Clin North Am. 1993;22:181-207.

3. **Genuth SM.** Diabetic ketoacidosis and hyperglycemic hyperosmolar coma. In: Bardin CW, ed. Current Therapy in Endocrinology and Metabolism. 6th ed. St. Louis: Mosby-Year Book; 1997;438-47.

4. **Wang LM, Tsai ST, Ho LT, Hu SC, Lee CH.** Rhabdomyolysis in diabetic emergencies. Diab Res Clin Pract. 1994;26:209-14.

Diabetes Mellitus Question 5
Answer: E

EDUCATIONAL OBJECTIVE: Determine the appropriate therapy for new-onset diabetes.

This patient has characteristics of both type 1 and type 2 diabetes mellitus. His obesity and age of onset are more typical of type 2 diabetes mellitus. His marked involuntary weight loss, ketosis, and negative family history favor type 1 diabetes mellitus. Although not required to be measured, the low C-peptide concentration adds confirmation to the clinical interpretation of his metabolic state as one of insulin deficiency. The presence of serum antibodies to glutamic acid decarboxylase or other islet antigens would add to the evidence for late onset of type 1 diabetes mellitus, but these are still largely research tools. There is nothing to suggest a secondary form of diabetes. As a practical matter, he should be treated promptly with insulin to eliminate his marked symptoms of hyperglycemia and to restore the significant lean body mass he has lost as indicated by his weakness. As normoglycemia is approached or frequent hypoglycemia occurs, and if the insulin requirement decreases to less than 40 units per day, a carefully monitored trial of a sulfonylurea drug in place of insulin may be considered. In such patients, removal of glucose toxicity with insulin may restore beta-cell responsiveness to a sulfonylurea drug. Therefore, permanent insulin therapy may not be required.

Patients who present in a metabolic state of true insulin deficiency only rarely respond promptly to weight reduction therapy alone; moreover, more lean body mass would be sacrificed. Metformin is not indicated for the treatment of ketotic diabetes because it does not stimulate secretion of insulin, which the patient clearly needs. Although there is a chance he would respond quickly to a maximum dose (for example, 20 mg of glyburide) but not a conventional low starting dose (for example, 2.5 mg of glyburide) of a sulfonylurea drug, this is not as certain as insulin to produce rapid improvement in his symptoms and biochemical abnormalities.

Bibliography

1. **Landin-Olsson M, Nilsson KO, Lernmark A, Sundkvist G.** Islet cell antibodies and fasting C-peptide predict insulin requirement at diagnosis of diabetes mellitus. Diabetologia. 1990;33:561-8.

2. **Genuth S.** Insulin in non–insulin-dependent patients. In: Mazzaferri EL, Bar RS, Kreisberg RA, eds. Advances in Endocrinology and Metabolism. Vol 3. St. Louis: Mosby-Year Book, Inc; 1992:89-116.

3. **Genuth S.** Clinical utility of C-peptide measurement in diabetes mellitus. Editorial. Endocr Pract. 1996;2:266-8.

4. **Peters AL, Davidson MB.** Maximal dose glyburide therapy in markedly symptomatic patients with type 2 diabetes: a new use for an old friend. J Clin Endocrinol Metab. 1996;81:2423-7.

5. **Stumvoll M, Nurjhan N, Perriello G, Dailey G, Gerich JE.** Metabolic effects of metformin in non–insulin-dependent diabetes mellitus. N Engl J Med. 1995;333:550-4.

Diabetes Mellitus Question 6
Answer: E

EDUCATIONAL OBJECTIVE: Educate patients about gestational diabetes.

This is a typical case of gestational diabetes discovered on routine screening. In most patients, follow-up glucose tolerance testing post partum indicates normal glucose tolerance. Some women exhibit impaired glucose tolerance (2-hour plasma glucose of 140 to 200 mg/dL) but are not diabetic. A very small percentage remain truly diabetic after delivery. If this woman requires insulin, it should be stopped at the time of delivery and no other therapy initiated unless or until monitoring indicates persistence of hyperglycemia.

All patients exhibiting gestational diabetes are at increased risk of developing permanent diabetes later in life. Obesity, a positive family history, or a previous history of obstetrical morbidity or gestational diabetes all increase the risk, but risk exists even without these factors. Failure to maintain normoglycemia in the third trimester increases the risk of macrosomia more than it does microsomia. There is no increased risk of neonatal diabetes. Her child will, however, be at increased risk for obesity in childhood and for type 2 diabetes mellitus in adulthood.

Bibliography

1. **Buchanan TA, Catalano PM.** The pathogenesis of GDM: implications for diabetes after pregnancy. Diab Rev. 1995;3:584-601.

2. **Kuhl C.** New approaches for the treatment of pregnant diabetic women. Diab Rev. 1995;3:621-31.

3. **Pettitt DJ, Baird HR, Aleck KA, Bennett PH, Knowler WC.** Excessive obesity in offspring of Pima Indian women with diabetes during pregnancy. N Engl J Med. 1983;308:242-5.

Diabetes Mellitus Question 7
Answer: E

EDUCATIONAL OBJECTIVE: Manage hypoglycemia resulting from sulfonylurea drugs or alcohol.

This 54-year-old man's hypoglycemia resulted from a combination of factors: 1) continued stimulation of excess insulin secretion by the sulfonylurea drug; 2) inhibition of gluconeogenesis by alcohol; and 3) prolonged fasting in the presence of the first two factors. Because sulfonylurea drugs can continue to act for several days and long beyond the time predicted by their plasma half-lives, it is mandatory to admit a patient like this for treatment and observation until it is certain that the effects of the sulfonylurea drug are dissipated. This is generally indicated when hyperglycemia reappears and is sustained (> 200 mg/dL) on glucose and carbohydrate intakes of approximately 250 g/d. Such patients should not be discharged from the emergency room soon after acute treatment with intravenous glucose has restored normoglycemia, because hypoglycemia is likely to recur. The regimen of 5% glucose in water at 80 mL/h provides only 4 g/h of glucose, which is insufficient to meet the usual needs of the central nervous system plus those of insulin-stimulated target tissues.

Because of the 24-hour period of fasting and because of alcohol inhibition of gluconeogeneseis, the patient's liver glycogen stores are almost certainly depleted. Therefore, the glycogenolytic effect of glucagon is unlikely to be sufficient to normalize plasma glucose. Hydrocortisone will cause resistance to the action of insulin but will require several hours before there is a significant impact on plasma glucose. Repeated high doses of prednisone or dexamethasone may be useful in such patients if normoglycemia cannot be maintained with amounts of glucose that can be conveniently administered. As much as 40 to 50 g/h of glucose may be needed for many hours, and concentrations of glucose greater than 10% may have to be administered through a central venous catheter. Treatment with diazoxide and octreotide has also been reported to be helpful in reducing the excess insulin secretion caused by sulfonylurea drugs. In addition to the aforementioned measures, parenteral thiamine should be administered prophylactically to this alcoholic patient who is being given large glucose loads.

Bibliography

1. **Freinkel N, Arky RA, Singer DL, Cohen AK, Bleicher SJ, Anderson JB, et al.** Alcohol hypoglycemia. IV. Current concepts of its pathogenesis. Diabetes. 1965;14:350.

2. **Johnson SF, Schade DS, Peake GT.** Chlorpropamide-induced hypoglycemia: successful treatment with diazoxide. Am J Med. 1977;63:799-804.

3. **Krentz AJ, Boyle PJ, Justice KM, Wright AD, Schade DS.** Successful treatment of severe refractory sulfonylurea-induced hypoglycemia with octreotide. Diabetes Care. 1993;16:184-6.

4. **Lecavalier L, Bolli G, Cryer P, Gerich J.** Contributions of gluconeogenesis and glycogenolysis during glucose counter-regulation in normal humans. Am J Physiol. 1989;256:E844-E51.

5. **Shorr RI, Ray WA, Daugherty JR, Griffin MR.** Individual sulfonylureas and serious hypoglycemia in older people. J Am Geriatr Soc. 1996;44:751-5.

Diabetes Mellitus Question 8
Answer: D

EDUCATIONAL OBJECTIVE: Identify appropriate management of diabetic gastroparesis.

This 43-year-old woman's early satiety, nausea, and vomiting are most likely caused by gastroparesis due to diabetic autonomic neuropathy with loss of coordinated gastric motility. Other evidence of autonomic neuropathy is her resting tachycardia, orthostatic blood pressure drop, and failure to show compensatory tachycardia. The delay in gastric emptying can cause retention of food for many hours, leading to vomiting. Metoclopramide, a prokinetic agent that increases acetylcholine release of the myenteric plexus, thereby stimulating gastric emptying, is the treatment of choice. It should be taken at least 30 minutes before eating. Another prokinetic agent that might alleviate this patient's symptoms is erythromycin.

Although nausea and vomiting may be symptoms of uremia, they are not usually this prominent until serum creatinine is considerably higher than 3.4 mg/dL. Ranitidine will block gastric acid secretion and might become useful later if she develops reflux esophagitis secondary to delayed gastric emptying at night. Verapamil may be contributing to her constipation but probably not her gastric symptoms; therefore, the constipation could be relieved by a change to another hypertensive agent. However, the combined α- and β-blocking agent, labetalol, could aggravate her orthostatic hypotension. The constipation could also be a result of diabetic enteropathy. Doxycycline is not a prokinetic antibiotic like erythromycin. Doxycycline could be tried if she developed diarrhea due to diabetic enteropathy. Her mild hyperkalemia suggests reducing the dose of angiotensin-converting enzyme inhibitor.

Bibliography

1. de Caestecker JS, Ewing DJ, Tothill P, Clarke BF, Heading RC, et al. Evaluation of oral cisapride and metoclopramide in diabetic autonomic neuropathy: an eight-week double-blind crossover study. Aliment Pharmacol Ther. 1989;3:69-81.
2. Erbas T, Varoglu E, Erbas B, Tastekin G, Akalin S. Comparison of metoclopramide and erythromycin in the treatment of diabetic gastroparesis. Diabetes Care. 1993;16:1511-4.
3. Feldman M, Schiller LR. Disorders of gastrointestinal motility associated with diabetes mellitus. Ann Intern Med. 1983;98:378-84.
4. McHugh S, Lico S, Diamant NE. Cisapride vs. metoclopramide. An acute study in diabetic gastroparesis. Dig Dis Sci. 1992;37: 997-1001.

Diabetes Mellitus Question 9
Answer: C

EDUCATIONAL OBJECTIVE: Identify methods of reducing the plasma glucose levels in patients with type 1 diabetes mellitus.

This 26-year-old man has marked swings in blood glucose, so that the overall long-term average is still too high, as shown by the hemoglobin A_{1c}. The combination of hypoglycemia before lunch and marked hyperglycemia after breakfast suggests that his regular insulin peak action is at 3 to 4 hours and past the time of absorption of his breakfast. This delayed regular insulin action is causing hypoglycemia before lunch. This may be complicated by the fact that patients with busy and irregular lifestyles often take regular insulin just before eating instead of at least 30 minutes before, as recommended. Therefore, a switch from regular insulin to lisproinsulin is likely to be helpful. Lisproinsulin has an onset of action 5 to 10 minutes after injection, a peak action 1 to 2 hours after injection, and a duration of only 4 hours. A change to lisproinsulin should reduce his postbreakfast and postsupper hyperglycemia and alleviate the hypoglycemia before lunch and bedtime. The need for a large 1600 h snack should disappear, along with the presupper hyperglycemia caused by the large snack.

Decreasing his morning NPH dose may increase his presupper blood glucose but will not correct the problems in the breakfast-to-lunch interval. Moving evening NPH to bedtime is not logical because his prebreakfast blood glucose is already satisfactory and prelunch hypoglycemia could be worsened by this maneuver. Increasing the regular insulin dose at lunch might reduce his presupper blood glucose level, but increasing regular insulin before breakfast and before supper will likely worsen hypoglycemia before lunch and at bedtime.

Bibliography

1. Anderson JH Jr, Brunelle RL, Koivisto VA, Pfutzner A, Trautmann ME, Vignati L, Dimarchi R. Reduction of postprandial hyperglycemia and frequency of hypoglycemia in IDDM patients on insulin-analog treatment. The Multicenter Insulin Lispro Study Group. Diabetes. 1997;46:265-70.
2. Binder C, Lauritzen T, Faber O, Pramming S. Insulin pharmacokinetics. Diabetes Care. 1984;7:188-99.
3. Hirsch IB, Farkas-Hirsch R, Skyler JS. Intensive insulin therapy for treatment of type 1 diabetes. Diabetes Care. 1990;13:1265-83.
4. Torlone E, Pampanelli S, Lalli C, Del Sindaco P, DiVincenzo A, Rambotti AM, et al. Effects of the short-acting insulin analog [Lys(B28), Pro(B29)] on postprandial plasma glucose control in IDDM. Diabetes Care. 1996;19:945-52.
5. Zinman B. The physiologic replacement of insulin. An elusive goal. N Engl J Med. 1989;321:363-70.

Diabetes Mellitus Question 10
Answer: A

EDUCATIONAL OBJECTIVE: Recognize the role of angiotensin-converting enzyme inhibitors and all receptor antagonists in the treatment and prevention of diabetic nephropathy.

Blockers of the renin-angiotensin system, especially angiotensin-converting enzyme (ACE) inhibitors, are widely used to treat or prevent the complications of diabetic nephropathy. In some diabetic conditions there is firm evidence of their value. In others, the rationale for their use relies on either animal data or supposition that many forms of diabetic renal disease will respond to therapy similarly.

In recent trials, use of ACE inhibitors in type I and type II non–insulin-dependent diabetic patients, when compared with other antihypertensive agents, has led to a slower decline in glomerular filtration rate (GFR) and delay in the progression of end-stage renal disease. In type II adult-onset diabetic patients with microalbuminuria who were normotensive, ACE inhibition led to preservation of GFR and less development of clinical proteinuria over 5 years. Cough occurs in up to 10% of patients treated with ACE inhibitors, because these medications inhibit kinase, leading to elevation of bradykinin levels, and at the same time they inhibit the converting enzyme. Hyperkalemia, rather than hypokalemia, is a common side effect of all ACE inhibitors, because they block the angiotensin II–mediated increase in serum aldosterone levels. Angiotensin II receptor antagonists do not lead to elevated bradykinin levels or cough. They have been shown to diminish proteinuria and slow the progression of glomerular damage in diabetic animals, but this has not yet been proven in humans.

Bibliography

1. **Maschio G, Alberti D, Janin G, Locatelli J, Mann JF, Motolese M, et al.** Effect of the angiotensin-converting-enzyme inhibitor benazepril on the progression of chronic renal insufficiency. The Angiotensin-Converting-Enzyme Inhibition in Progressive Renal Insufficiency Study Group. N Engl J Med. 1996;334:939-45.
2. **Lewis EJ, Hunsicker L, Bain RP, Rohde RD.** The effect of angiotensin-converting enzyme inhibition on diabetic nephropathy. The Collaborative Study Group. N Engl J Med. 1993;329:1456-62.
3. **Ravid M, Savin H, Jutrin I, Bental T, Katz B, Lishner M.** Long-term stabilizing effect of ACE inhibition on plasma creatinine and on proteinuria in normotensive type II diabetic patients. Ann Intern Med. 1993;118:577-81.
4. **Remuzzi A, Perico N, Amuchastegui CS, Malanchini B, Mazerska M, Battaglia C, et al.** Short- and long-term effect of angiotensin II receptor blockade in rats with experimental diabetes. J Am Soc Nephrol. 1993;4:40-9.

Diabetes Mellitus Question 11
Answer: A

EDUCATIONAL OBJECTIVE: Recognize appropriate techniques for the measurement of microalbuminuria and recall its utility.

In normal persons the excretion of 10 to 30 mg/d of albumin makes up only a small portion of what is considered the normal daily excretion of proteins—up to 150 mg/d. Microalbuminuria refers to the urinary excretion of albumin specifically and is considered to be abnormal when the daily excretion is greater than 30 mg. Accurate measurement of urine albumin requires sensitive immunoassay. Standard colorimetric dipstick methods (used for routine urinalysis) are not sensitive or specific enough. In many longitudinal studies the presence of abnormal microalbuminuria in a juvenile-onset diabetic patient predicts future development of diabetic nephropathy.

New dipstick methods are available for screening for microalbuminuria. In a recent study (Marshall, 1992), the sensitivity of the Micral dipstick method was greater than 90% and the specificity was 91% in patients with urinary albumin greater than 20 mg/L by radioimmunoassay. Failure of this dipstick method to detect significant microalbuminuria occurred when the dipstick was not exposed to the urine for the recommended 5 seconds. Also, reading the dipstick before the recommended 5 minutes waiting time led to underestimation of albuminuria. Confirmation of a positive dipstick analysis for microalbumin should be done on a timed urine specimen.

Bibliography

1. **Bennett PH, Haffner S, Kasiske BL, Keane WF, Mogensen CE, Parving HH, et al.** Screening and management of microalbuminuria in patients with diabetes mellitus: recommendations to the Scientific Advisory Board of the National Kidney Foundation from an ad hoc committee of the Council on Diabetes Mellitus of the National Kidney Foundation. Am J Kidney Dis. 1995;25:107-12.
2. **Marshall SM, Shearing PA, Alberti KG.** Micral-test strips evaluated for screening for albuminuria. Clin Chem. 1992;38:588-91.

Diabetes Mellitus Question 12
Answer: D

EDUCATIONAL OBJECTIVE: Recognize the most common cause of end-stage renal disease in the United States.

Diabetic nephropathy now accounts for nearly 40% of all new cases of end-stage renal disease (ESRD) in the United States, with hypertension being the second most common cause. The higher representation of minority races in patients with ESRD is in part explained by a higher incidence and prevalence of both hypertension and diabetes mellitus in these groups, as well as a greater susceptibility to renal injury from these causes. Insulin-dependent diabetes mellitus has a greater effect on the incidence of ESRD in white patients, whereas non–insulin-dependent diabetes mellitus has a greater effect on the incidence in black patients. Many of the diabetic patients have proliferative retinopathy and later develop worsening hypertension and fluid accumulation as ESRD progresses.

As mentioned previously, hypertension is the second most common cause of ESRD, followed by chronic glomerulonephritis, renal cystic disease, and chronic interstitial nephritis, which are important but less common causes of ESRD.

Bibliography

1. US Renal Data Systems: USRDS 1996 Annual Data Report. The National Institutes of Health, National Institute of Diabetes and Digestive and Kidney Disorders, Bethesda MD 1995. Am J Kidney Dis. 1996;28(suppl 2):S34-S47.

2. **Eberhardt MS, Wagener DK, Herman WH, Tomlinson-Marshall LA, Hawthorne VM.** Trends in renal disease morbidity and mortality in the United States, 1979 to 1990. Am J Kidney Dis. 1995;26:308-20.

3. **Perneger TV, Brancati FL, Whelton PK, Klag MJ.** End-stage renal disease attributable to diabetes mellitus. Ann Intern Med. 1994;121:912-8.

4. **Parving HH, Hommel E, Mathiesen E, Skott P, Edsberg B, Bahnsen M, et al.** Prevalence of microalbuminuria, arterial hypertension, retinopathy and neuropathy in patients with insulin dependent diabetes. Br Med J. 1988;296:156-60.

DEEP VENOUS THROMBOSIS

Deep Venous Thrombosis Question 1
Answer: B

EDUCATIONAL OBJECTIVE: Manage deep venous thrombosis during pregnancy.

This patient has unmistakable symptoms and signs of deep venous thrombosis that has occurred during pregnancy. Although the precise cause of this condition in pregnancy is uncertain, especially in the absence of trauma or pelvic compression by the uterus of the large veins from the lower extremities, a perturbation of the intrinsic clotting and fibrinolytic systems is believed to be important. This woman should receive intravenous heparin in therapeutic doses for the remainder of the pregnancy, followed by conversion to warfarin for a period of about 3 months. Warfarin crosses the placental barrier and causes embryopathy in 4% to 14% of pregnant women. Although the greatest risk of this complication occurs between weeks 6 and 12 of gestation, warfarin can induce intracranial hemorrhage during delivery. Both subcutaneous heparin (with mid-dosing interval partial thromboplastin time [PTT] adjusted at two to three times baseline PTT) and low–molecular-weight heparin are attractive alternatives to intravenous heparinization. However, neither of these approaches has been studied in a large number of pregnant patients.

There is no indication in this patient to do a venogram because the diagnosis seems well established on the basis of history, physical examination, and noninvasive studies. Furthermore, an inferior vena cava filter is not indicated because the patient has not received a trial of medical therapy and has not suffered any adverse consequences of her venous thrombophlebitis.

Bibliography

1. **Hirsh J, Raschke R, Warkentin TE, Dalen JF, Deykin D, Poller L.** Heparin: mechanism of action, pharmacokinetics, monitoring, efficacy, and safety. Chest. 1995; 108:258S-275S.
2. **Elkayam E.** Anticoagulation in pregnant women with prosthetic heart valves: a double jeopardy. J Am Coll Cardiol. 1996;27:1704-6.

Deep Venous Thrombosis Question 2
Answer: A

EDUCATIONAL OBJECTIVE: Recommend an appropriate duration of oral anticoagulant therapy for a patient with a venous thromboembolism.

This patient developed an apparently spontaneous (unprovoked) deep venous thrombosis following a business trip. A 1-hour airplane flight is unlikely to provoke a thrombosis in a healthy individual. Although his family history indicates that an uncle had a thrombosis following hip surgery, this does not necessarily indicate a familial disorder, given the high frequency of thromboembolism following lower-extremity orthopedic surgery. The patient seems otherwise well, with no symptoms to suggest cancer or a myeloproliferative disease. The laboratory studies show no evidence of a hereditary or acquired hypercoagulable state. The low-normal levels of protein C, protein S, and antithrombin III are most likely due to the effects of an acute deep venous thrombosis. Thus, this patient has a single spontaneous proximal venous thrombosis.

Two studies have now suggested that at least 6 months of therapy would be indicated. A standard international normalized ratio (INR) of 2 to 3 would be appropriate. A shorter duration of therapy, for example, 6 weeks, might be considered in a patient with an obviously provoked thrombosis, such as that following a leg injury or major surgery. Three months of treatment are probably insufficient based on the studies of Schulman and associates and Prandoni and coworkers. Higher intensities of warfarin (INR, 2.5 to 3.5) are usually reserved for patients with antiphospholipid antibodies or patients with artificial cardiac valves. Lifelong therapy might be considered in a patient with a single spontaneous unprovoked major venous thrombosis but clearly not at low INRs with the addition of aspirin. Two studies have shown that low-INR warfarin plus low-dose aspirin failed to prevent systemic emboli after atrial fibrillation (SPAF-3), and this therapy had no effect in the secondary prevention of myocardial infarction (CARS).

Laboratory tests for a hypercoagulable state are normal, although protein C, protein S, and antithrombin III activities were all at the low end of the normal range. These results are most likely due to the impact of an acute thrombosis. Optimally, laboratory testing should be obtained a few weeks after anticoagulant therapy is stopped to reduce the chance of false-positive results.

Bibliography

1. **Hirsh J.** The optimal duration of anticoagulant therapy for venous thrombosis. N Engl J Med. 1995;332:1710-1.

2. **Hirsh J, Fuster V.** Guide to anticoagulant therapy. Part 2: Oral anticoagulants. Circulation. 1994;89:1469-80.

3. **Levine MN, Hirsh J, Gent M, Turpie AG, Weitz J, Ginsberg J, et al.** Optimal duration of oral anticoagulant therapy: a randomized trial comparing four weeks with three months of warfarin in patients with proximal deep vein thrombosis. Thromb Haemost. 1995;74:606-11.

4. **Prandoni P, Lensing AW, Cogo A, Cuppini S, Villalta S, Carta M, et al.** The long-term clinical course of acute deep venous thrombosis. Ann Intern Med. 1996;125:1-7.

5. **Schulman S, Rhedin AS, Lindmarker P, Carlsson A, Larfars G, Nicol P, et al.** A comparison of six weeks with six months of oral anticoagulant therapy after a first episode of venous thromboembolism. N Engl J Med. 1995;332:1661-5.

Deep Venous Thrombosis Question 3
Answer: E

EDUCATIONAL OBJECTIVE: Treat a patient with a proximal deep venous thrombosis with low–molecular-weight heparin in an outpatient setting.

Therapeutic doses of low–molecular-weight heparin have been repeatedly shown to be safe and effective for treatment of patients with proximal deep venous thrombosis. Enoxaparin, 1 mg/kg every 12 h, and dalteparin, 200 U/kg daily, have been used in clinical trials. Outpatient treatment of patients with thrombosis with low–molecular-weight heparin has been shown to be safe and effective. The success of outpatient therapy hinges on patient education and cooperation. Visiting nurses or other health care providers should be available to visit patients in their homes and obtain daily prothrombin times to monitor the effects of warfarin.

Therapeutic doses of low–molecular-weight heparin without laboratory monitoring would be an appropriate treatment for this patient. As long as the patient is cooperative and accessible, he will be a good candidate for outpatient treatment because he has no serious illness.

Some of the other alternatives would be far less likely to prevent recurrent thromboembolism. Subcutaneous heparin in prophylactic doses would be insufficient to prevent a recurrent thrombosis in a patient with a documented deep system lesion. Aspirin has not been shown to be effective in patients with deep venous thrombosis, and low–molecular-weight heparin in prophylactic doses would be insufficient treatment. Finally, monitoring is not necessary in patients treated with low–molecular-weight heparin unless long-term treatment (> 1 week) is required or the patient is at high risk of hemorrhage or thrombosis.

Outpatient treatment of deep venous thrombosis with low–molecular-weight heparin is very attractive, particularly because of the expected cost savings and patient acceptance. In practice, it will be important to obtain a sufficient overlap of low–molecular-weight heparin therapy with warfarin before discontinuing the heparin. Loading doses of warfarin are not necessary and may even increase the risk of thrombosis. The international normalized ratio should be in the therapeutic range (2 to 3) for at least 24 hours before the heparin is stopped. One study has suggested that at least 60% of patients with proximal deep venous thrombosis will be candidates for outpatient treatment.

Bibliography

1. **Koopman MM, Prandoni P, Piovella F, Ockelford PA, Brandjes DP, van der Meer J, et al.** Treatment of venous thrombosis with intravenous unfractionated heparin administered in the hospital as compared with subcutaneous low-molecular-weight heparin administered at home. N Engl J Med. 1996;334:682-7.

2. **Lensing AW, Prins MH, Davidson BL, Hirsh J.** Treatment of deep venous thrombosis with low-molecular-weight heparins. A meta-analysis. Arch Intern Med. 1995;155:601-7.

3. **Levine M, Gent M, Hirsh J, Leclerc J, Anderson D, Weitz J, et al.** A comparison of low-molecular-weight heparin administered primarily at home with unfractionated heparin administered in the hospital for proximal deep-vein thrombosis. N Engl J Med. 1996;334:677-81.

4. **Harrison L, Johnston M, Massicotte MP, Crowther M, Moffat K, Hirsh J.** Comparison of 5-mg and 10-mg loading doses in initiation of warfarin therapy. Ann Intern Med. 1997;126:133-6.

Deep Venous Thrombosis Question 4
Answer: B

EDUCATIONAL OBJECTIVE: Select an optimal therapeutic regimen for a patient with heparin-induced thrombocytopenia and thrombosis.

This patient clearly has heparin-induced thrombocytopenia, as evidenced by the acute onset of thrombocytopenia, a positive heparin-induced thrombocytopenia test, and a pulmonary embolus. Venous thromboembolism is common in patients with heparin-induced thrombocytopenia, occurring in more than 50% of patients. In this instance, his initial exposure to heparin during his coronary angiography may have sensitized him to heparin, so that the heparin-induced thrombocytopenia antibody developed in just 3 days after readministering heparin. A heparinoid (danaparoid) has been shown to be safe and effective in patients with heparin-induced thrombocytopenia and has recently been approved for use in the United States. Other candidates include specific thrombin inhibitors, such as recombinant hirudin and argatroban.

The use of an inferior vena cava filter, danaparoid, and warfarin would be the most reasonable approach in this setting. Using intravenous heparin along with platelet transfusions would very likely incite further thromboses. High titers of patient antibody could combine with platelet factor 4 and heparin to promote platelet aggregation, activation of endothelial cells, and thrombosis.

Intravenous streptokinase might be considered but would be associated with a very high risk of hemorrhaging in this postoperative patient. Moreover, his blood pressure is normal, and he is otherwise stable. Antiplatelet therapy can prevent in vitro platelet aggregation but has not been shown to be effective in patients with heparin-induced thrombocytopenia. If given in concert with thrombolytic agents, hemorrhaging could be severe.

Low–molecular-weight heparin should not be used in patients with established heparin-induced thrombocytopenia because it cross-reacts with the heparin-induced thrombocytopenia antibody 90% to 95% of the time. Low–molecular-weight heparin is much less likely than standard heparin to provoke heparin-induced thrombocytopenia but cannot be used as therapy once the syndrome has developed.

Finally, stopping all antithrombotic therapy and treating with antiplatelet drugs is unlikely to prevent further thrombi in this high-risk patient with a recent pulmonary embolism. There is no evidence that antiplatelet drugs such as aspirin or ticlopidine can prevent thrombocytopenia or thrombosis in patients with heparin-induced thrombocytopenia. Heparin-coated catheters have been reported to produce persistent thrombocytopenia in patients with heparin-induced thrombocytopenia and should be replaced with non–heparin-coated lines, if possible.

Bibliography

1. **Chong BH.** Heparin-induced thrombocytopenia. Br J Haematol. 1995;89:431-9.
2. **Kelton JG, Smith JW, Warkentin TE, Hayward CP, Denomme GA, Horsewood P.** Immunoglobulin G from patients with heparin-induced thrombocytopenia binds to a complex of heparin and platelet factor 4. Blood. 1994;83:3232-9.
3. **Visentin GP, Aster RH.** Heparin-induced thrombocytopenia and thrombosis. Curr Opin Hematol 1995;2:351-57.
4. **Warkentin TE, Levine MN, Hirsh J, Horsewood P, Roberts RS, Gent M, et al.** Heparin-induced thrombocytopenia in patients treated with low-molecular-weight heparin or unfractionated heparin. N Engl J Med. 1995;332:1330-5.
5. **Warkentin TE, Kelton JG.** A 14-year study of heparin-induced thrombocytopenia. Am J Med. 1996;101:502-7.
6. **Warkentin TE.** Danaparoid (Orgaran) for the treatment of heparin-induced thrombocytopenia (HIT) and thrombosis: effects on in vivo thrombin and cross-linked fibrin generation, and evaluation of the clinical significance of in vitro cross-reactivity (XR) of danaparoid for HIT-IgG. Blood. 1996;88:626a.

Deep Venous Thrombosis Question 5 Answer: B

EDUCATIONAL OBJECTIVE: Identify patients who require a heparin (anti-Xa) assay rather than an activated partial thromboplastin time to monitor intravenous heparin therapy.

Approximately 40% of patients with systemic lupus erythematosus (SLE) will show laboratory evidence of a lupus anticoagulant on testing. This patient's activated partial thromboplastin time (aPTT) was clearly increased at 43 seconds, and her prothrombin time was also slightly prolonged. In addition, she had mild thrombocytopenia, which has been shown to be a predictor for thrombosis in patients with SLE and antiphospholipid antibodies.

In this situation, the lupus anticoagulant makes monitoring heparin using the aPTT difficult, if not impossible. Even small amounts of heparin will greatly prolong the aPTT in the presence of a lupus anticoagulant, so that the test is no longer reflective of heparin concentrations in the blood. Accordingly, a heparin assay, which does not depend on phospholipid, is needed to assure that therapeutic levels of the anticoagulant agent are administered. If aPTT measurements are used, then substantial undertreatment is likely to occur.

Option A suggests decreasing the rate of infusion of heparin and rechecking the aPTT. However, as noted above, the aPTT will not accurately reflect the heparin concentration when a lupus anticoagulant is present. It is possible that an aPTT range of 80 to 100 seconds might reflect a heparin level of 0.35 to 0.7 U/mL, but this relationship must be documented using the appropriate test. Stopping heparin and inserting an inferior vena cava filter may help prevent pulmonary emboli, but extension of the deep venous thrombosis and progression of a postthrombotic syndrome are likely in the absence of adequate anticoagulant therapy. Finally, administration of low–molecular-weight heparin in therapeutic doses might be an effective alternative treatment, but the aPTT is insensitive to low–molecular-weight heparin and will not accurately reflect plasma concentrations of the drug.

Heparin assays are considered the gold standard for monitoring therapeutic concentrations of heparin. Medical conditions that prolong the aPTT (for example, lupus anticoagulant, warfarin therapy, liver disease, thrombolytic treatment) frequently make the aPTT unreliable as a guide to heparin therapy. In contrast, patients are often refractory to heparin therapy because of a large thromboembolism or associated inflammatory or malignant disease owing to marked elevations of factor VIII or other acute-phase reactants. In this situation an aPTT will be too short when compared with heparin concentrations in the plasma. Patients who require more than 40,000 units of heparin per day should be monitored using a heparin assay rather than the aPTT.

Bibliography

1. **Brill-Edwards P, Ginsberg JS, Johnston M, Hirsh J.** Establishing a therapeutic range for heparin therapy. Ann Intern Med. 1993;119:104-9.
2. **Goodnight SH.** Antiphospholipid antibodies and thrombosis. Curr Opin Hematol. 1994;1:354-61.
3. **Levine MN, Hirsh J, Gent M, Turpie AG, Cruickshank M, Weitz J, et al.** A randomized trial comparing activated thromboplastin time with heparin assay in patients with acute venous thromboembolism requiring large daily doses of heparin. Arch Intern Med. 1994;154:49-56.

Deep Venous Thrombosis Question 6
Answer: C

EDUCATIONAL OBJECTIVE: Manage thrombosis of the greater saphenous vein.

The presence of a superficial thrombosis can be detected by physical examination, but noninvasive testing is required for evaluation of the deep system. Noninvasive testing is reserved for superficial phlebitis involving the greater saphenous vein above the knee in order to assess for extension into the saphenofemoral junction and the greater risk for embolization.

Surgical consultation is an option, but ligation of the greater saphenous vein would be indicated only if the patient could not receive heparin therapy. The best

management for this patient is repeated ultrasonography in 7 to 10 days and full heparin therapy if the clot propagates into the deep system. Local therapy, which might include analgesics, hot compresses, and elevation, could be used for symptomatic relief.

Bibliography

1. **Weinman EE,** Salzman EW. Deep vein thrombosis. N Engl J Med. 1994;331:1630-41.

Deep Venous Thrombosis Question 7
Answer: B

EDUCATIONAL OBJECTIVE: Select the appropriate diagnostic test for investigation of clinically suspected acute pulmonary embolism.

Compression ultrasonography is the appropriate and cost-effective diagnostic test for the investigation of clinically suspected acute pulmonary embolism in this patient. The risk factors (age, recent surgical resection of adenocarcinoma, and chronic congestive heart failure) and the clinical presentation (new onset of dyspnea) both strongly suggest acute pulmonary embolism. Although pulmonary edema represents an alternative diagnosis, the pretest clinical suspicion for acute pulmonary embolism must be high or intermediate, and it would be inappropriate to treat pulmonary edema without excluding acute pulmonary embolism. A low-probability ventilation-perfusion lung scan pattern combined with a high or an intermediate a priori clinical suspicion cannot exclude acute pulmonary embolism. Compression ultrasonography, if positive for deep venous thrombosis, allows treatment to begin. If compression ultrasonography is negative, pulmonary angiography, a more expensive and invasive procedure, is necessary.

Serial impedance plethysmography or serial compression ultrasonography is not appropriate because this patient has serious cardiopulmonary disease. Deep venous thrombi may be missed with the initial study, and fatal recurrence is possible. Surface echocardiography can provide clues to the diagnosis of acute pulmonary embolism (for example, regional right ventricular dysfunction), but unless intracardiac thrombi are seen, echocardiography cannot confirm the diagnosis of acute pulmonary embolism.

Bibliography

1. **Stein PD, Hull RD, Saltzman HA, Pineo G.** Strategy for diagnosis of patients with suspected acute pulmonary embolism. Chest. 1993;103:1553-9.

2. **Oudkerk M, van Beek EJ, van Putten WL, Buller HR.** Cost-effectiveness analysis of various strategies in the diagnostic management of pulmonary embolism. Arch Intern Med. 1993;153:947-54.

3. **Hull RD, Raskob GE, Ginsberg JS, Panju AA, Brill-Edwards P, Coates G, et al.** A noninvasive strategy for the treatment of patients with suspected pulmonary embolism. Arch Intern Med. 1994;154:289-97.

4. **McConnell MV, Solomon SD, Rayan ME, Come PC, Goldhaber SZ, Lee RT.** Regional right ventricular dysfunction detected by echocardiography in acute pulmonary embolism. Am J Cardiol. 1996;78:469-73.

Deep Venous Thrombosis Questions 8-11
Answers: 8(A); 9(C); 10(E); 11(B)

EDUCATIONAL OBJECTIVE: Manage patients with acute deep venous thrombosis.

Acute proximal deep venous thrombosis (DVT) and acute pulmonary embolism are common disorders. Inadequate initial therapy increases the likelihood of recurrent DVT and pulmonary embolism. Furthermore, increasing evidence suggests that the risk for recurrent venous thromboembolism is substantial when warfarin is discontinued, especially when the DVT is not associated with a reversible risk factor such as recent trauma or surgery.

The 15-year-old boy illustrates juvenile onset of venous thrombosis in the absence of risk factors. The occurrence of venous thromboembolism at such an early age is unusual, and because he was adopted, the family history is limited. Thus, a search for an inherited predisposition is appropriate to guide the duration of warfarin management, although deficient or dysfunctional protein C, protein S, or antithrombin III is identified infrequently even when juvenile idiopathic venous thromboembolism is accompanied by a positive family history. Testing for factor V Leiden followed by lifetime warfarin therapy is not appropriate because this is a very young man to commit to indefinite therapy with warfarin after a first episode of symptomatic DVT. Because he is young, otherwise healthy, and has a supportive family, this patient can be managed with low–molecular-weight heparin (enoxaparin) for at least 5 days overlapped with warfarin (international normalized ratio [INR] of 2.0 to 3.0) for 4 days, with warfarin continued for 6 months. Early outpatient management results in substantial cost savings.

The 35-year-old woman has acute proximal DVT that is secondary to her knee arthroplasty and oral contraceptives. She is not a candidate for outpatient management with low–molecular-weight heparin and warfarin because of her wound hematoma. Also, she should have human chorionic gonadotropin (β-HCG) checked before initiating warfarin, because warfarin has severe fetopathic effects during the first trimester of a pregnancy. This is a first episode of DVT accompanied by a reversible risk factor; warfarin can be discontinued after 3 months because the risk of recurrence is low (approximately 5% over 2 years).

The 74-year-old woman has recurrent idiopathic DVT. This patient's risk for recurrent venous thromboembolism is substantial (approximately 20% over 2 years). In the absence of compelling risk factors for bleeding, she should receive warfarin indefinitely.

The previously healthy 80-year-old man has acute DVT that presumably is secondary to his age and the immobility associated with extended air travel. However, his unexplained anemia and thrombocytopenia raise the question of an occult lymphoproliferative malignancy. Inpatient management with therapeutic doses of heparin overlapped with warfarin is appropriate. Six months of warfarin also is appropriate in this patient.

Bibliography

1. **Hirsh J, Hoak J.** Management of deep venous thrombosis and pulmonary embolism. A statement for healthcare professionals. Council on Thrombosis (in consultation with the Council on Cardiovascular Radiology), American Heart Association. Circulation. 1996;93:2212-45.

2. **Schulman S, Rhedin AS, Lindmarker P, Carlsson A, Larfars G, Nicol P, et al.** A comparison of six weeks with six months of oral anticoagulant therapy after a first episode of venous thromboembolism. Duration of Anticoagulation Trial Study Group. N Engl J Med. 1995;332:1661-5.

3. **Ridker PM, Miletich JP, Stampfer MJ, Goldhaber SZ, Lindpaintner K, Hennekens CH.** Factor V Leiden and risks of idiopathic venous thromboembolism. Circulation. 1995;92:2800-2.

4. **Hyers TM, Hull RD, Weg JG.** Antithrombotic therapy for venous thromboembolic disease. Chest. 1995;108:335S-51S.

5. **Levine M, Gent M, Hirsh J, Leclerc J, Anderson D, Weitz J, et al.** A comparison of low-molecular-weight heparin administered primarily at home with unfractionated heparin administered in the hospital for proximal deep-vein thrombosis. N Engl J Med. 1996;334:677-81.

DYSPNEA

Dyspnea Question 1
Answer: D

EDUCATIONAL OBJECTIVE: Diagnose constrictive pericarditis in patients with rheumatoid arthritis.

Constrictive pericarditis is the most common clinically important cardiac manifestation of rheumatoid arthritis, but it is relatively rare. These patients usually present with an insidious illness, and Kussmaul's sign is often positive, as it is in this patient. Evaluation should begin with echocardiography, although in patients with constrictive pericarditis, echocardiography may not be diagnostic and right heart catheterization may be required. The treatment is surgery.

Pulmonary hypertension can present with right heart failure, but an increased pulmonic second sound would be expected as well as other findings such as a right ventricular gallop. Bronchiolitis obliterans does not cause right heart failure. Cardiomyopathies generally cause left heart failure, cardiac enlargement, and pulmonary congestion. Cirrhosis causes edema, but the venous pressure is generally low or normal because the edema is due to a combination of increased portal pressure and hypoalbuminemia.

Bibliography

1. **Escalante A, Kaufman RL, Quismorio FP Jr, Beardmore TD, et al.** Cardiac compression in rheumatoid pericarditis. Semin Arthritis Rheum. 1990;20:148-63.

Dyspnea Question 2
Answer: B

EDUCATIONAL OBJECTIVE: Treat the patient with minimally symptomatic heart failure due to left ventricular systolic dysfunction.

This young man shows evidence of an idiopathic dilated cardiomyopathy. The absence of an S_3 is not unexpected because left ventricular function is only modestly depressed. The echocardiographic features of biventricular dysfunction and dilatation are characteristic of a primary myopathic process. Angiotensin-converting enzyme (ACE) inhibition is the initial treatment of choice for asymptomatic or minimally symptomatic left ventricular dysfunction, regardless of the cause of the disorder. Results from the SOLVD Prevention Trial of enalapril in patients with asymptomatic left ventricular dysfunction confirm a 29% risk reduction in either death or development of overt symptomatic heart failure over a 3-year time period. Although most patients in this study had ischemic left ventricular dysfunction, the beneficial effects of enalapril appear to be independent of disease origin.

A diuretic agent, such as furosemide, has no role in the treatment of patients without evidence of volume overload, because it may increase renin and angiotensin II production. Digoxin's role should be limited to patients with persistently symptomatic heart failure who are already receiving treatment with optimal doses of an ACE inhibitor and diuretic. The Digoxin Investigation Group (DIG) trial showed that chronic digoxin therapy improved symptoms but did not result in a survival benefit. The suppression of asymptomatic premature ventricular contractions by amiodarone has not been convincingly shown to lower sudden death risk in patients with impaired left ventricular function. The role of β-blockade in minimally symptomatic patients with dilated cardiomyopathy remains speculative.

This patient should also be advised to limit his physical activities and avoid running during the acute phase of his illness.

Bibliography

1. The SOLVD Investigators. Effect of enalapril on mortality and the development of heart failure in asymptomatic patients with reduced left ventricular ejection fractions. N Engl J Med. 1992;237:685-91.

2. **Konstam MA, Kronenberg MW, Rousseau MF, Udelson JE, Melin J, Stewart D, et al.** Effect of the angiotensin converting enzyme inhibitor enalapril on the long-term progression of left ventricular dilatation in patients with asymptomatic systolic dysfunction. SOLVD (Studies of Left Ventricular Dysfunction) Investigators. Circulation. 1993;88:2277-83.

3. **Singh SN, Fletcher RD, Fisher SG, Singh BN, Lewis HD, Deedwania PC, et al.** Amiodarone in patients with congestive heart failure and asymptomatic ventricular arrhythmia. Survival Trial of Antiarrhythmic Therapy in Congestive Heart Failure. N Engl J Med. 1995;333:77-82.

Dyspnea Question 3
Answer: A

EDUCATIONAL OBJECTIVE: Identify congenital heart disease in an adult.

The patient's history, physical examination, and laboratory findings most likely suggest an atrial septal defect, ostium secundum in location. If this were a ventricular septal defect, one would expect the murmur to radiate to the right of the sternum and possibly to be associated with a systolic thrill. In patients with uncomplicated, small ventricular septal defects, the chest radiograph does not show enlargement of the pulmonary arteries or increased pulmonary blood flow. Pulmonic stenosis is excluded by the absence of an ejection sound (that is, a sharp early systolic sound occurring just after the S_1). Furthermore, the electrocardiogram of isolated pulmonic stenosis usually shows evidence for right ventricular hypertrophy, and the chest radiograph does not show increased pulmonary blood flow in the absence of other cardiac lesions. Finally, the murmur of a patent ductus arteriosus should be continuous in the age group of this patient, for there is little likelihood that pulmonary hypertension (leading to reversal of the shunt and loss of the continuous quality of the murmur) would have occurred at this young age. Because a patent ductus arteriosus usually does not place a strain on the right heart in the absence of pulmonary hypertension, the electrocardiogram is most often normal in such patients.

Bibliography

1. **Perloff JK.** Clinical Recognition of Congenital Heart Disease. Philadelphia: WB Saunders; 1987:188-220, 272-350, 365-404, 467-98.

Dyspnea Questions 4-7
Answers: 4(B); 5(D); 6(C); 7(E)

EDUCATIONAL OBJECTIVE: Distinguish pleural fluid characteristics associated with different disorders.

Patients with nephrotic syndrome commonly develop pleural effusions caused by hypoalbuminemia or pulmonary thromboembolism. Pleural effusions associated with hypoalbuminemia are usually serous, bilateral, of equal size, and subpulmonic. Protein concentration is less than 1 g/dL, and lactate dehydrogenase (LDH) concentration is less than 100 U/L. Pleural effusion due to thromboembolic disease is usually exudative, unilateral, hemorrhagic pleural effusion or bilateral effusions of disparate size. In a series of 36 patients with nephrotic syndrome, 22% had pulmonary emboli. In addition, the nephrotic syndrome may be due to or complicated by renal vein thrombosis, in which the incidence of pulmonary emboli is about 50%. The pathogenic mechanisms underlying vascular thrombosis under these circumstances are uncertain, but urinary loss of clotting inhibitors, hemoconcentration due to edema and diuretics, increased platelet aggregation, and heightened hepatic synthesis of fibrinogen and other clotting factors probably combine to cause a hypercoagulable state. Hemorrhagic pleural effusions can also be caused by malignancy or trauma. If the LDH is greater than two thirds the serum upper limit of normal, if the fluid-to-serum LDH ratio is greater than 0.6 or the fluid-to-serum protein ratio is greater than 0.5, the pleural effusion is an exudate with 99% sensitivity and 80% specificity.

Neoplasms of any type can metastasize to the pleura, but carcinoma of the lung and breast and lymphomas account for 75% of all malignant pleural effusions. Ovarian carcinoma is the fourth leading cause and accounts for 8% of all malignant pleural effusions. In the 56-year-old woman with widely metastatic ovarian carcinoma who develops exertional dyspnea and bilateral pleural effusions over several months, pleural effusion due to metastatic carcinoma is the most likely diagnosis. Malignant pleural effusions may be serous, serosanguineous, or grossly bloody. A serous effusion can result from either lymphatic obstruction or an endobronchial lesion with atelectasis. A grossly bloody effusion suggests direct pleural involvement with tumor. Malignant pleural effusions are usually exudates but up to 10% are transudates, and the protein concentration ranges from 1.5 g/dL to 8 g/dL. At times, the pleural fluid–to–serum protein ratio may be low, but the fluid qualifies as an exudate by LDH criteria. When pleural fluid qualifies as an exudate by LDH criteria alone, as in this case, it is highly suggestive of malignancy. One third of malignant pleural effusions have a pleural fluid pH of less than 7.3, and these low-pH effusions have been noted to have low glucose concentrations as well (less than 60 mg/dL). Patients with low-pH, low-glucose pleural effusions usually have large tumor burdens and significantly shorter mean survival (2.5 months) than those with normal pH and glucose (11.5 months). An elevated pleural fluid amylase (greater than the upper limits of normal for serum or pleural fluid:serum ratio greater than 1) can occur with acute pancreatitis, pancreatic pseudocyst, esophageal rupture, malignancy, and ruptured ectopic pregnancy. About 10% of malignant pleural effusions have high amylase concentrations, and although these effusions are usually due to pancreatic, lung, or ovarian cancer, any carcinoma can cause an elevated pleural fluid amylase.

In the case of the 60-year-old man who presents with painful swollen joints and an asymptomatic pleural effusion, rheumatoid pleurisy is a likely diagnosis. Pleural involvement probably is the most common thoracic manifestation of rheumatoid disease. Clinical rheumatoid pleurisy occurs in approximately 5% of patients with rheumatoid disease and has a striking male predominance. The chest radiograph usually shows a small to moderate unilateral effusion. The effusion may appear turbid with a yellow/green tint, and sometimes the fluid contains debris due to breakdown of necrotic nodules from the visceral pleura. Effusions are exudative by protein (up to 7.3 g/dL) and LDH criteria (frequently with concentrations greater than 1000 U/L). The most striking and consistent features of rheumatoid pleural effusions are a low pleural fluid glucose and pH and a high LDH.

Esophageal perforation most commonly arises as a complication of esophagoscopic examination. Patients with spontaneous rupture of the esophagus commonly have a history of retching or vomiting followed by severe chest pain and develop a pleural effusion that is usually left-sided. The pleural fluid findings depend on the degree of perforation and the timing of the thoracentesis in relation to the injury. Minor perforations without mediastinal pleural tears or early thoracentesis will show a serous-sterile exudate with a predominance of polymorphonuclear cells and a normal pleural fluid amylase concentration and pH. Once the mediastinal pleura tears, amylase of salivary origin appears in the fluid in high concentration and the pH rapidly and progressively falls. The reason that the pleural fluid is so markedly acid (in the range of 6) is that glucose, the substrate for acid generation, tends to be readily available in the pleural fluid. Other findings in the pleural fluid suggestive of esophageal rupture include the presence of squamous epithelial cells and food particles. In this case, the pleural fluid finding most compatible with esophageal rupture is an exudative, purulent fluid with a normal glucose, very low pH, and elevated amylase. This is in contrast to a patient with an empyema in whom the glucose is diminished with a normal amylase.

Bibliography

1. **Sahn SA.** State of the art. The pleura. Am Rev Respir Dis. 1988;138:184-234.

2. **Rodriguez-Panadero F, Lopez-Mejias J.** Survival time of patients with pleural metastatic carcinoma predicted by glucose and pH studies. Chest. 1989;95:320-4.

3. **Light RW.** Pleural Disease. Malvern, PA: Lea & Febiger; 1990.

Dyspnea Question 8
Answer: E

EDUCATIONAL OBJECTIVE: Recognize the signs and symptoms of altitude sickness.

Travelers to areas of elevation higher than that they are accustomed to may experience difficulty in acclimatization. This is particularly true when ascending from sea level to 9500 feet and participating in vigorous physical exertion, as this patient did. The findings are consistent with pulmonary edema in a young man at low risk for cardiac decompensation. This scenario should raise suspicion of noncardiogenic pulmonary edema, in this case due to high altitude. The precise factors that place a patient at risk of this phenomenon are not known. Return to a lower altitude often results in prompt and dramatic recovery.

In the absence of volume depletion, which is not suggested in this patient, normal saline is unlikely to be therapeutic and may worsen gas exchange. Furosemide would be appropriate for pulmonary edema associated with congestive heart failure or other volume overload states. The pathophysiologic mechanism in noncardiogenic pulmonary edema is primarily a capillary leak phenomenon, and furosemide may not be as effective. Corticosteroids or acetazolamide (through carbonic anhydrase inhibition) may be effective when descent to a lower altitude is not immediately feasible.

Bibliography

1. High altitude sickness. Med Lett. 1988;30:89-91.

Dyspnea Question 9
Answer: A

EDUCATIONAL OBJECTIVE: Recognize the interrelation of clinical factors that determine oxygen transport.

The delivery of oxygen (Do_2) to metabolizing cells is a fundamentally important function of the pulmonary and cardiovascular systems. Do_2 is determined by the amount of oxygen contained in blood (termed oxygen capacity or Cao_2) and the rate at which blood flows to the periphery, which is measured as cardiac output (CO). A patient's Cao_2 can be calculated by measuring the hemoglobin content of blood (Hb) in units of g/dL and multiplying it by the fractional oxygen saturation of Hb (Sa_{O_2}). This term is then multiplied by 1.34, which is the volume of oxygen that can combine with 1 g of fully saturated Hb. A small proportion of oxygen is delivered to cells in solution via blood; this amount is calculated by multiplying the partial pressure of oxygen (Pa_{O_2}) by the constant 0.003. Delivery of oxygen is then calculated by multiplying Ca_{O_2} by CO (L/min). A factor of 10 dL/L is used to multiply the final result to convert units to mL/min. The final equation for D_{O_2}, therefore, is:

$$D_{O_2} = (Pa_{O_2} \times 0.003 + [Hb\ g/dL \times Sa_{O_2} \times 1.34\ mL/g]) \times CO\ L/min \times 10\ dL/L$$

This equation has clinical utility because it predicts the magnitude of effect on D_{O_2} of various interventions that alter Pa_{O_2}, Hb, Sa_{O_2}, and CO. For instance, changes in Pa_{O_2} have little effect on the quantity of O_2 in solution because of the small value of the multiplier factor 0.003. Increasing Hb from 9 to 10 g/dL represents only an 11% increase in Hb as a multiplier of the low numerical values for the example patient of Sa_{O_2} (0.85) and CO (3 L/min). Similarly, increasing Sa_{O_2} from 0.85 to 0.95 is only a 12% increase in its multiplier effect on the other terms in the equation. Increasing CO from 3 to 4 L/min, however, increases the multiplier effect of CO by 33% and would, therefore, have the largest effect on increasing D_{O_2}. When uncertain as to the relative benefits of maximizing Hb, Sa_{O_2}, or CO, clinicians can put values for each into the equation and compare the calculated results for D_{O_2}. Option A would increase D_{O_2} from 312.5 to 416.6 mL/min, as shown below:

$$(55\ mm\ Hg \times 0.003 + [9\ g/dL \times 0.85 \times 1.34\ mL/g]) \times 3\ L/min \times 10\ dL/L = 312.5\ mL/min$$

$$(55\ mm\ Hg \times 0.003 + [9\ g/dL \times 0.85 \times 1.34\ mL/g]) \times 4\ L/min \times 10\ dL/L = 416.6\ mL/min$$

Increasing the pH of the example patient would actually decrease the availability of oxygen to metabolizing tissue because the oxyhemoglobin dissociation curve would shift to the left. This leftward shift indicates that the affinity of Hb for oxygen increases, thereby decreasing the unloading of oxygen to metabolically active cells.

Bibliography

1. **Snyder JV.** Oxygen transport: the model and reality. In: Snyder JV, Pinsky MR, eds. Oxygen Transport in the Critically Ill. Chicago: Yearbook Medical Publishers, Inc.; 1987:3-15.

2. **Watkins GM, Rabelo A, Pizak LF, Sheldon GF.** The left shifted oxyhemoglobin curve in sepsis: a preventable defect. Ann Surg. 1974;180:213-20.

3. **Glauser FL, Polatty RC, Sessler CN.** Worsening oxygenation in the mechanically ventilated patient. Causes, mechanisms, and early detection. Am Rev Respir Dis. 1988;138:458-65.

Dyspnea Question 10
Answer: D

EDUCATIONAL OBJECTIVE: Recognize the features of severe pulmonary hypertension and select the appropriate initial diagnostic study.

This young woman presents with a classic history for severe pulmonary hypertension. The first test should be an echocardiogram to establish the presence of severe pulmonary hypertension and to exclude significant mitral stenosis. Although she has risk factors (obesity and oral contraceptives) for pulmonary embolism and chronic large-vessel thromboemboli, pulmonary angiography is not appropriate as an initial diagnostic test. Ventilation-perfusion lung scanning should be done after pulmonary hypertension has been established by echocardiography and before pulmonary angiography is considered. A normal perfusion lung scan obviates the need for pulmonary angiography in this situation.

Her youth and healthy appearance are characteristic of patients with this condition and often mislead the physician when severe pulmonary hypertension is present. Thus, recommending an exercise test without first excluding severe pulmonary hypertension is not appropriate. Similarly, spirometry, although appropriate for the evaluation of known pulmonary hypertension, is not helpful for the initial detection of clinically suspected pulmonary hypertension. Antinuclear antibody is an appropriate screening test for collagen vascular disease, but it is not useful as an initial laboratory study when the clinician suspects pulmonary hypertension.

Bibliography

1. **Rubin LJ.** Primary pulmonary hypertension. Chest. 1993;104:236-50.

Dyspnea Question 11
Answer: D

EDUCATIONAL OBJECTIVE: Recognize epiglottitis in an adult and use appropriate diagnostic procedures.

The most common symptoms in adults presenting with epiglottitis are sore throat (95%), odynophagia (94%), and muffled voice (54%). The patient in this case presents with dyspnea in the setting of a sore throat and voice change. Thromboembolism can occur in a small minority of patients taking oral contraceptive pills, but this patient's presentation does not suggest a pulmonary embolism. A direct approach for diagnosis of suspected epiglottitis is most appropriate. Either indirect or direct laryngoscopy in a setting where intubation is available is the appropriate diagnostic test. The patient has dyspnea and is anxious. Lateral neck films have a sensitivity of only 79% and sending a patient with dyspnea and likely epiglottitis for lateral neck films poses a risk to the patient. Neck computed tomography scanning has not been evaluated for the diagnosis of epiglottitis and is not recommended.

Bibliography

1. **Frantz TD, Rasgon BM, Quesenberry CP Jr.** Acute epiglottitis in adults. Analysis of 129 cases. JAMA. 1994;272:1358-60.

Dyspnea Question 12
Answer: C

EDUCATIONAL OBJECTIVE: Identify the pharmacologic approach in the risk management of the pregnant patient with asthma.

The management of asthma during pregnancy necessitates consideration of the risk and the potential benefits of therapy. Maternal respiratory compromise may cause fetal hypoxia, leading to increased perinatal mortality and low birth weight. Patients with moderately severe asthma require terbutaline or albuterol along with inhaled cromolyn sodium or beclomethasone. Cromolyn sodium administered parenterally to pregnant rodents has shown no evidence of increased fetal malformations compared with controls. Observational studies of 296 women taking cromolyn also showed no increased rates of fetal malformations. In a controlled trial of 40 women with severe asthma, neonatal mortality, spontaneous abortion, and congenital malformations were not increased in users of inhaled beclomethasone. Breast-feeding is not contraindicated for patients taking inhaled glucocorticoids because these drugs are not present in milk. Ipratropium bromide should be used during pregnancy only if clearly needed.

Although some patients respond well to theophylline, inhaled β-agonists as needed are preferred due to the toxicity and monitoring requirements of theophylline. Allergen immunotherapy for the atopic pregnant patient who does not wish to use other oral medications may be continued at the same current dose without escalation as long as the patient does not have frequent reactions. In asthmatic patients with extreme sensitivity, the risk versus benefit must be weighed because anaphylactic reaction could adversely effect the fetus. Oral steroids would not be indicated without first trying inhaled cromolyn or lower-dose inhaled corticosteroids.

Bibliography

1. **Schatz M, Hoffman CP, Zeiger RS.** The course and management of asthma and allergic diseases during pregnancy. In: Middleton E, ed. Allergy: Principles and Practice. 4th ed. St. Louis: Mosby-Year Book; 1993:1301-42.
2. **Clark SL.** Asthma in pregnancy. Obstet Gynecol. 1993;82:1036-40.
3. **Barnes PJ.** Inhaled glucocorticoids for asthma. N Engl J Med. 1995;332:868-75.
4. **Greenberger PA, Patterson R.** Beclomethasone dipropionate for severe asthma during pregnancy. Ann Intern Med. 1983;98:478-80.

Dyspnea Questions 13-15
Answers: 13(D); 14(A); 15(C)

EDUCATIONAL OBJECTIVE: Choose appropriate asthma treatment modalities depending on presentation and severity of the disease.

The 35-year-old man in the first item requires urgent attention, systemic corticosteroid therapy, and close follow-up for evidence of either improvement with treatment or respiratory failure; he may have to be admitted to the medical intensive care unit, if available.

Mild intermittent asthma or acute asthmatic episodes predictably associated only with specific events or exposure such as exercise (as in the 18-year-old male athlete) or allergen exposure (for example, cat) can ordinarily be treated with a β₂-agonist metered-dose inhaler (MDI) as needed. Exercise-induced asthma can often be prevented by the use of the MDI before exercise.

A patient presenting with a history of chronic obstructive pulmonary disease (COPD) and significant respiratory impairment deserves an adequate therapeutic trial with systemic corticosteroids, provided that there is no other cause of an exacerbation of COPD, such as bacterial bronchitis or pneumonia, cor pulmonale, or congestive heart failure. The patient denied purulent sputum production, was afebrile, and the chest radiograph was clear; therefore, antibiotic therapy is not indicated. A full, adequate trial of prednisone, 60 mg daily for 7 to 14 days, is needed, followed by tapering quickly by 5-mg/d decrements to 20 mg/d and subsequent slower taper and follow-up spirometry. Divided daily doses are considered by some experts to be more effective during the initial high-dose regimen.

Adequate follow-up will document the extent of reversibility, if any, and help establish goals for continuing care.

Bibliography

1. Guidelines for the diagnosis and management of asthma. Highlights of the expert panel report 2. National Asthma Education Program. Bethesda, MD: National Heart, Lung and Blood Institutes. NIH Publication #97-4051A, 1997.
2. **Kaliner M, Lemanske R.** Rhinitis and asthma. JAMA. 1992;268:2807-29.
3. **Kay AB.** Asthma and inflammation. J Allergy Clin Immunol. 1991;87:893-910.
4. **McFadden ER Jr, Gilbert IA.** Asthma. N Engl J Med. 1992;327:1928-37.
5. **Weinberger SE.** Recent advances in pulmonary medicine. N Engl J Med. 1993;328:1389-97, 1462-70.

together with the appropriate history, the diagnosis of asthma.

Bibliography

1. **Chan-Yeung M, Harber P, Bailey W, Balmes J, Barnhart S, Hargreave FE, et al.** Guidelines for the evaluation of impairment disability in patients with asthma. Am Rev Respir Dis. 1993;147:1056-61.
2. **McFadden ER Jr, Gilbert IA.** Asthma. N Engl J Med. 1992;327:1928-37.
3. **Hargreave FE, Dolovich J, Newhouse, M.** The assessment and treatment of asthma: a conference report. J Allergy Clin Immunol. 1990;85:1097-111.
4. Guidelines for the diagnosis and management of asthma. Highlights of the expert panel report 2. National Asthma Education Program. Bethesda, MD: National Heart, Lung and Blood Institute. NIH Publication #97-4051A, 1997.

Dyspnea Question 16
Answer: D

EDUCATIONAL OBJECTIVE: Recall the essential criterion for the definitive diagnosis of asthma.

Although items A through E may all be associated with asthma or lead toward a clinical diagnosis of asthma, only the documentation of the reversibility of airways obstruction is definitive. To establish a diagnosis of asthma, a physician must show that episodic symptoms of air flow obstruction are present, air flow obstruction is at least partially reversible, and alternative diagnoses have been excluded. Patients with atopic asthma, allergic rhinitis, or no disease may have positive skin tests to inhalant allergens ("demonstrated atopic status"). Nonatopic patients have other forms of asthma (occupational or idiopathic). Relief of symptoms with bronchodilator therapy may occur in chronic obstructive pulmonary disease (COPD) or other conditions, is subjective and is insufficient evidence for a diagnosis of asthma without documented spirometric evidence of concurrent reversed obstruction. Decreased FEV_1/FVC simply denotes obstructed airways, and evidence of improved FEV_1 is necessary to diagnose asthma. A positive methacholine challenge is supportive of the diagnosis, but overlap with nonasthmatic individuals makes it nondefinitive.

The degree of reversibility required for a definitive diagnosis of asthma has been much debated. A committee report (Chan-Yeung et al.) has suggested that an improvement in FEV_1 of 12% or greater, with an absolute change of at least 200 mL from the baseline level, confirms that there is significant reversibility and,

Dyspnea Questions 17-19
Answers: 17(C); 18(B); 19(D)

EDUCATIONAL OBJECTIVE: Differentiate various categories of occupational lung disorders.

A careful and complete occupational history allows a clinician to differentiate among occupational disorders with common clinical features. The first case is irritant-induced asthma or reactive airways dysfunction syndrome (RADS) that is caused by airway injury after inhalation of toxic levels of a respiratory irritant (ammonia, caustic acids, smoke). Symptoms begin almost immediately after the inciting exposure and can persist for years. The diagnosis is based on a compatible history and confirmed by a positive methacholine test. Spirometry and physical examination are often normal in affected patients.

In addition to diagnosing RADS, methacholine testing is clinically useful. The test is considered positive if the provocative dose of methacholine required to cause a 20% decrease from baseline FEV_1 (PD_{20}) is 10 mg/mL or less. Because of the good predictive value of a negative test, a normal methacholine test can effectively exclude current occupational and nonoccupational asthma. Therefore, methacholine testing is often used to exclude cough-variant asthma in patients with a chronic cough. However, a positive test is nonspecific, that is, methacholine sensitivity is present not only in most patients with active asthma but also in a large proportion of patients with chronic bronchitis, as well as atopic and asymptomatic patients. Thus, in order to prove occupational asthma in a worker who has a positive methacholine test, the clinician must prove that airway obstruction is work-related and that it improves when the patient is away from work. This requires serial monitoring of peak flow rates at work or, if possible, a specific inhalation test performed by a specialist.

Bronchiolitis obliterans is an inflammatory and fibrotic obliterative disorder of the terminal bronchioles that can be caused by injury to the airways after inhalation of toxic irritants and is characterized by airway obstruction and diffusion abnormalities. In contrast, the diffusing capacity for carbon monoxide (DLco) in RADS is normal. Bronchiolitis obliterans is also a sequela of viral respiratory infections, is a rare feature of rheumatoid arthritis, and has been documented as a complication of autologous bone marrow transplantation.

The second case is a classic presentation of acute hypersensitivity pneumonitis with characteristic systemic symptoms, dyspnea, bilateral crackles, a diffusion abnormality, and spirometry pattern consistent with a restrictive ventilatory pattern. The chest radiograph can be normal but more often reveals bilateral pulmonary infiltrates. Serum precipitins to *Bacillus subtilis* and *Aspergillus* enzymes and clinical resolution after leaving the work environment would confirm the diagnosis.

The third case is a typical presentation of IgE-mediated occupational asthma caused by microbial enzymes used by bakers as dough conditioners. Baker's asthma is also caused by cereal proteins (wheat, rye) and mold contaminants (*Aspergillus, Alternaria*) in flour. This patient exhibited a dual-phase asthmatic response after inhaling enzyme powder at work. Serial changes in peak expiratory flow rate at work and home and a positive skin prick test to the extracted enzyme would confirm a diagnosis of occupational asthma.

Organic toxic dust syndrome refers to conditions such as grain fever, which is a toxic noninfiltrative disorder caused by inhalation of high levels of endotoxin or mycotoxin in grain dust. Typical symptoms include fever, myalgias, dyspnea, cough, and airways obstruction but without diffusion abnormalities or parenchymal involvement.

Bibliography

1. **Salvaggio JE.** The identification of hypersensitivity pneumonitis. Hosp Pract. 1995;30:57-66.

2. **Fink JN.** Hypersensitivity pneumonitis. In: Middleton E, ed. Allergy: Principles and Practice. 4th ed. St. Louis: Mosby-Year Book; 1993.

3. **Chan Yeung M, Malo JL.** Occupational asthma. N Engl J Med. 1995;333:107-12.

Dyspnea Question 20
Answer: B

EDUCATIONAL OBJECTIVE: Diagnose deconditioning as a cause of dyspnea in patients with chronic cardiopulmonary disease.

This 52-year-old man has congestive heart failure that is well-compensated and is suffering from ongoing dyspnea after a protracted illness. Deconditioning is an important, often neglected cause of dyspnea, especially in patients with underlying chronic illness. Recent studies have shown that deconditioning frequently contributes to the sense of breathlessness and fatigue felt by patients with chronic congestive heart failure. It is a potentially reversible process that significantly interferes with the functional capacity of patients with compensated heart failure. Distinguishing deconditioning from cardiac disease may be difficult.

Cardiopulmonary exercise testing can be useful in determining the cause of dyspnea in patients with chronic cardiopulmonary disease. Deconditioning is characterized by a decrease in maximal exercise capacity with normal gas exchange, heart rate, and cardiac output in response to exercise. Exercise is not limited by respiratory factors assessed by relating maximum ventilation at peak exercise to the maximal voluntary ventilation (often reported as the "dyspnea index"). Deconditioned patients may have a mild decrease in the anaerobic threshold (the threshold where anaerobic metabolism supplements energy production). Patients with cardiac disease have a reduced cardiac output and may experience a mild increase in the alveolar-arterial O_2 (A–aO_2) gradient in response to exercise. The anaerobic threshold is typically reduced. This patient has a diminished anaerobic threshold, which is seen in either condition. However, the congestive heart failure is well-compensated on his current medication, and deconditioning is the most likely cause of the persistent symptoms.

The A-aO_2 gradient during exercise is usually markedly increased in patients with pulmonary vascular disease such as chronic pulmonary emboli and in patients with pulmonary fibrosis or interstitial lung disease. Obstruction to airflow should be evident on the spirometry parameters in patients with chronic obstructive pulmonary disease. In addition, the breathing reserve is inadequate and the dyspnea index is elevated, which correlates with the severity of disease.

Bibliography

1. **Gillespie DJ, Staats BA.** Unexplained dyspnea. Mayo Clin Proc. 1994;69:657-63.

2. **Weisman IM, Zeballos RJ.** An integrated approach to the interpretation of cardiopulmonary exercise testing. Clin Chest Med. 1994;15:421-45.

Dyspnea Questions 21-23
Answers: 21(C); 22(D); 23(E)

EDUCATIONAL OBJECTIVE: Recognize the clinical presentation and management of patients with interstitial lung disease.

This is a common clinical scenario in a patient with idiopathic pulmonary fibrosis. Often at the onset of the illness, superficial questioning may not reveal real complaints. However, a history of progressive breathlessness or cough and a reduction in the patient's level of activity (from 1 to 5 years before presentation) is obtained. The differential diagnosis in this case includes idiopathic pulmonary fibrosis, chronic hypersensitivity pneumonitis, chronic idiopathic bronchiolitis obliterans with organizing pneumonia, connective tissue disease such as rheumatoid arthritis or progressive systemic sclerosis, and chronic sarcoidosis.

A lung biopsy establishes the diagnosis and the extent and severity of disease. Fiberoptic bronchoscopy with transbronchial lung biopsy may be the initial procedure when sarcoidosis, lymphangitic carcinomatosis, eosinophilic pneumonia, Goodpasture's syndrome, or infection is suspected. However, in this setting, an open lung biopsy by limited thoracotomy or thoracoscopy is preferred. Lung biopsy is indicated because it provides an accurate diagnosis, excludes neoplastic and infectious processes that occasionally mimic progressive interstitial disease, occasionally identifies a more treatable process than originally suspected (for example, chronic hypersensitivity pneumonitis), and provides a better assessment of disease activity. Because this patient has no significant underlying disease other than his lung disease, there is no contraindication to open lung biopsy.

Pulmonary function tests in patients with diffuse interstitial lung disease most often reveal a restrictive pattern with reduced lung volumes, reduced diffusing capacity for carbon monoxide, and arterial hypoxemia that is often exaggerated or elicited by exercise. In general, as the disease progresses and the lung becomes stiffer, lung compliance decreases and lung volumes fall. The presence of an obstructive ventilatory defect would be distinctly uncommon, especially in a non-smoker without concomitant chronic obstructive pulmonary disease (COPD). Resting PaO_2 may be normal, but the alveolar-arterial oxygen gradient is usually elevated because the patient is hyperventilating.

Gallium lung scanning has no role in the diagnosis and staging of idiopathic pulmonary fibrosis. The inferior group of deep cervical lymph nodes, particularly those lying medially on the scalenus anterior muscle and below the omohyoid muscle (the so-called *scalene nodes*), become involved in various inflammatory, infectious, or neoplastic processes that originate within the thorax. Consequently, a scalene lymph node biopsy is used as a diagnostic procedure in the evaluation of pulmonary disease, especially if the nodes are palpable or noted to be enlarged by radiographic imaging of the superior mediastinum. The technique may be employed to diagnose lung cancer (up to 90% positive when the nodes are palpable) or sarcoidosis (with an 84% rate of positive scalene node biopsies in confirmed cases of the disease). Scalene lymph node biopsy is not indicated in this patient. Percutaneous renal biopsy with immunofluorescence may be indicated in the diagnostic evaluation of a patient with diffuse alveolar hemorrhage or vasculitis, such as in Goodpasture's syndrome.

Repeating the chest radiographs and pulmonary function studies at 6-month intervals may be useful to follow the course of the patient's disease. At this time, the best approach is to begin treatment. Spontaneous remissions do not occur in idiopathic pulmonary fibrosis, and the disease is invariably progressive. A trial of corticosteroid therapy is indicated once the diagnosis is confirmed. A favorable clinical response occurs in approximately one third of patients. Therapy is often initiated with prednisone, 1.0 to 1.5 mg/kg per day (using ideal body weight), and not to exceed a total dose of 100 mg per day. This is given as a single, oral dose in the morning. Alternate-day therapy is not recommended. After approximately 2 to 3 months of daily prednisone therapy, chest radiographs and pulmonary physiologic studies are re-evaluated. If the patient is responsive, that is, improved or stabilized, the daily dosage of prednisone is tapered (by 5 to 10 mg each week) until a maintenance dosage of 0.5 mg/kg per day is reached. This dosage is continued for an additional 3 to 6 months with the realization that, with clinical and physiologic deterioration, the dosage may have to be raised to previous levels. In general, it is unlikely that corticosteroid therapy can be discontinued, and patients are usually maintained on 0.25 mg/kg per day. In fact, no clear-cut guidelines exist for the length of therapy in idiopathic pulmonary fibrosis. At least 1 year of therapy with or without another immunosuppressive agent and then a gradual tapering with regular follow-up (3 to 6 months) have been advocated. Many clinicians believe that lifelong treatment is required in patients who respond to the initial therapy. Cyclophosphamide, azathioprine, and colchicine are alternative agents used in treatment. Current methods are inadequate to predict response to treatment. Penicillamine has not been shown to be effective.

Lung transplantation is an encouraging treatment modality for patients with end-stage lung disease. However, this patient's age as well as his current status would be contraindications to lung transplantation. The criteria for recipient selection include (1) age less than 55 years, (2) poor functional status with limited life expectancy (less than 12 to 18 months), (3) no current treatment or health problem that will increase the risk of the operation or limit its long-term success, (4) ineffectiveness or unavailability of medical therapy, (5) sta-ble psychological profile, (6) absence of illicit drug use and no tobacco use or alcohol abuse, and (7) no other evidence of major organ dysfunction or contraindications to immunosuppressive therapy.

Bibliography

1. **du Bois RM.** Idiopathic pulmonary fibrosis. Annu Rev Med. 1993;44:441-50.

2. **Haslam PL.** Cryptogenic fibrosing alveolitis. In: Baughman RP (ed). Bronchoalveolar Lavage. St. Louis: Mosby-Year Book; 1992:116-36.

3. **King TE Jr, Mortenson RL.** Syndromes that mimic idiopathic pulmonary fibrosis. Immunol Clin North Am. 1992;12:461-89.

4. **Mortenson RL, King TE Jr.** Idiopathic pulmonary fibrosis. In: Lichtenstein LM, Fauci AS (eds). Current Therapy in Allergy, Immunology, and Rheumatology. Philadelphia: BC Decker, Inc; 1992:233-41.

5. **Wade JF III, King TE Jr.** Infiltrative and interstitial lung disease in the elderly. Clin Chest Med. 1993;14:501-21.

DYSURIA

Dysuria Question 1
Answer: B

EDUCATIONAL OBJECTIVE: Recognize drugs that are contraindicated in patients taking methotrexate.

Trimethoprim-sulfamethoxazole inhibits dihydrofolate reductase and has been known to enhance methotrexate toxicity. None of the other drugs are associated with a drug–drug interaction. Patients taking methotrexate should notify their practitioners. Patients should be told to give a complete list of medications they are receiving to other physicians they visit to avoid drug–drug interactions.

Bibliography

1. **al-Awadhi A, Dale P, McKendry RJ.** Pancytopenia associated with low dose methotrexate therapy. A regional survey. J Rheumatol. 1993;20:1121-5.

Dysuria Question 2
Answer: D

EDUCATIONAL OBJECTIVE: Manage a patient with urethritis.

The urethral Gram stain is diagnostic for gonococcal infection. Gonorrhea and syphilis are often transmitted together. In addition, when gonorrhea is diagnosed, the presence of *Chlamydia* should be assumed, and both conditions should be treated. Penicillin, amoxicillin, and tetracycline are no longer used for treatment because the prevalence of gonococcal resistance has become too high. Single doses of cefixime, ceftriaxone, and ofloxacin are recommended in the United States. Fluoroquinolone resistance was reported in Asia and Australia as early as 1990 and has begun to appear in the United States. In 1995, outbreaks of fluoroquinolone-resistant gonococcal infection were reported from Seattle and Denver; both outbreaks involved commercial sex workers. Because 15% to 25% of heterosexual men and 30% to 50% of women with gonorrhea are co-infected with *Chlamydia*, all patients with gonococcal infection should also be treated for chlamydial infection. Ofloxacin given for a week, not as a single dose, is effective treatment for *Chlamydia*. A 7-day course of doxycycline is highly effective against *Chlamydia* but not gonorrhea. However, a single 2-g dose of azithromycin is equally effective against both gonorrhea and *Chlamydia*, assures compliance, and, in one study, was more cost effective than doxycycline; treated patients, however, should be warned about possible gastrointestinal side effects, such as nausea and abdominal cramping. Cefixime has no activity against *Chlamydia*. Even though the overall incidence of syphilis is declining in the United States, obtaining a serum VDRL or other nontreponemal test (for example rapid plasma reagin or serum thymic factor) is still recommended.

The responsibility of the physician does not end with treatment of the patient. The physician is obligated to counsel the patient about high-risk behaviors and ensure that the patient's sexual partner(s) is (are) identified and treated. In this case, the patient's wife deserves examination and treatment for gonococcal and chlamydial infection. Testing the patient for antibodies to HIV may provide relief from anxiety and negative reinforcement toward his behavior, but is not recommended routinely for the 1 to 4 million patients who contract gonorrhea or chlamydial infections annually.

Bibliography

1. **Centers for Disease Control and Prevention.** 1993 sexually transmitted diseases treatment guidelines. MMWR. 1993;42(RR-14):1-102.

2. Fluoroquinolone resistance in *Neisseria gonorrhoeae*–Colorado and Washington, 1995. MMWR. 1995;44:761-4.

3. **Magid D, Douglas JM Jr, Schwartz JS.** Doxycycline compared with azithromycin for treating women with genital *Chlamydia trachomatis* infections: an incremental cost-effectiveness analysis. Ann Intern Med. 1996;124:389-99.

Dysuria Question 3
Answer: D

EDUCATIONAL OBJECTIVE: Manage a patient with primary herpes simplex virus infection.

Primary genital herpes simplex virus type 2 (HSV-2) infection can present with significant systemic symptoms including headache, fever, sore throat, and generalized lymphadenopathy. Treatment of primary herpes simplex infections with acyclovir within the first 3 days is effective in shortening the duration and severity of illness. Therefore, this patient should be treated. In contrast, acyclovir treatment for established, recurrent genital herpes infection has minimal impact on symptoms. Sexual partners of patients with HSV-2 infection do not warrant immediate treatment unless they also have systemic symptoms of primary HSV-2 infection. Transmission of HSV-2 to neonates exposed during vaginal delivery from women who are experiencing first-episode HSV-2 infection can be as high as 50%. On the other hand, the transmission risk is minimal in a general population of previously infected, HSV-2 seropositive women. If a recurrent outbreak occurs near the time of delivery, the risk of transmission is about 3%.

Of course, it is appropriate to discuss with the patient and her sexual partner the ramifications of HSV-2 infection and the means of preventing transmission and suppressing frequent or severe recurrences. Although HSV-2 infection can be transmitted when active lesions are present, most transmission actually occurs when the infected partner is asymptomatic. Asymptomatic shedding occurs in more than one half of women taught to do daily cultures for HSV-2 at home and recognize lesions of HSV-2 infection. Careful, prospective studies of HSV-2 acquisition among discordant couples have shown that most transmission occurs as a result of asymptomatic viral shedding. Most, but not all, asymptomatic shedding occurs in the days immediately before and after symptomatic recurrences. Acyclovir prophylaxis can suppress most asymptomatic shedding but may be incompletely successful in preventing transmission. Patients should be counseled that condom use at all times as well as abstinence during symptomatic recurrences is the best means of preventing HSV-2 transmission. Only patients with frequent recurrences (more than five per year) or those with infrequent but severe recurrences should receive continuous acyclovir prophylaxis.

Bibliography

1. **Bryson YJ, Dillon M, Lovett M, Acuna G, Taylor S, Cherry JD, et al.** Treatment of first episodes of genital herpes simplex virus infection with oral acyclovir. A randomized double-blind controlled trial in normal subjects. N Engl J Med. 1983;308:916-21.

2. **Frenkel LM, Garratty EM, Shen JP, Wheeler N, Clark O, Bryson YJ.** Clinical reactivation of herpes simplex virus type 2 infection in seropositive pregnant women with no history of genital herpes. Ann Intern Med. 1993;118:414-8.

3. **Wald A, Zeh J, Selke S, Ashley RL, Corey L.** Virologic characteristics of subclinical and symptomatic genital herpes infections. N Engl J Med. 1995;333:770-5.

4. **Wald A, Zeh J, Barnum G, Davis LG, Corey L.** Suppression of subclinical shedding of herpes simplex virus type 2 with acyclovir. Ann Intern Med. 1996;124:8-15.

Dysuria Questions 4-8
Answers: 4(C); 5(B); 6(B); 7(D); 8(A)

EDUCATIONAL OBJECTIVE: Manage urinary tract infections in various clinical situations.

The successful therapy of urinary tract infections (UTIs) is dependent upon the site of infection (upper or lower tract), the presence or absence of complicating factors such as urinary stones, and the selection of antimicrobial agents that are concentrated in the urine with good activity against the responsible organism. Cure is defined as the clearance of clinical symptoms and signs and eradication of the responsible organisms without relapse. In general, uncomplicated lower tract disease responds more rapidly to treatment and with a lower rate of relapse than upper tract disease; cure rates of more than 95% are expected with appropriate regimens given for 3 days. With upper tract disease the same 3-day regimen may lead to relapses in 30% to 40% of patients, unless treatment is extended to at least 2 weeks. With complicated UTIs the failure rate is also high unless treatment is prolonged. In the case of UTIs complicating chronic indwelling catheterization, the eradication of organisms is difficult, and therapy must be tempered by the knowledge of the development of colonization with resistant strains.

The first patient has uncomplicated UTI with symptoms referable only to the lower tract. Short-course therapy with trimethoprim-sulfamethoxazole or a quinolone should cure more than 95% of compliant patients. It is not cost-effective to obtain a urine culture, because the vast majority of these infections will be caused by *Escherichia coli* that are susceptible to trimethoprim-sulfamethoxazole or a quinolone. Urine cultures are indicated only when there is a failure to respond to treatment by 48 hours or, in the case of recurrence, within weeks after completion of therapy.

The second patient has recurrent UTIs despite repeated bouts of short-course treatment. There is an increased likelihood of infection with resistant organisms because of the previous history of antibiotic exposure. A urine culture is indicated at the start of treatment, and the treatment must be prolonged to reduce the incidence of relapse or persistent colonization and reinfection by the original organism.

Older men with spontaneously developing UTI have a much higher likelihood of having structural or functional abnormalities of the urinary tract or coexisting prostatitis than women. These patients should have the urine cultured, should receive from 2 to 4 weeks of treatment with antimicrobial agents, and in most cases should be evaluated urologically. An exception to the latter rule may be seen in young sexually active men with first episode cystitis, particularly if they are uncircumcised, homosexual, or have a sexual partner with vaginal colonization with uropathogens.

Patients with the syndrome of acute pyelonephritis like the 24-year-old woman may be quite ill constitutionally, have infection that leads to bacteremia and sepsis or septic shock, and may be unable to take oral medications because of nausea and vomiting. Given the potentially dangerous nature of this infection, patients with severe manifestations should be admitted to the hospital for close observation and hydration, in addition to treatment with parenteral broad-spectrum antibiotics. Because many *E. coli* are now resistant to ampicillin by virtue of a β-lactamase activity, the use of β-lactamase-resistant β-lactam (for example, ampicillin-sulbactam) or the combination of ampicillin and gentamicin may provide better initial coverage against both *E. coli* and enterococci. Other options for therapy might include a third-generation cephalosporin or a fluoroquinolone.

Asymptomatic bacteruria or pyuria is the rule in patients with chronic indwelling Foley catheters, such as the 78-year-old woman. Treatment should be reserved for symptomatic episodes only and should be of a sufficient duration to relieve the symptoms.

Bibliography

1. **Stamm WE, Hooten TM.** Management of acute uncomplicated urinary tract infection in adults. N Engl J Med. 1993;329:1328-34.

2. **Lipsky BA.** Urinary tract infections in men. Epidemiology, pathophysiology, diagnosis, and treatment. Ann Intern Med. 1989;110:138-50.

3. **Stamm WE.** Catheter-associated urinary tract infections: epidemiology, pathogenesis and prevention. Am J Med. 1991;91:65-71.

4. **Neu HC.** Urinary tract infections. Am J Med. 1992;92:63-70.

Dysuria Question 9
Answer: E

EDUCATIONAL OBJECTIVE: Know the pathogenesis of reactive arthritis.

This patient's history is compatible with a double infection with *Neisseria* and *Chlamydia*. The antibiotic treatment eradicated only the former pathogen. Following his episode of nonspecific urethritis, the patient developed reactive arthritis or Reiter's syndrome. Although the cause of this condition is not clear, there is strong evidence that the disease is associated with venereal or gut infections. Recent studies have detected antigenic material derived from *Chlamydia, Yersinia,* and *Salmonella* in synovial fluids and tissues from many patients with Reiter's syndrome and reactive arthritis. Other studies involving attempts to culture the bacteria have yielded inconclusive or negative results. Thus, the role of live microorganisms in the induction and maintenance of inflammatory arthritis is still unknown. There is, however, evidence that prolonged treatment with antibiotics of the tetracycline or erythromycin class significantly decreases the duration of illness in *Chlamydia*-triggered disease, but patients with nonchlamydial reactive arthritis do not respond to the treatment. In another study, antibiotic treatment was associated with a significant reduction in the rate of postvenereal arthritic flares.

Bibliography

1. **Inman RD.** Reactive arthritis, Reiter's syndrome, and enteric pathogens. In: Espinosa L, Goldenberg D, Arnett F, Alarcon G, eds. Infections in the Rheumatic Diseases: A Comprehensive Review of Microbial Relations to Rheumatic Disorders. Orlando: Grune & Stratton; 1988:273-9.

2. **Lauhio A, Leirisalo-Repo M, Lahdevirta J, Saikku P, Repo H.** Double-blind, placebo-controlled study of three month treatment with lymecycline in reactive arthritis, with special reference to *Chlamydia* arthritis. Arthritis Rheum. 1991;34:6-14.

GASTROINTESTINAL BLEEDING

Gastrointestinal Bleeding Question 1
Answer: E

EDUCATIONAL OBJECTIVE: Begin medical management of a patient with advanced decompensated cirrhosis presenting with hematemesis.

This man with advanced decompensated cirrhosis presents with several complications of portal hypertension, including variceal hemorrhage, ascites, and renal insufficiency. The immediate concern is volume resuscitation. Colloid is appropriate in view of the low serum albumin and renal insufficiency, and should aid in improved renal perfusion and resolution of hyponatremia.

Octreotide, a synthetic analogue of somatostatin that shares the four amino acids that are responsible for its biological activity, has a much longer half-life (1 to 2 h) than somatostatin (1 to 2 min). Unlike somatostatin, octreotide is available in the United States and is used at a dose of 50 μg/h. Randomized clinical trials have shown that octreotide is more effective than placebo, vasopressin, and balloon tamponade in controlling acute variceal bleeding. Octreotide has also been shown to be as effective as sclerotherapy for the control of active bleeding and to decrease early rebleeding over 5 days when combined with endoscopic treatment. Because octreotide has minimal side effects octreotide infusion should be initiated before endoscopic evaluation in patients suspected of variceal hemorrhage.

Empiric prophylactic therapy with broad-spectrum antibiotics would be appropriate because of the increased risk for bacterial infection during hospitalization for upper gastrointestinal tract hemorrhage in patients with cirrhosis and advanced hepatic decompensation. Panendoscopy should be performed to identify the source of bleeding and to initiate endoscopic therapy for esophageal varices, if identified, by band ligation or sclerotherapy. Less likely sources of bleeding (such as peptic ulcer, Mallory-Weiss tear, and portal hypertensive gastropathy) could be identified and potentially treated.

After hemodynamic stabilization, large-volume paracentesis of tense ascites is recommended for symptomatic relief and to decrease portal pressure and con-sequently reduce the risk for continued or recurrent variceal bleeding. Lactulose therapy is appropriate to treat hepatic encephalopathy; however, patients such as this should not be given anything by mouth until active bleeding has stopped and endoscopic evaluation has been completed. Gastric contents, including blood and medications, will frustrate endoscopic procedures and will predispose to aspiration in a somnolent patient with upper gastrointestinal bleeding. It is appropriate to consider endotracheal intubation for airway protection prior to endoscopic procedures in such patients.

Bibliography

1. **Beeson I, Ingrand P, Person B, Boutroux D, Heresbach D, Bernard P, et al.** Sclerotherapy with and without octreotide for acute variceal bleeding. N Engl J Med. 1995;333:555-60.

2. **Pauwels A, Mostefa-Kara N, Debenes B, Degoutte E, Levy VG.** Systemic antibiotic prophylaxis after gastrointestinal hemorrhage in cirrhotic patients with a high risk of infection. Hepatology. 1996;24:802-6.

3. **Kravetz D, Romero G, Argonz J, Guevara M, Suarez A, Abecasis R, et al.** Total volume paracentesis decreases variceal pressure, size, and variceal wall tension in cirrhotic patients. Hepatology. 1997;25:59-62.

Gastrointestinal Bleeding Question 2
Answer: E

EDUCATIONAL OBJECTIVE: Recognize potential complications of NSAIDs, especially in the large and small bowel.

NSAIDs may cause small-bowel perforation, ulcers, and strictures; similar findings may occur in the large bowel. Inflammatory bowel disease re-exacerbations may occur in patients taking NSAIDs. The majority of reported lesions occur in the cecum and ascending colon. Most patients with colonic ulcers are over 50 years old. The mechanism by which NSAIDs cause ulcers is unknown, but it may be a combination of a local mucosal reaction and increased intestinal permeability. Discontinuation of NSAID therapy usually causes healing of the lesion in 6 to 8 weeks. The patient should be reevaluated in 4 to 6 weeks.

Bibliography

1. **Stamm C , Burkhalter CE, Pearce W, Larsen B, Willis M, Kikendall JW, et al.** Benign colonic ulcers associated with nonsteroidal anti-inflammatory drug ingestion. Am J Gastroenterol. 1994;89:2230-3.

2. **Hayllar J, Smith T, Macpherson A, Price AB, Gumpel M, Bjarnason I.** Nonsteroidal antiinflammatory drug-induced small intestinal inflammation and blood loss. Effects of sulfasalazine and other disease-modifying drugs. Arthritis Rheum. 1994;37:1146-50.

Gastrointestinal Bleeding Question 3
Answer: B

EDUCATIONAL OBJECTIVE: Recognize the need for vigorous volume resuscitation in acute upper gastrointestinal bleeding.

This patient has a hemodynamically significant upper gastrointestinal bleed. His resting tachycardia and orthostatic blood pressure changes suggest that he has lost significant intravascular volume. Vital signs are a more reliable indicator of acute volume loss than the hemoglobin concentration or hematocrit, which may be normal even with severe acute gastrointestinal bleeding.

The initial approach to this patient should be restoration of intravascular volume, which should be done with crystalloid solutions, such as saline or lactated Ringer's solution given at a rapid rate until the vital signs normalize. Blood products should be reserved for patients with profound anemia followed by crystalloid volume replacement. Nasogastric aspiration is not required to determine the level of bleeding because the history of hematemesis establishes the level of bleeding proximal to the ligament of Treitz. It is helpful, however, in determining whether the bleeding is continuing and in identifying the need for gastric lavage using a large-bore gastric tube in preparation for endoscopy. Although endoscopy will identify the bleeding site, estimate the risk for rebleeding, and allow treatment of bleeding lesions, it should be delayed until the patient is hemodynamically stable.

Bibliography

1. **Laine L, Peterson WL.** Bleeding peptic ulcer. N Engl J Med. 1994;331:717-27.

2. **Lieberman D.** Gastrointestinal bleeding: initial management. Gastroenterol Clin North Am. 1993;22:723-36.

3. **Freeman ML, Cass OW, Peine CJ, Onstad GR.** The non-bleeding visible vessel versus the sentinel clot: natural history and risk of rebleeding. Gastrointest Endosc. 1993;39:359-66.

4. **Laine L, Cohen H, Brodhead J, Cantor D, Garcia F, Mosquera M.** Prospective evaluation of immediate versus

delayed refeeding and prognostic value of endoscopy in patients with upper gastrointestinal hemorrhage. Gastroenterology. 1992;102:314-6.

5. **Longstreth GF, Feitelberg SP.** Outpatient care of selected patients with acute non-variceal upper gastrointestinal haemorrhage. Lancet. 1995;345:108-11.

6. **Rockall TA, Logan RF, Devlin HB, Northfield TC.** Variation in outcome after acute upper gastrointestinal haemorrhage. The National Audit of Acute Upper Gastrointestinal Haemorrhage. Lancet. 1995;346:346-50.

Gastrointestinal Bleeding Question 4
Answer: B

EDUCATIONAL OBJECTIVE: Recognize that therapy for *Helicobacter pylori* infection alters the clinical course of ulcer disease.

Although many gastrointestinal diseases have been associated with *H. pylori* infection, including gastric lymphoma, gastric adenocarcinoma, and peptic ulcers, other gastrointestinal diseases such as nonulcer dyspepsia, gastroesophageal reflux disease, Barrett's esophagus, and NSAID-induced ulcers have had conflicting data as to their association as well as response to therapy.

At this time, the only convincing clinical evidence that therapy alters the clinical course of a disease is with peptic ulcer. There are substantial data regarding the treatment of nonulcer dyspepsia in *H. pylori*, but the data are inconclusive as to whether there is any benefit. There are no data whether the treatment of patients infected with *H. pylori* prevents the later development of gastric cancer.

NSAID ulcers do not appear to be more common in patients infected with *H. pylori*. However, in patients with peptic ulcers, the concomitant use of NSAIDs may increase the risk for ulcer complications. In a patient taking NSAIDs presenting with an ulcer and infected with *H. pylori*, it is impossible to determine whether the ulcer is an NSAID-induced or *H. pylori*–induced ulcer; treatment should be directed at both causes.

Bibliography

1. **Fendrick AM, Chernew ME, Hirth RA, Bloom BS.** Alternative management strategies for patients with suspected peptic ulcer disease. Ann Intern Med. 1995;123:260-8.

2. **Laine L, Cominelli F, Sloane R, Casini-Raggi V, Marin-Sorensen M, Weinstein WM.** Interaction of NSAIDs and *Helicobacter pylori* on gastrointestinal injury and prostaglandin production: a controlled double-blind trial. Aliment Pharmacol Ther. 1995;9:127-35.

3. **Sonnenberg A, Townsend WF.** Costs of duodenal ulcer therapy with antibiotics. Arch Intern Med. 1995;155:922-8.

Gastrointestinal Bleeding Question 5
Answer: E

EDUCATIONAL OBJECTIVE: Institute appropriate treatment of bleeding ulcer disease.

This patient bled from a duodenal ulcer. Endoscopy can assess the patient's risk for rebleeding. If a vessel is observed at the base of the ulcer, the risk for rebleeding is highest, with more than half of such patients having rebleeding. If the ulcer base is clean, the risk for rebleeding is <5%. Patients such as the one in this question who have adherent clots have a 15% to 25% risk for rebleeding. Therefore, the risk not high enough to warrant active intervention at this time. If he were to start bleeding again, endoscopic treatment with thermal contact devices, injection therapy, or laser photocoagulation would be indicated.

If these measures fail then surgical intervention is indicated. The success rate of intra-arterial vasopressin is low and should be reserved for poor surgical candidates who fail to respond to endoscopic therapy. Although the rate of rebleeding is not high enough to warrant active intervention at this time, it is too high to justify discharging the patient.

Bibliography

1. Laine L, Cohen H, Brodhead J, Cantor D, Garcia F, Mosquera M. Prospective evaluation of immediate versus delayed refeeding and prognostic value of endoscopy in patients with upper gastrointestinal hemorrhage. Gastroenterology. 1992;102:314-6.
2. Cook DJ, Guyatt GH, Salena BJ, Laine LA. Endoscopic therapy for acute nonvariceal upper gastrointestinal hemorrhage: a meta-analysis. Gastroenterology. 1992;102:139-48.

Gastrointestinal Bleeding Question 6
Answer: C

EDUCATIONAL OBJECTIVE: Start prophylactic treatment of bleeding from portal hypertension.

The presence of portal hypertensive gastropathy indicates portal hypertension, probably from cirrhosis secondary to chronic hepatitis C infection. The patient should receive prophylactic therapy with propranolol, which has been shown to reduce bleeding from esophageal varices and portal hypertensive gastropathy.

Interferon-α has not been studied in these circumstances, and sclerotherapy, though useful for varices, cannot be used for portal hypertensive gastropathy. TIPS is currently limited to treating acute variceal bleeding. Portacaval shunts are not used prophylactically because of the high incidence of hepatic encephalopathy. The patient may ultimately need a liver transplant but not for prophylaxis for the first variceal hemorrhage.

Bibliography

1. Pagliaro L, D'Amico G, Sorensen TI, Lebrec D, Burroughs AK, Morabito A, et al. Prevention of first bleeding in cirrhosis. A meta-analysis of randomized trials of nonsurgical treatment. Ann Intern Med. 1992;117:59-70
2. Poynard T, Cales P, Pasta L, Ideo G, Pascal JP, Pagliaro L, et al. Beta-adrenergic-antagonist drugs in the prevention of gastrointestinal bleeding in patients with cirrhosis and esophageal varices. An analysis of data and prognostic factors in 589 patients from four randomized clinical trials. Franco-Italian Multicenter Study Group. N Engl J Med. 1991;324:1532-8.
3. Perez-Ayuso RM, Pique JM, Bosch J, Panes J, Gonzalez A, Perez R, et al. Propranolol in the prevention of recurrent bleeding from severe portal hypertensive gastropathy in cirrhosis. Lancet. 1991;338:509-10.

Gastrointestinal Bleeding Question 7
Answer: C

EDUCATIONAL OBJECTIVE: Recognize coagulopathy associated with chronic liver disease.

This patient has cryptogenic cirrhosis with portal hypertension and esophageal varices. The platelet count of 75,000/μL is consistent with the presence of splenomegaly and a redistribution of 80% of the circulating platelets into the red pulp of the spleen. The activated partial thromboplastin time (aPTT) and prothrombin time (PT) were both prolonged and corrected with the addition of normal plasma, which is consistent with the presence of deficiency (rather than an inhibitor) of coagulation proteins that affect both the aPTT and the PT. Although the aPTT and PT may be prolonged in patients with vitamin K deficiency and may correct with the addition of normal plasma, patients with vitamin K deficiency do not have splenomegaly unless it is associated with severe nontropical sprue with splenomegaly (occurs 10% to 20% of the time). The hemostatic defects seen in chronic liver disease are multiple in origin and include decreased synthesis of coagulation factors, thrombocytopenia due to portal hypertension, prolonged bleeding time due to acquired platelet dysfunction of unknown etiology, systemic fibrinolysis due to a combination of elevated levels of tissue plasminogen activator, decreased levels of plasminogen activator inhibitor, and decreased levels of alpha-2-plasmin inhibitor.

Although patients with disseminated intravascular coagulation may present with thrombocytopenia, prolonged aPTT, and prolonged PT, D-dimer levels are usually elevated, and the fibrinogen level would probably be lower.

Although acquired factor V inhibitors typically prolong the aPTT and PT, the presence of a factor V inhibitor could not be corrected by the addition of normal plasma to either test. Moreover, most factor V inhibitors result from recent exposure to topical thrombin (or fibrin glue) because of the presence of bovine factor V, which can cause the development of cross-reacting antibodies to human factor V.

Systemic fibrinolysis should always be considered in patients with chronic liver disease because it is present in 50% of the patients. However, if this patient had systemic fibrinolysis, the fibrinogen level would normally be even lower than 165 mg/dL. However, it is conceivable that this patient does have systemic fibrinolysis, and the clot lysis time should be done to rule out this complicating problem.

Bibliography

1. **Francis RB Jr.** Clinical disorders of fibrinolysis: a critical review. Blut. 1989;59:1-14.

2. **Francis CW, Marder VJ.** Physiologic regulation and pathologic disorders of fibrinolysis. In: Colman RW, Hirsh J, Marder VJ, Salzman EW, eds. Hemostasis and Thrombosis: Basic Principles and Clinical Practice. 3rd ed. Philadelphia: JB Lippincott Co; 1994:1076-103.

3. **Hathaway WE, Goodnight, SH Jr.** Liver diseases. In: Hathaway WE, Goodnight SH Jr, eds. Disorders of Hemostasis and Thrombosis: A Clinical Guide. New York: McGraw-Hill, Inc; 1993:211-8.

4. **Hathaway WE, Goodnight, SH Jr.** Systemic fibrinolysis. In: Hathaway WE, Goodnight SH Jr, eds. Disorders of Hemostasis and Thrombosis: A Clinical Guide. New York: McGraw-Hill, Inc; 1993:230-6.

5. **Hersch SL, Kunelis T, Francis RB.** The pathogenesis of accelerated fibrinolysis in liver cirrhosis: a critical role for tissue plasminogen activator inhibitor. Blood. 1987;69:1315-9.

6. **Joist JH.** Hemostatic abnormalities in liver disease. In: Colman RW, Hirsh J, Marder VJ, Salzman EW, eds. Hemostasis and Thrombosis: Basic Principles and Clinical Practice. 3rd ed. Philadelphia: JB Lippincott Co; 1994:906-20.

Gastrointestinal Bleeding Question 8
Answer: A

EDUCATIONAL OBJECTIVE: Manage a patient with lower gastrointestinal bleeding.

In patients of this age, the most likely causes of lower gastrointestinal bleeding are diverticular disease and vascular malformations. NSAIDs may also cause such bleeding. A colon neoplasm usually presents with occult blood in the stool rather than vigorous bleeding. Inflammatory bowel disease rarely presents with bleeding in the absence of other symptoms. The absence of blood in the nasogastric aspirate makes an upper gastrointestinal source of bleeding unlikely but not impossible.

The procedure with the greatest diagnostic yield and greatest potential for therapeutic intervention in this patient is colonoscopy. Patients with persistent lower gastrointestinal tract bleeding should have a rapid purge of the colon to remove as much blood as possible and immediately thereafter they should undergo colonoscopy. If a source of bleeding cannot be identified on colonoscopy, the lesion may occasionally be identified and treated with angiography. Radionuclide scans can identify bleeding of insufficient volume to be detected by angiography, but such scans are imprecise for localizing the site of bleeding and cannot be used for therapy. Barium studies should be avoided; their yield in this situation is low, and retained barium will prevent colonoscopy or angiography.

Surgery should be reserved for lesions identified by colonoscopy or angiography. that have failed to respond to vigorous therapy. Empiric hemicolectomy should be used only in extraordinary circumstances.

Bibliography

1. **Richter JM, Christensen MR, Kaplan LM, Nishioka NS.** Effectiveness of current technology in the diagnosis and management of lower gastrointestinal hemorrhage. Gastrointest Endosc. 1995;41:93-8.

THE HEALTHY PATIENT

The Healthy Patient Question 1
Answer: E

EDUCATIONAL OBJECTIVE: Evaluate the preventive health screening options for a healthy college-bound adolescent.

The patient is a healthy adolescent with no health risks. Screening mammography is not recommended before the age of 30 years even for women with first-degree relatives with breast cancer. Although her father has a lipid disorder, the patient has no other cardiovascular risk factors, and the treatment of lipid disorders in adolescents is controversial. If the patient had requested to be placed on oral contraceptives, a baseline cholesterol level may be warranted because of the lipid changes that can occur with some oral contraceptives. Many college health forms request a hematocrit or hemoglobin level, but the cost-effectiveness of random testing is questionable. Screening an asymptomatic patient for hypothyroidism is not cost effective.

Teaching breast self-examination is an important element of the adolescent physical examination. In this patient's case, the positive family history should prompt the clinician to emphasize its importance.

Bibliography

1. **Hulley SB, Newman TB, Grady D, Garber AM, Baron RB, Browner WS.** Should we be measuring blood cholesterol levels in young adults? JAMA. 1993;269:1416-9.

The Healthy Patient Questions 2-3
Answers: 2(E); 3(B)

EDUCATIONAL OBJECTIVE: Recognize the reliability of screening tests in population groups with different disease prevalence.

The reliability of a screening test is influenced by its sensitivity and specificity and by the prevalence of disease in the population under consideration. The positive predictive value of a test refers to the ability of a positive test result to identify disease (true-positive rate). Because the pretest probability of disease in this patient is so low (1/10,000) even a specificity of 98% results in 200 false-positive results and a positive predictive value of only about 0.5% (0.98/200.98 in a hypothetic population of 10,000). Stated another way, of the approximately 201 positive results, only one is a true positive.

	HIV Infection	**No HIV Infection**	
Positive HIV ELISA	0.98 true positive	200 false positive	Post-test probability of HIV infection given a positive HIV ELISA is 0.98/200.98 ≈ 0.5%
Negative HIV ELISA	0.02 false negative	9799 true negative	Post-test probability of HIV infection given a negative HIV ELISA is 0.02/9799.02 ≈ 0.0002%
	Patients infected with HIV = 1	Patients without HIV infection = 9999	

When prevalence rises to 50%, the ability of the test to distinguish between normal and diseased populations rises. Without changing the operating characteristics of the test (sensitivity and specificity), the positive predictive value increases to 98% (4900/5000). The negative predictive value also rises to 98%, meaning 2% of patients with negative HIV ELISA tests would be infected. This phenomenon underscores the need for specific confirmatory tests (Western blot in this case) and the hazards of screening for diseases in a population at low risk.

	HIV Infection	No HIV Infection	
Positive HIV ELISA	4900 true positive	100 false positive	Post-test probability of HIV infection given a positive HIV ELISA is 4900/5000 = 98%
Negative HIV ELISA	100 false negative	4900 true negative	Post-test probability of HIV infection given a negative HIV ELISA is 100/5000 = 2%
	Patients infected with HIV = 5000	Patients without HIV infection = 5000	

Bibliography

1. **Pauker SG, Eckman MH.** Principles of diagnostic testing. In: Kelley WN, ed. Textbook of Internal Medicine. Philadelphia: Lippincott; 1991:16-7.

The Healthy Patient Question 4
Answer: B

EDUCATIONAL OBJECTIVE: Counsel a traveler on vaccination for viral hepatitis.

The Immunization Practices Advisory Committee (ACIP) of the Centers for Disease Control and Prevention recommends pre-exposure hepatitis A vaccination for the following persons: (1) persons planning to travel to countries with high or intermediate endemicity of hepatitis A virus (HAV) infection, including Mexico; (2) sexually active homosexual and bisexual men; (3) injection drug users or persons who use noninjection street drugs; and (4) persons with chronic liver disease.

For optimal, sustained protection against HAV infection, it is recommended that a booster injection be given to adults at 6 to 12 months after the initial vaccination. However, within 4 weeks after an initial vaccination, antibody responses occur, and persons can assume to be protected. To be certain of vaccine-induced immunity in travelers leaving within a short period, simultaneous administration of immune globulin and HAV vaccine, at separate deltoid sites, may be appropriate.

In the United States, previous HAV exposure is sufficiently low in most children and middle-aged adults who are not members of high-risk populations, that it is cost-effective to recommend hepatitis A vaccination without previous antibody testing. The current strategy of HBV control in the United States includes screening pregnant women for HBsAg and administration of hepatitis B immune globulin and HBV vaccine to their neonates, universal vaccination of all infants, catch-up vaccination of preteenagers (11 and 12 year olds), and continuing vaccination of high-risk populations. In monogamous, heterosexual couples without high-risk behavior, the risk for HBV infection is very low and vaccination is not recommended.

Bibliography

1. CDC. Licensure of inactivated hepatitis A vaccine and recommendations for use among international travelers. MMWR 1995;44:559-650.
2. **Balistreri WF.** A new vaccine for an old disease. Viral hepatitis. 1996;2:49-59.
3. **Dobson S, Scheifele D, Bell A.** Assessment of a universal, school-based hepatitis B vaccination program. JAMA. 1995;274:1209-13.

The Healthy Patient Questions 5-10
Answers: 5(B); 6(A); 7(C); 8(B); 9(B); 10(E)

EDUCATIONAL OBJECTIVE: Understand the indications for screening patients for colon malignancies.

The patient with no risk factors should begin screening flexible sigmoidoscopy at age 50 years, having repeat procedures every 3 to 5 years. A history of colon cancer at age 70 years in a patient's father does not increase the patient's risk for colon cancer. The presence of hyperplastic polyps does not increase the risk for colon carcinoma; therefore, the 50-year-old man with one hyperplastic polyp should continue with flexible sigmoidoscopy every 3 to 5 years. A patient with a single adenoma 10 mm in diameter or larger has an increased risk for other polyps or colon cancer and should undergo colonoscopy. Data are conflicting about the need to perform colonoscopy on single adenomas smaller than 10 mm in diameter.

The patient with a family history of familial adenomatous polyposis (FAP) should have annual flexible sigmoidoscopy beginning shortly before the earliest time a member of the family was found to have polyps or age 25 years, whichever is earlier. Many experts recommend surveillance beginning by age 12 years in those at risk. The polyps in familial adenomatous polyposis begin to develop in the distal colon first, and therefore flexible sigmoidoscopy is all that is needed. Soon genetic screening may predict who is at risk and therefore who would need annual sigmoidoscopy.

The patient with familial nonpolyposis colon cancer should undergo regular colonoscopy every 2 to 3 years beginning at age 20 to 25 years or at an age 5 years younger than the age of the earliest colon cancer diagnosis in the family. The polyps in this syndrome are less numerous and occur more frequently in the left colon; therefore, regular full colonoscopy is needed in these high-risk patients.

Bibliography

1. **Bond JH.** Polyp guideline: diagnosis, treatment and surveillance for patients with nonfamilial colorectal polyps. Ann Intern Med. 1993;119:836-43.

2. **Winawer SJ, Zauber AG, Gerdes H, O'Brien MJ, Gottlieb LS, Sternberg SS, et al.** Risk of colorectal cancer in families of patients with adenomatous polyps. N Engl J Med. 1996;334:82-7.

The Healthy Patient Question 11
Answer: B

EDUCATIONAL OBJECTIVE: Recognize the importance of familial colon cancer syndromes.

This patient has three first-degree family members with colorectal cancer (one under age 50 years) and two members with extracolonic tumors; the patient is therefore likely a member of a Lynch II kindred. Flexible sigmoidoscopy would exclude familial adenomatous polyposis but not hereditary nonpolyposis colorectal cancer (HNPCC). Therefore, screening regimens that include only fecal occult blood testing and/or sigmoidoscopy are inadequate. A single colonoscopy

also is insufficient; the absence of polyps at this time does not mean that the patient is not at risk. A lifetime colonoscopy surveillance program is needed. If a colorectal cancer develops, a complete colectomy should be performed because of the high likelihood of recurrent colorectal cancers.

A family history of colorectal cancer is present in 25% of patients with colorectal cancer. Families at increased risk may be divided into those with well-delineated inherited syndromes and those with common or "sporadic" cancer in which there is one or more affected first-degree relatives. Case-control studies show that first-degree relatives of patients with common colon cancer have a 2.1-fold increased risk for colon cancer. With two affected first-degree relatives, the risk is sixfold. The risk for noncolorectal malignancies in relatives of patients with sporadic colon cancer does not appear to be increased.

Up to 5% of cases of colorectal cancer may be due to inherited cancer syndromes. The polyposis syndromes are well recognized, but these dramatic syndromes account for <1% of cases. These include the adenomatous polyposis syndromes (familial adenomatous polyposis and its variants Gardner's and Turcot syndrome) and the hamartomatous syndromes (Peutz-Jeghers syndrome and familial juvenile polyposis). The adenomatous polyposis syndromes are characterized by the development of thousands of adenomatous polyps that appear in the second decade and virtually always by age 30 years. Colon cancer is virtually inevitable unless the colon is removed. The mean age at which colon cancer develops in these patients is 39 years. Familial adenomatous polyposis is an autosomal dominant condition, which in 87% of cases can be linked to a defect in the *APC* gene on chromosome 5q21. With molecular genetic methods, the abnormal protein products from the mutated *APC* gene can now be detected, which will allow for genetic screening. Peutz-Jeghers syndrome is an autosomal dominant condition characterized by hamartomas throughout the gastrointestinal tract but predominantly in the small intestine. In addition, perioral melanin deposits are present in >90% of affected patients. Up to 50% of patients with Peutz-Jeghers syndrome develop cancer of the gastrointestinal tract and other organs, especially the breast and gonads.

HNPCC (or Lynch syndromes I and II) is an autosomal dominant condition that may account for up to 5% of cases of colon cancer. Lynch syndrome I is characterized by the development of colon cancer, often at an early age, which has a predilection for the right colon. Unlike patients with the polyposis syndromes, patients with Lynch syndrome I may have few or no adenomatous polyps. Lynch syndrome II shares all these features but also is associated with extracolonic tumors, particularly cancer of the ovary, uterus, urologic tract, and stomach. Because affected patients do not develop diffuse polyposis or other unusual physical findings, it is difficult to distinguish these families from other families with "sporadic" colon cancer. A thorough family history is critical for the identification of these families and the institution of appropriate screening tests. At present, the diagnosis is based on three criteria: (1) three or more first-degree relatives with colorectal cancer; (2) colorectal cancer involving at least two generations; and (3) one or more cases of colorectal cancer diagnosed before age 50 years. These stringent criteria likely exclude many affected families. Recently, many patients with HNPCC have been found to have a genetic defect linked to chromosomes 2, 3 (familial), or 7. Mutations recently identified in the genes *RMSH2, RMLHTI, RPMS1,* and *RPMS2* can be found in the majority of HNPCC kindreds. These genes appear to be an integral part of a complex that is responsible for detecting and repairing base-pair mismatches that occur during DNA replication. In the near future, it may be possible to screen families with an increased prevalence of colorectal cancer and/or extracolonic tumors for these mutations. In the meantime, it is recommended that patients who appear to be members of HNPCC kindreds undergo colonoscopy at least every 2 years beginning at age 25 or 5 years younger than the earliest occurrence of colorectal cancer in the family. Women in Lynch II families should undergo careful gynecologic evaluation.

Bibliography

1. **St. John DJ, McDermott FT, Hopper JL, Debney EA, Johnson WR, Hughes ES.** Cancer risk in relatives of patients with common colorectal cancer. Ann Intern Med. 1993;118:785-90.

2. **Powell SM, Peterson GM, Krush AJ, Booker S, Jen J, Giardiello FM, et al.** Molecular diagnosis of familial adenomatous polyposis. N Engl J Med. 1993;329:1982-7.

3. **Lynch HT, Smyrk TC, Watson P, Lanspa SJ, Lynch JF, Lynch PM, et al.** Genetics, natural history, tumor spectrum, and pathology of hereditary nonpolyposis colorectal cancer: an updated review. Gastroenterology. 1993;104:1535-49.

4. **Leach FS, Nicolaides NC, Papadopoulos N, Liu B, Jen J, Parsons R, et al.** Mutations of a mutS homologue in hereditary nonpolyposis colorectal cancer. Cell. 1993;75:1215-25.

5. **Bronner CE, Baker SM, Morrison PT, Warren G, Smith LG, Lescoe MK, et al.** Mutation in the DNA mismatch repair gene homologue hMLH1 is associated with hereditary non-polyposis colon cancer. Nature. 1994;368:258-61.

The Healthy Patient Question 12
Answer: A

EDUCATIONAL OBJECTIVE: Evaluate the use of exercise testing in the diagnosis of coronary artery disease.

Noninvasive stress testing for the diagnosis of coronary artery disease is most helpful when there is an intermediate pre-test likelihood of disease. The middle-aged man with atypical angina falls in this category. A positive stress electrocardiogram (ECG) result in a patient with a low likelihood of disease, such as the 31-year-old woman, is most likely to be a false-positive. Patients with unstable angina, such as the 55-year-old man, should not have exercise testing because of the risk of myocardial infarction.

Resting ST-segment changes, left ventricular hypertrophy, left bundle branch block, and digitalis make exercise repolarization changes difficult to interpret. Therefore, if patients likely to have left ventricular hypertrophy need testing, such as the 69-year-old woman, an exercise ECG would not be an appropriate study. If patients are symptomatic, an exercise imaging test (for example, thallium scintigraphy) would be appropriate. Stress testing is not likely to provide diagnostic information in asymptomatic patients following coronary angioplasty. Results do not correlate closely with the presence of restenosis.

Bibliography

1. **Ellestad MH.** Stress Testing: Principles and Practice. 3rd ed. Philadelphia: F. A. Davis Company;1986.

2. **Cheitlin MD.** Finding the high-risk patient with coronary artery disease. JAMA. 1988;259:2271-7.

3. **Gershlick A, Brack MJ, More RS, Syndercombe-Court D, Balcon R.** Angiographic restenosis after angioplasty: comparison of definitions and correlation with clinical outcome. Coron Artery Dis. 1993;4:73-81.

The Healthy Patient Question 13
Answer: C

EDUCATIONAL OBJECTIVE: Identify the advantages and disadvantages of noninvasive techniques in the evaluation of suspected familial hypertrophic cardiomyopathy.

The evolution of molecular genetics has helped decipher the genetic basis of many inherited cardiac disorders. Familial hypertrophic cardiomyopathy is inherited as an autosomal dominant disease that is characterized by hypertrophy, typically of the left ventricle, that predominantly involves the interventricular septum and occurs in the absence of known causes for hypertrophy such as hypertension or valvular heart disease. Although an autosomal dominant pattern has been recognized for approximately 50% of cases, there is a highly variable degree of penetrance. Genetic techniques have identified at least three distinct chromosomal loci responsible for familial cases of hypertrophic disease: 14q1, 1q3, and 15q2. The responsible genes result in mutations in the β-myosin heavy-chain, cardiac troponin T, and α-tropomyosin, respectively. At least 36 distinct mutations in the β-myosin heavy-chain gene alone have been reported, and their clinical presentations and natural histories vary greatly. Mutations of the β-myosin heavy-chain gene occur in approximately 20% to 30% of familial cases of hypertrophic cardiomyopathy; the exact incidence of mutations in troponin T and α-tropomyosin remains unknown. Abnormalities of myosin-binding protein C have also been recently reported in hypertrophic disease. As with other autosomal dominant disorders, spontaneous mutations may also occur, and in many individual cases no familial pattern may be identified.

Echocardiography remains the most cost-effective method for evaluating family members suspected of having asymptomatic hypertrophic disease. Despite echocardiography's high degree of sensitivity and specificity, it is important to recognize that the morphologic expression of this disease may not be complete or even evident until well into adolescence. Thus, a normal echocardiogram in childhood does not definitively exclude the possibility of preclinical disease. In asymptomatic young children with a positive family history of hypertrophic disease and a normal echocardiogram, serial echocardiography should be done. Echocardiography will identify the vast majority of adults with hypertrophic disease, but a normal echocardiogram does not entirely exclude a mild variant of disease or the small possibility of sudden cardiac death.

Screening of family members suspected for hypertrophic disease has increased in importance as better diagnostic methods have evolved. Physical examination is neither sensitive nor specific for establishing the correct diagnosis because physical examination may be entirely normal. If outflow tract obstruction is absent, a systolic murmur is typically absent. Although electrocardiographic evidence for unexplained hypertrophy is specific as a marker, its sensitivity is quite low. A detailed family pedigree is important in trying to establish a hereditary basis for the disorder in a particular family. However, even a detailed family history cannot detect with certainty whether a particular individual has inherited the disease, because only one half of all offspring will be affected. Genetic characteriza-

tion remains a research technique used in families with suspected hereditary hypertrophic cardiomyopathy. Identification of the precise genetic mutation in one proband can permit rapid evaluation of all family members by means of peripheral blood analysis. Despite its sensitivity and specificity, this technique is not yet widely available.

Bibliography

1. **Marian AJ, Roberts M.** Recent advances in the molecular genetics of hypertrophic cardiomyopathy. Circulation. 1995;92:1336-47.

2. **Rosenzweig A, Watkins H, Hwang DS, Miri M, McKenna W, Traill TA, et al.** Preclinical diagnosis of familial hypertrophic cardiomyopathy by genetic analysis of blood lymphocytes. N Engl J Med. 1991;325:1753-60.

3. **Maron BJ, Spirito P, Wesley Y, Arce J.** Development and progression of left ventricular hypertrophy in children with hypertrophic cardiomyopathy. N Engl J Med. 1986;315:610-4.

4. **Panza JA, Maron BJ.** Relation of electrocardiographic abnormalities to evolving left ventricular hypertrophy in hypertrophic cardiomyopathy during childhood. Am J Cardiol. 1989;63:1258-65.

5. **Solomon SD, Wolff S, Watkins H, Ridker PM, Come P, McKenna WJ, et al.** Left ventricular hypertrophy and morphology in familial hypertrophic cardiomyopathy associated with mutations of the beta-myosin heavy chain gene. J Am Coll Cardiol. 1993;22:498-505.

The Healthy Patient Questions 14-17
Answers: 14(A); 15(A); 16(D); 17(D)

EDUCATIONAL OBJECTIVE: Distinguish among different patient types at risk for pneumonia and select the correct preventive approach.

Preventive approaches that have proven valuable in community-acquired pneumonia include pneumococcal and influenza vaccines. In nosocomial pneumonia, there is no systematic approach to prevention that has been proven effective, but there are multiple experimental approaches in limited use.

Pneumococcal vaccine is effective and should be given to patients who are older than 65 years, have chronic heart or lung disease, have other chronic medical illnesses, reside in chronic care facilities, or who have immunosuppressive illnesses such as Hodgkin's disease, chronic lymphocytic leukemia, multiple myeloma, and HIV infection. In addition, those with splenic dysfunction, caused by splenectomy or illness (such as sickle cell anemia), should be vaccinated to prevent overwhelming pneumococcal pneumonia and sepsis. The efficacy of the vaccine has been proved in case-control studies to be 60% to 70%; its efficacy may be greater if the vaccine is given to patients earlier in the course of chronic illness. The protective efficacy may wane in patients with immunosuppressive illness and in others with chronic disease who may not sustain high levels of antibody for prolonged periods; these individuals should be revaccinated after 6 years. One potentially effective application of the vaccine is its use as part of a hospital-based program, because up to 60% of all patients admitted for community-acquired pneumonia have been hospitalized for some reason in the preceding 4 years. Thus, if all hospitalized patients are considered for vaccination before discharge, immunizations will be given to a clearly high-risk population.

Influenza vaccine should be given to patients who qualify for pneumococcal vaccine because of chronic medical illness, advanced age, or immunosuppressive illness, but it does not need to be given to patients whose only indication is splenic dysfunction. Influenza vaccine must be repeated yearly and is effective only if given in the late fall in anticipation of the high-risk period. Efficacy in preventing deaths has been reported to be as high as 80% in the nursing home elderly population. Others who also qualify for influenza vaccine include those who can transmit the illness to high-risk individuals as well as those with high levels of exposure. Thus, health care workers, those who provide care to or live with chronically ill patients, and those who work in day-care centers should be immunized.

There are no other vaccines that are of proven efficacy in community-acquired pneumonia. *Haemophilus influenzae* type b vaccine has prevented pediatric meningitis and other invasive infections due to this organism, but it is not routinely recommended for adults. However, use of this vaccine should be considered (although not absolutely recommended) in certain high-risk adults such as those with HIV infection, those with an organ transplant, those receiving immunosuppressive therapy, patients with certain hematologic malignancies, and patients with anatomic or functional asplenia.

There is no vaccine against *Pseudomonas*. The 65-year-old man with chronic obstructive pulmonary disease in the spring should receive pneumococcal vaccine, but influenza vaccine should not be given until the fall. The 37-year-old woman who has had a splenectomy is otherwise well, has already electively received *Haemophilus influenzae* type b vaccine and now only needs pneumococcal vaccine. The 68-year-old man and 45-year-old woman should receive only influenza vaccine. The 68-year-old man qualifies because it is the fall, he has chronic cardiac disease,

and he does not need pneumococcal vaccine at this time because he received it 4 years ago. The woman working in a nursery school, who is being seen in the fall, should be immunized against influenza because of her high level of exposure to infection.

Bibliography

1. **Arunabh, Niederman MS.** Prevention of community-acquired pneumonia. Semin Respir Crit Care Med. 1996;17:273-82.

2. **Bassin AS, Niederman MS.** Prevention of ventilator-associated pneumonia. An attainable goal? Clin Chest Med. 1995;16:195-208.

The Healthy Patient Question 18
Answer: D

EDUCATIONAL OBJECTIVE: Choose the most appropriate strategy for exercise counseling.

The most important factor to lasting success of an exercise program is that it is an activity that the person enjoys and that fits into his or her lifestyle. In addition, patient input is essential to determine a realistic frequency, time, and type of activity. Therefore, making a specific recommendation of both where and when a person should exercise is not as likely to be successful.

The exercise treadmill test (ETT) is a poor screening tool in an asymptomatic patient. It is not necessary in anyone starting a low to moderate level of exercise. Although ETT might be considered in a 45-year-old man with multiple cardiac risk factors who wants to begin vigorous exercise, the patient described in this question is sedentary and should not begin exercising at a vigorous level. Sedentary persons should start off slowly with a moderate level of activity, which will decrease the risk for orthopedic and cardiovascular morbidity.

This patient should start off at a low to moderate level (50% to 70% of maximum heart rate) and be advised to report any early warning signs of coronary artery disease. Education and motivation are appropriate for a patient not yet ready to consider exercising but not for this patient who is already motivated and ready to make a plan.

Bibliography

1. **Schlant RC, Blomqvist G, Branenburg RO, DeBusk R, Ellestad MH, Fletcher GF, et al.** Guidelines for exercise testing: A report of the Joint American College of Cardiology/American Heart Association Task Force on Assessment of Cardiovascular Procedures (Subcommittee on Exercise Testing). Circulation. 1986;74:653A-667A.

2. **Peterson DM.** Exercise and physical activity in the adult population: a general internist's perspective. J Gen Intern Med. 1993;8:149-59.

The Healthy Patient Question 19
Answer: C

EDUCATIONAL OBJECTIVE: Counsel patients about life style modifications that lower blood pressure.

Excessive alcohol consumption can raise blood pressure. In a controlled trial examining the effects of hygienic interventions, higher alcohol intake was the characteristic most strongly associated with an elevated blood pressure. Up to 10% of all cases of hypertension are attributable to the use of alcohol. This patient admits to regular alcohol use and has a mildly elevated γ-glutamyltransferase. Limiting his intake of alcohol to less than two drinks per day will likely lower his blood pressure. Weight reduction in patients more than 10% above their ideal body weight will significantly lower their blood pressure. This patient is at his ideal body weight, and weight loss is unlikely to be effective and should not be recommended.

Stopping smoking does not lower blood pressure. With the initial exposure to nicotine, new smokers may have an acute rise in their blood pressure. However, tolerance quickly develops to the hypertensive effects of nicotine. Similarly, the habitual use of caffeine does not increase blood pressure, and eliminating caffeine from the diet does not substantially alter the blood pressure. Smoking cessation, however, is an important lifestyle intervention because of the synergistic effect of nicotine and hypertension on the risk for cardiovascular disease. Results from randomized trials examining the effect of relaxation therapy on lowering blood pressure have been inconsistent and fail to provide convincing evidence that it is beneficial.

Bibliography

1. The sixth report of the Joint National Committee on Detection, Evaluation, and Treatment of High Blood Pressure (JNC-VI). Arch Intern Med. 1997;157:2413-46. (also available at http://www.nhlbi.nih.gov/guidelines/hypertension/jnc.htm)
2. National High Blood Pressure Education Program Working Group report on primary prevention of hypertension. Arch Intern Med. 1993;153:186-208.
3. **Stamler R, Stamler J, Grimm R, Gosch FC, Elmer P, Dyer A, et al.** Nutritional therapy for high blood pressure. Final report of a four-year randomized controlled trial — the Hypertension Control Program. JAMA. 1987;257:1484-91.

The Healthy Patient Question 20
Answer: D

EDUCATIONAL OBJECTIVE: Prescribe calcium supplementation to fulfill a patient's calcium requirement.

This patient is postmenopausal and is not taking hormone replacement therapy. Her recommended daily calcium intake is 1500 mg a day, which can be achieved through dietary and supplemental sources. Her dietary calcium intake is approximately 600 mg of calcium (two dairy servings) a day. She needs 900 mg more in the form of supplementation, and therefore administering 900 mg of calcium gluconate will fulfill her requirement.

Calcium carbonate, citrate, lactate, and gluconate are all effective calcium supplements. Calcium carbonate is the only one that needs to be chewed and taken with food. Dolomite or oyster shell calcium, however, should not be recommended as it has been found to contain potentially harmful levels of lead. Fifteen hundred milligrams of calcium carbonate is more than she needs, and 400 mg of calcium citrate is not enough. Green leafy vegetables are a rich source of calcium but do not contain enough to fulfill her daily needs (for example, a half cup of cooked spinach contains 88 mg of calcium).

Bibliography

1. **Nuhlicek DN, Schubot DB, Midtling JE, eds.** A Physician's Guide to Nutrition Patient Education. Milwaukee, Wisconsin; Medical College of Wisconsin, Department of Family Medicine: 1991.
2. **Goodhart R, Shils M, eds.** Modern Nutrition in Health and Disease. 6th ed. Philadelphia: Lea & Febiger; 1987.

The Healthy Patient Question 21
Answer: C

EDUCATIONAL OBJECTIVE: Recognize an inadequate Pap screening test result and differentiate the clinical profile and early symptoms of cervical cancer from endometrial and ovarian cancers.

The concern in this case is that an absence of endocervical cells on a Pap smear represents an inadequate Pap screening test for cancer of the cervix, which commonly presents with irregular vaginal bleeding such as the onset of menometrorrhagia in a premenopausal woman. "Breakthrough bleeding" is unlikely in this patient who has been taking oral contraceptives uneventfully for 6 years. Oral contraceptives actually provide a protective effect against ovarian and even endometrial cancer.

Ovarian cancer is often associated with elevated CA-125 and an abnormal transvaginal ultrasound; but 15% or less of affected patients present with vaginal bleeding and the disorder is unusual in a woman younger than 35 years. Endometrial cancer, which commonly presents with vaginal bleeding, is best diagnosed by either endometrial biopsy (an office procedure) or dilatation and curettage under general anesthesia; however, the vast majority of all endometrial cancers occur in women over age 50 years.

Up to 30% of premenopausal women presenting with invasive cervical cancer have had a normal Pap smear within the past year, indicating a high rate of false-negative screening tests. This is largely explained by the overall high frequency of Pap smears that are described by cytologists as lacking endocervical cells, presumably due to poor examiner technique and inadequate sampling of cells from the squamocolumnar junction of the endocervix. Use of an endocervical brush in addition to cervical spatula and cotton-tipped applicator enhance the likelihood of adequate sampling, but colposcopic biopsy may still be required, especially if a cervical abnormality is observed or if the patient is at high risk for cervical cancer. Particular attention must be given to HIV-positive women (even if asymptomatic) because they have been shown to have a markedly increased incidence of high-grade intraepithelial neoplasia and more rapid development of aggressive cervical cancer.

Bibliography

1. **Rose PG.** Screening for gynecologic malignancies in primary care: cervical cancer. Emerg Med. 1993;133-40.
2. **Northfelt DW.** Cervical and anal neoplasia and HPV infection in persons with HIV infection. Oncology. 1994;8:33-7.

The Healthy Patient Questions 22-26
Answers: 22(C); 23(C); 24(C); 25(A); 26(B)

EDUCATIONAL OBJECTIVE: Distinguish the use of various breast cancer detection strategies.

Men are also at risk for breast cancer, and mammography can be associated with a false-negative result. Observation is clearly not indicated in the 56-year-old man, and neither thermography nor ultrasound can exclude the possibility of malignancy; therefore, biopsy is indicated.

A negative mammogram cannot rule out malignancy in the 36-year-old woman with the palpable lump. Breast cancer is the leading cause of death in women this age. Observation is clearly not indicated. The mass has already been present through two menstrual cycles. Ultrasound cannot exclude the possibility of cancer. Failure to pursue a persistent mass in the breast (normal imaging studies notwithstanding) is one of the most common, and potentially serious errors that can be made in such situations; biopsy is indicated here also.

Neither thermography nor ultrasound is likely to exclude the diagnosis of cancer in a patient in whom no apparent mass is found. Clustered microcalcifications have a significant association with both invasive and noninvasive breast cancer, and therefore a needle localization procedure for a definitive diagnosis is required.

The likelihood of breast cancer in a 18-year-old is very small. A lump of 1 week's duration is most probably associated with fluid accumulation in a cyst. Although ultrasound or cyst aspiration is a reasonable possibility, the lump will most likely disappear with observation alone.

However, a persistent lump in the breast of an 18-year-old woman cannot be ruled out as malignancy on clinical grounds. Because a mammogram in this young woman will likely be uninterpretable and the larger theoretical but potential risk of radiation, ultrasound to diagnose the cyst is the appropriate approach to this patient.

Bibliography

1. **Donegan WL.** Evaluation of a palpable breast mass. N Engl J Med. 1992;327:937-42.
2. **Kinne DW, Kopans DB.** Physical examination and mammography in the diagnosis of breast disease. In: Harris JR, Hellman S, Henderson IC, Kinne DW. eds. Breast Disease. Philadelphia: JB Lippincott Co.; 1991:81-106.

The Healthy Patient Question 27
Answer: E

EDUCATIONAL OBJECTIVE: Recognize and treat Paget's disease of bone.

Patients with Paget's disease (osteitis deformans) may present with asymptomatic elevations of serum alkaline phosphatase. Urinary hydroxyproline levels may be elevated, and roentgenograms will show characteristic changes of bone, such as a mottled increase of bone density, coarse trabeculation, incomplete fractures, and "tufts of cotton wool" in the skull. Serum calcium and phosphate levels are usually normal. In asymptomatic patients with limited disease, such as this patient, no therapy is warranted.

Indications for treatment include bone pain, fracture, hearing loss or vertigo, progressive deformity, extensive involvement of weight-bearing bones (such as the femoral neck), and high-output cardiac failure. In patients requiring therapy, the safety, efficacy and lower cost of bisphosphonates make them the therapy of choice over the alternative, calcitonin.

Bibliography

1. **Stewart GO, Nicholson GC.** Treatment of osteoporosis and Paget's disease. Curr Opin Rheumatol. 1991;3:380-7.

2. **Hosking DJ.** Advances in the management of Paget's disease of bone. Drugs. 1990;40:829-40.

The Healthy Patient Question 28
Answer: E

EDUCATIONAL OBJECTIVE: Identify physiological and pathological conditions that may affect antibody responses.

Although patients with HIV disease often have polyclonal activation of B lymphocytes and hyperglobulinemia, they are poor producers of specific antibodies after immunizations. Bacterial pneumonias are common in these patients.

A report demonstrates that vitamin B_{12} deficiency in elderly persons is a risk factor for poor responses to pneumococcal vaccine. Patients aged 65 to 87 years were immunized with 23-valent pneumococcal vaccine. Persons with subnormal serum vitamin B_{12} levels (range 80 to 185 pg/mL; normal > 200 pg/mL) had poor responses to immunization; persons with normal serum vitamin B_{12} levels had good responses. This finding is similar to that in patients with deficiency of transcobalamin II in whom antibody responses are poor.

Common variable immunodeficiency is the most common disorder of immunodeficiency in adults. Post-splenectomy patients may have poor responses to pneumococcal vaccine and multiple immunizations may be required.

Bibliography

1. **Fata FT, Herzlich BC, Schiffman G, Ast AL.** Impaired antibody responses to pneumococcal polysaccharide in elderly patients with low serum B_{12} levels. Ann Intern Med. 1996;124:299-304.

2. **Hirschtick RE, Glassroth J, Jordan MC, Wilcosky TC, Wallace JM, Kvale PA, et al.** Bacterial pneumonia in persons infected with the human immunodeficiency virus. N Engl J Med. 1995;333:845-51.

The Healthy Patient Question 29
Answer: D

EDUCATIONAL OBJECTIVE: Recognize the association between cervical neoplasia and human papillomavirus infection.

This patient has lesions typical for human papillomavirus (HPV) infection. HPV infection is generally a clinical diagnosis, and therefore, biopsy is usually not indicated. Identification of HPV lesions can be enhanced by the application of 3% to 5% acetic acid to mucosal and skin surfaces. After acetic acid application, tissues infected with HPV may turn white and appear shiny and raised.

Because women with certain serotypes of HPV infection (for example, HPV 16 and 18) have a 50- to 300-fold increased risk for development of cervical intra-epithelial neoplasia and invasive cervical cancer, screening with a Papanicolaou smear is indicated. Papanicolaou smears showing inflammation should be repeated within 3 months. Colposcopic examination of the cervix for HPV infection is required for patients whose Papanicolaou smears indicate high-grade squamous intra-epithelial lesions (moderate dysplasia/cervical intra-epithelial neoplasia 2, severe dysplasia/cervical intra-epithelial neoplasia 3, or carcinoma in situ). Some experts would do colposcopy on patients with low-grade squamous epithelial lesions (mild dysplasia/cervical intra-epithelial neoplasia 1) as well. Cultures for *Neisseria gonorrhoeae* and *Chlamydia trachomatis* and a VDRL (condylomata lata from secondary syphilis can rarely be confused with HPV infection) should be obtained for this patient.

HIV testing is not required unless such testing would allay fears of the patient. Serologic testing for exposure to genital herpes is similarly unwarranted.

Bibliography

1. **Barton SE.** Viral infections of the genital tract. Curr Opin Infect Dis. 1996;9:48-51.

2. **Galloway DA.** Navigating the descent in papillomavirus hell. J Infect Dis. 1994;170:1075-6.

3. **Coker R, Desmond N, Tomlinson D, Bretherton K, Byrne M.** Screening for cervical abnormalities in women with anogenital warts in an STD clinic: an inappropriate use of colposcopy. Int J STD AIDS. 1994;5:442-4.

4. **Falagas ME, Gorbach SL.** IDCP Guidelines: sexually transmitted diseases, part III. Infect Dis Clin Pract. 1996;5:85-93.

HIV DISEASE

HIV Disease Question 1
Answer: C

EDUCATIONAL OBJECTIVE: Recognize the clinical presentation of bacillary angiomatosis in a patient with HIV infection.

This 27-year-old man with HIV infection has lesions most consistent with the diagnosis of bacillary angiomatosis. A distinct infection most commonly seen in patients infected with HIV, bacillary angiomatosis can present in the skin but also may involve the viscera and bones. It is most probably caused by *Bartonella henselae*. In the skin, the morphology of the lesions varies, and the number of lesions ranges from one to many. Unlike Kaposi's sarcoma, these lesions commonly bleed.

Kaposi's sarcoma can present in the skin with lesions similar to those seen in patients with bacillary angiomatosis. It is therefore essential to biopsy any purple lesion that may arise in the skin of HIV-infected patients, because bacillary angiomatosis is treatable and if undiagnosed, can be progressive and potentially fatal.

Histologically, the lesions of bacillary angiomatosis may resemble those of pyogenic granuloma, but silver stains often show organisms in the tissue of patients with bacillary angiomatosis. Although pyogenic granulomas may occur in any setting, the rapid onset of multiple pyogenic granulomas is rare.

Secondary syphilis is commonly seen in the setting of HIV. The lesions can vary, and a granulomatous form of this disease is recognized. Skin biopsies distinguish these two entities, and special silver stains show the presence of spirochetes in secondary syphilis.

Cutaneous cryptococcosis is an important manifestation of AIDS. The most common lesions in cutaneous cryptococcosis, however, are either scattered papules and nodules with central crusting resembling molluscum contagiosum or brown to purple nodules.

Bibliography

1. **Koehler JE, Quinn FD, Berger TG, Le Boit PE, Tappero JW.** Isolation of *Rochalimaea* species from cutaneous and osseous lesions of bacillary angiomatosis. N Engl J Med. 1992;327:1625-31.

2. **Tompkins DC, Steigbigel RT.** *Rochalimaea*'s role in cat scratch disease and bacillary angiomatosis. Ann Intern Med. 1993;118:388-90.

HIV Disease Question 2
Answer: C

EDUCATIONAL OBJECTIVE: Identify the appropriate treatment strategy and regimen for early HIV disease.

Treatment for HIV infection should be considered for patients who have symptoms, a CD4 cell count under 500/μL, or a plasma HIV RNA level above 5000 copies/mL. This patient's recent history of mild fatigue and varicella zoster infection should raise concerns about possible early disease progression and need for antiretroviral therapy. Although the CD4 cell count is over 500/μL, the patient's HIV RNA level is elevated; he is, therefore, at an increased risk for disease progression and should be considered for antiretroviral therapy. The prognostic utility of the CD4 cell count appears to be strongest for short-term outcomes, particularly with advancing HIV disease. Therefore, HIV RNA levels are increasing used to evaluate patients and judge both the need for and the adequacy of antiretroviral therapy.

Studies have shown that combination regimens are superior to zidovudine monotherapy at all stages of disease, and zidovudine monotherapy should not be chosen as an option. Based on the goals of maximizing viral suppression during therapy and the desire to block or delay drug resistance, combination regimens with two or more drugs are widely recommended for the treatment of HIV infection. Several combination regimens, including zidovudine with either didanosine, zalcitabine, or lamivudine, are associated with clinical and survival benefits. Didanosine and zalcitabine have overlapping toxicities with reference to peripheral neuropathy and are not recommended because of the potential risk for serious peripheral neuropathy. The use of combination regimens with protease inhibitors in early HIV disease is not well defined, and some clinicians would defer treatment with a protease inhibitor until the patient exhibited a high viral load. Viral load should be monitored in this setting. Although some physicians might treat the patient more aggressively, there are no data from controlled clinical trials to support this approach.

Bibliography

1. **Mellors JW, Rinaldo CR Jr, Gupta P, White RM, Todd JA, Kingsley LA.** Prognosis in HIV-1 infection predicted by the quantity of virus in plasma. Science. 1996;272:1167-70.

2. **Hammer SM, Katzenstein DA, Hughes MD, Gundaker H, Schooley RT, Haubrich RH, et al.** A trial comparing nucleoside monotherapy with combination therapy in HIV-infected adults with CD4 cell counts from 200 to 500 per cubic millimeter. AIDS Clinical Trials Group Study 175 Study Team. N Engl J Med. 1996;335:1081-90.

3. **Bartlett JA, Benoit SL, Johnson VA, Quinn JB, Sepulveda GE, Ehmann WC, et al.** Lamivudine plus zidovudine compared with zalcitabine plus zidovudine in patients with HIV infection. A randomized, double-blind, placebo-controlled trial. North American AIDS Working Party. Ann Intern Med. 1996;125:161-72.

4. **Carpenter CC, Fischl MA, Hammer SM, Hirsch MS, Jacobsen DM, Katzenstein DA, et al.** Antiretroviral therapy for HIV infection in 1996. Recommendations of an international panel. JAMA. 1996;276:146-54.

HIV Disease Question 3
Answer: C

EDUCATIONAL OBJECTIVE: Identify causes of esophageal ulceration in patients with HIV disease.

Esophagitis due to *Candida* or herpes simplex virus is associated with acute or subacute symptoms of odynophagia, retrosternal chest pain, and nausea, with or without fever. Upper gastrointestinal endoscopy confirms the presence of shallow ulceration with overlying exudate. *Candida* esophagitis is more likely to be associated with patchy white plaques lining the mucosal surface of the esophagus; however, these plaques are not always seen. In addition, in severe cases of esophagitis due to herpes simplex virus, exudates may be extensive and may mimic the whitish plaques seen with *Candida* infection. Biopsy of the lesions and demonstration of organisms in culture or by histopathologic examination will distinguish between the two entities. Recurrent mucocutaneous candidiasis and the presence of oral candidiasis may be a clue to the diagnosis of candidiasis, but their absence does not rule out this diagnosis. In a patient whose symptoms are not severe or debilitating, clinical response to a trial of therapy with oral fluconazole, 100 mg/d for 7 to 14 days, may provide a presumptive diagnosis without resorting to upper gastrointestinal endoscopy or biopsy. A lack of response after 7 days argues against candidiasis.

Cytomegalovirus (CMV) may also cause esophagitis and esophageal ulceration. Organ disease due to CMV, however, is usually a complication of late-stage HIV disease in patients with CD4 cell counts of less than 50/μL. It would be unusual for a patient with a CD4 cell count of 150/μL to present with extensive CMV ulceration of the esophagus. The gastrointestinal tract may be involved at any level with CMV, although the two most common locations are the colon, where CMV produces an enterocolitis with mucosal ulceration, bleeding, and diarrhea, and the esophagus, where CMV may be more likely to present with single large ulcers. Tissue biopsy and demonstration of organisms in culture or by histopathologic examination may be necessary; the latter may be the more specific of the two diagnostic tests in that reactivation of CMV can occur in the setting of profound immunosuppression, resulting in positive CMV cultures of oropharyngeal or respiratory secretions, urine, or blood in the absence of end-organ disease.

Anecdotal case reports suggest that retained pills or capsules, in particular of zidovudine, may cause esophageal ulceration in patients with HIV disease. The symptoms induced by this complication are the same as those of esophagitis due to other causes. Upper gastrointestinal endoscopy generally reveals only a single ulcer, often with evidence of the retained fragments of the pill or capsule. Treatment is usually supportive and the ulcers spontaneously remit with removal of the offending agent and symptomatic therapy.

Idiopathic esophageal ulcers are thought to be immunologically mediated. In the esophagus they more often tend to be localized rather than diffuse and may enlarge and coalesce to form a "giant" esophageal ulcer. Spontaneous healing is uncommon; short-term corticosteroid therapy and thalidomide have both been used successfully to treat idiopathic esophageal ulceration.

Bibliography

1. **Bonacini M, Young T, Laine L.** The causes of esophageal symptoms in human immunodeficiency virus infection. A prospective study of 110 patients. Arch Intern Med. 1991;151:1567-72.

2. **Paterson DL, Georghiou PR, Allworth AM, Kemp RJ.** Thalidomide as treatment of refractory aphthous ulceration related to human immunodeficiency virus infection. Clin Infect Dis. 1995;20:250-4.

3. **Wilcox CM, Diehl DL, Cello JP, Margaretten W, Jacobson MA.** Cytomegalovirus esophagitis in patients with AIDS. A clinical, endoscopic, and pathologic correlation. Ann Intern Med. 1990;113:589-93.

4. **Edwards P, Turner J, Gold J, Cooper DA.** Esophageal ulceration induced by zidovudine. Ann Intern Med. 1990;112:65-6.

HIV Disease Question 4
Answer: B

EDUCATIONAL OBJECTIVE: Determine when *Pneumocystis carinii* pneumonia (PCP) prophylaxis should be instituted in a patient with a CD4 cell count above 200/μL.

Although a CD4 cell count of 200/μL is generally used as the threshold for beginning primary prophylaxis against PCP, PCP occurs in patients with CD4 cell counts above that level, and other evidence of immunosuppression or progressive disease may appropriately prompt PCP prophylaxis. Such evidence includes unexplained fever lasting more than 2 weeks, oral candidiasis, any AIDS-defining infection, or Kaposi's sarcoma. In this patient, the oral candidiasis is an indication to start PCP prophylaxis with the usual first-line agent, trimethoprim-sulfamethoxazole.

Despite the presence of oral candidiasis, the CD4 cell count is too high to consider *Mycobacterium avium* complex (MAC) prophylaxis or to raise the concern of MAC bacteremia. Clotrimazole troches should be adequate treatment for episodes of candidiasis in this patient; systemic anticandidal treatment is reserved for failures of local treatment. Candidemia is a rare complication of HIV, and is not suggested by this patient. Infrequent episodes of herpes simplex do not warrant daily prophylaxis.

Bibliography
1. Simonds RJ, Hughes WT, Feinberg J, Navin TR. Preventing *Pneumocystis carinii* pneumonia in persons infected with the human immunodeficiency virus. Clin Infect Dis. 1995;21:S44-8.

HIV Disease Question 5
Answer: B

EDUCATIONAL OBJECTIVE: Identify the threshold for initiation of tuberculosis prophylaxis in a patient with HIV and exclude active tuberculosis as the first step in response to positive purified protein derivative (PPD).

Reactivation tuberculosis is an important co-infection in patients with HIV, particularly in the eastern part of the United States. Clinical tuberculosis occurs at a rate of 5.4 cases per 100 person-years among documented converters, and is only slightly less common among HIV-seropositive PPD reactors. In patients with HIV infection, induration of 5 mm or more in response to PPD is regarded as positive. This patient should receive isoniazid prophylaxis after exclusion of active tuberculosis by chest radiography.

Administration of a second booster dose of PPD may be appropriate in elderly patients with an initially negative test, but this is not reasonable in a patient whose first PPD is positive. The patient has natural immunity to hepatitis B, obviating the need for hepatitis B immunization, and has not yet reached the CD4 threshold for initiation of *Pneumocystis carinii* prophylaxis, since he does not have oral candidiasis or systemic symptoms. Anergy testing using batteries of skin test antigens has recently been demonstrated to yield poorly reproducible results in patients with HIV.

Bibliography
1. Markowitz N, Hansen NI, Hopewell PC, Glassroth J, Kvale PA, Mangura BT, et al. Incidence of tuberculosis in the United States among HIV-infected persons. The Pulmonary Complications of HIV Infection Study Group. Ann Intern Med. 1997:126:123-32.

2. Chin DP, Osmond D, Page-Shafer K, Glassroth J, Rosen MJ, Reichman LB, et al. Reliability of anergy skin testing in persons with HIV infection. The Pulmonary Complications of HIV Infection Study Group. Am J Resp Crit Care Med. 1996;153:1982-4.

HIV Disease Question 6
Answer: D

EDUCATIONAL OBJECTIVE: Select an appropriate management strategy for HIV-related thrombocytopenia.

Thrombocytopenia in HIV-seropositive patients may reflect impaired production due to HIV infection of megakaryocytes, accelerated peripheral destruction mediated by antibodies, hypersplenism, or a combination of these mechanisms. In this untreated patient with no evidence of marrow infiltration, a trial of an antiviral regimen containing high-dose zidovudine is the appropriate first step. Intravenous immunoglobulin may be effective, but it is costly and does not affect the HIV viral load. Prednisone will cause further immunosuppression and is therefore undesirable. Splenectomy is reserved for patients in whom medical treatment fails. Lymph node biopsy and bone marrow biopsy are unnecessary in this patient with isolated thrombocytopenia and no systemic signs.

Bibliography
1. Najean Y, Rain JD. The mechanism of thrombocytopenia in patients with HIV infection. J Lab Clin Med. 1994;123:415-20.

2. **Landonio G, Cinque P, Nosari A, Gafa S, Rizzo F, Coen M, et al.** Comparison of two dose regimens of zidovudine in an open, randomized, multicenter study for severe HIV-related thrombocytopenia. AIDS. 1993;7:209-12.

3. **Jahnke L, Applebaum S, Greenberger PA, Green D.** An evaluation of intravenous immunoglobulin in the treatment of human immunodeficiency virus-associated thrombocytopenia. Transfusion. 1994;34:759-64.

4. **Marroni M, Gresele P, Landonio G, Lazzarin A, Coen N, Vezza R, et al.** Interferon-alpha is effective in the treatment of HIV-1-related, severe, zidovudine-resistant thrombocytopenia. A prospective, placebo-controlled, double-blind trial. Ann Intern Med. 1994;121:423-9.

HIV Disease Question 7
Answer: B

EDUCATIONAL OBJECTIVE: Assess benefits and side effects of *Mycobacterium avium* complex (MAC) prophylaxis and recognize the potential for drug interactions.

MAC prophylaxis has been controversial. Although prophylaxis has been demonstrated to decrease the incidence of MAC bacteremia in patients with advanced immunosuppression, there are concerns about efficacy, cost, side effects, and the development of resistance, particularly when monotherapy is used. However, recent studies have demonstrated the effectiveness of a simple azithromycin or clarithromycin regimen, both of which reduced the incidence of disseminated MAC by 60% compared with historical controls and by 50% compared with rifabutin prophylaxis. A combined regimen of rifabutin and azithromycin was somewhat more effective but increased side effects.

Clarithromycin may not be useful for this patient, because it requires daily dosing and is more likely to interact with ritonavir, which may enhance drug side effects.

Bibliography
1. **Havlir DV, Dube MP, Sattler FR, Forthal DN, Kemper CA, Dunne MW, et al.** Prophylaxis against disseminated *Mycobacterium avium* complex with weekly azithromycin, daily rifabutin, or both. N Engl J Med. 1996;335:392-8.

2. **Pierce M, Crampton S, Henry D, Heifets L, LaMarca A, Montecalvo M, et al.** A randomized trial of clarithromycin as prophylaxis against disseminated *Mycobacterium avium* complex infection in patients with advanced acquired immunodeficiency syndrome. N Engl J Med. 1996;335:384-91.

HIV Disease Question 8
Answer: B

EDUCATIONAL OBJECTIVE: Diagnose and manage anal condylomata in an HIV-infected man.

The lesions described in this patient may represent condyloma acuminatum (human papillomavirus infection) or condyloma latum (a manifestation of secondary syphilis). The former are more often dry and verrucous in appearance and sometimes pedunculated, while condyloma lata may be more sessile and moist in appearance; however, the two entities may be clinically indistinguishable from one another based on appearance. Recurrent anal human papillomavirus infection or recurrent manifestations of syphilis are not unusual in previously infected patients with advanced immunosuppression. Unless a specific diagnosis of syphilis is made, presumptive treatment with benzathine penicillin is inappropriate.

The incidence of anal carcinoma among HIV-infected homosexual men with anal human papillomavirus infection is 100 times that in the general population. The rapidity with which anal human papillomavirus lesions progress to dysplasia or neoplasia is unknown. For this reason, careful visual examination and treatment of human papillomavirus-associated lesions are recommended. Histopathologic or cytopathologic examination is required to confirm the diagnosis of condylomata due to human papillomavirus and should be performed to detect the presence of dysplasia or anal carcinoma before ablative therapy for human papillomavirus is undertaken. Lesions demonstrating dysplastic or neoplastic changes should be resected. Although it may be reasonable to repeat an examination in 3 months if the diagnosis has been firmly established and high-risk human papillomavirus DNA types such as 16 and 18 are not present, this strategy is not appropriate in this setting.

Bibliography
1. **Palefsky JM, Holly EA, Gonzales J, Lamborn K, Hollander H.** Natural history of anal cytologic abnormalities and papillomavirus infection among homosexual men with group IV HIV disease. J Acquir Immune Defic Syndr. 1992;5:1258-65.

2. **Kiviat NB, Critchlow CW, Holmes KK, Kuypers J, Dunphy C, Surawicz C, et al.** Association of anal dysplasia and human papillomavirus with immunosuppression and HIV infection among homosexual men. AIDS. 1993;7:43-9.

3. **Vernon SD, Holmes KK, Reeves WC.** Human papillomavirus infection and associated disease in persons infected with human immunodeficiency virus. Clin Infect Dis. 1995;21:S121-4.

HIV Disease Question 9
Answer: C

EDUCATIONAL OBJECTIVE: Select routine health care maintenance for an HIV-seropositive patient.

Good care of HIV-seropositive patients requires attention to detail and careful follow-up, even when the patient has a high CD4 cell count and does not require specific treatment for HIV. The rapid plasma reagin assay should be repeated annually. Serial determination of serum cryptococcal antigen is not recommended as a screening test in asymptomatic patients. Because this patient's hepatitis B surface antibody is positive at baseline, there is no need to repeat it. The patient should be counseled on minimizing the risk of exposure to toxoplasmosis. A repeat *Toxoplasma* antibody measurement is not required until immunosuppression is advanced enough to put the patient at risk if she has been exposed.

Women with HIV who have not undergone a hysterectomy should have a pelvic examination and Papanicolaou smear annually. The finding of atypical squamous cells of uncertain significance, which in some patients leads eventually to dysplastic changes, should prompt earlier repeat of the Papanicolaou smear. The frequency of repeat CD4 determination depends on the initial level and the proximity to CD4-based decision points, such as the threshold of 200/μL for initiation of prophylactic therapy for *Pneumocystis carinii* pneumonia. At this level, repeat determination in 6 months is reasonable. Because results of the initial purified protein derivative (PPD) test are positive, additional PPD testing is not appropriate.

Bibliography

1. **Freedberg KA, Malabanan A, Samet JH, Libman H.** Initial assessment of patients infected with human immunodeficiency virus: the yield and cost of laboratory testing. J Acquir Immune Defic Syndr. 1994;7:1134-40.
2. **Jewett JF, Hecht FM.** Preventive health care for adults with HIV infection. JAMA. 1993;269:1144-53.

HIV Disease Question 10
Answer: A

EDUCATIONAL OBJECTIVE: Select appropriate initial laboratory and clinical testing in a patient newly diagnosed with HIV disease.

Serologic testing for syphilis is indicated in all persons with HIV, as syphilis is a common sexually transmitted disease and may be more virulent in the presence of HIV infection. Since this patient believes that his HIV infection was sexually acquired, he is clearly at risk for syphilis. HIV-1 p24 antigen may have usefulness in the early diagnosis of HIV seroconversion disease, but it has no clinical utility for either prognosis or for monitoring the impact of therapy.

Direct measures of viral load by either branched DNA (bDNA) or polymerase chain reaction (PCR) methods are more accurate and possess greater clinical utility. Hepatitis C antibody may be important in evaluating elevated liver function tests found in patients with HIV infection, but it is not required in the initial evaluation. Tuberculin skin testing is not indicated in this man who has previously tested positive. β_2-microglobulin is nonspecific in HIV infection and does not have any clinical utility. Other indicated tests are *Toxoplasmosis gondii* IgG, cytomegalovirus IgG, and hepatitis B serology.

Bibliography

1. **Kaplan JE, Masur H, Holmes KK, Wilfert CM, Sperling R, Baker SA, et al.** USPHS/IDSA guidelines for the prevention of opportunistic infections in persons infected with human immunodeficiency virus: an overview. Clin Infect Dis. 1995;21:S12-31.
2. **O'Brien WA, Hartigan PM, Martin D, Esinhart J, Hill A, Benoit S, et al.** Changes in plasma HIV-1 RNA and CD4+ lymphocyte counts and the risk of progression to AIDS. Veterans Affairs Cooperative Study Group on AIDS. N Engl J Med. 1996;334:426-31.

HIV Disease Question 11
Answer: A

EDUCATIONAL OBJECTIVE: Diagnose oral hairy leukoplakia.

This patient's lesions are typical of oral hairy leukoplakia, a lesion associated with mucosal epithelial infection with Epstein-Barr virus. The lesions can be distinguished from those due to *Candida* species by their more linear frondlike appearance and their adherence to the mucosa, such that material cannot be scraped off with a tongue blade. The finding of a few yeast forms in a scraping of mucosal cells from these lesions reflects colonization of the oral mucosa with *Candida* species and is not diagnostic of oral thrush. A biopsy of the lesion would yield histopathologic changes consistent with Epstein-Barr virus, which can be demonstrated with monoclonal antibody, immunohistochemical staining techniques, or electron microscopy. Oral hairy leukoplakia can wax and wane over time, may resolve spontaneously, or may respond to acyclovir or zidovudine. It is likely that the anecdotally reported response to zidovudine is a reflection of improved immune function induced by reduction of HIV replication; if so, oral hairy leukoplakia may also resolve with aggressive antiretroviral therapy with other agents. The lack of resolution with therapies directed at oropharyngeal candidiasis is sometimes used as a diagnostic clue for oral hairy leukoplakia.

Although aphthous stomatitis may begin with white buccal mucosal lesions, they are not frondlike and they quickly progress to painful, shallow mucosal ulcers. These may be single or multiple and may be seen at all stages of HIV disease. They are a common side effect reported with zalcitabine therapy. In severe cases they may coalesce to form large ulcers that interfere with hydration or nutrition. Mild cases generally resolve spontaneously or respond to symptomatic topical therapy with a solution containing a local anesthetic agent to reduce pain, an oral corticosteroid preparation to reduce inflammation, and a narrow-spectrum antibiotic to reduce the likelihood of secondary bacterial infection of the ulcers. For severe episodes, a short course of systemic corticosteroids or thalidomide may reduce symptoms and accelerate healing.

A whitish exudate with surrounding erythema and superficial ulceration may be found on the gingiva (interdental papillae) in patients with bacterial gingivitis. The acute necrotizing form may be associated with severe mouth pain, progressive erosion of gums, and ultimately tooth loss. This complication is seen more often in patients with advanced immunosuppression. Treatment requires local debridement, frequent use of antiseptic mouthwash, and short courses of systemic antibiotics, such as metronidazole, amoxicillin, or clindamycin.

Bibliography

1. **Greenspan JS, Greenspan D, Winkler JR.** Oral complications of HIV infection. In: Sande MA, Volberding PA, eds. Medical Management of AIDS. 3rd ed. Philadelphia, PA: WB Saunders Co; 1992:161-75.

2. **Greenspan D, Greenspan JS, Hearst NG, Pan LZ, Conant MA, Abrams DI, et al.** Relation of oral hairy leukoplakia to infection with the human immunodeficiency virus and the risk of developing AIDS. J Infect Dis. 1987;155:475-80.

HIV Disease Question 12
Answer: D

EDUCATIONAL OBJECTIVE: Respond to a patient at apparently low risk who requests HIV testing.

Patient requests for HIV testing are opportunities for HIV education and for candid discussion of risk behaviors, but even if the risk by history appears to be low, the physician should not attempt to dissuade the patient from testing, as some patients will not divulge risky behaviors. (An exception to this general rule is the patient with a mental health disorder, such as AIDS phobia, obsessive/compulsive disorder, or anxiety or neuroses, who has already been tested.) HIV antibody detection by ELISA with confirmatory Western blot is the most reliable way to screen for HIV infection. Both sensitivity and specificity are excellent.

The CD4 cell count is appropriate for assessing the impact of chronic HIV infection on the immune system, but it is neither sensitive nor specific for detection of infection. A positive test for viral RNA would be specific for HIV infection, but some infected persons may have nondetectable viral RNA, making this test a poor choice for screening.

Bibliography

1. **Barbacci M, Repke JT, Chaisson RE.** Routine prenatal screening for HIV infection. Lancet. 1991;337:709-11.

HIV Disease Question 13
Answer: A

EDUCATIONAL OBJECTIVE: Select the best management approach for a patient with symptoms of cerebral toxoplasmosis.

Cerebral toxoplasmosis is the most common opportunistic process occurring in the central nervous system among AIDS patients. Therefore, patients who have or have had positive results to a serologic test should be assumed to have toxoplasmosis, and a trial of antitoxoplasmosis therapy should be initiated empirically. The treatment of choice for cerebral toxoplasmosis is combination therapy with sulfadiazine and pyrimethamine; a combination of pyrimethamine and clindamycin is usually effective in patients who cannot tolerate sulfa medications. If the patient does not demonstrate a response to treatment after 7 to 10 days, further diagnostic workup, including brain biopsy, should be performed.

Although the lesions can usually be seen on a contrast-enhanced CT scan (as in this case), MRI is usually more sensitive and is useful in patients who have negative results on CT scan but a clinical presentation consistent with toxoplasmosis. In this patient, magnetic resonance imaging may be helpful in preparing for brain biopsy if the lesions do not respond to empiric therapy; however, it is best used either as the initial diagnostic procedure (in lieu of the CT scan) or when results of an initial CT scan with contrast are negative.

Several research studies have demonstrated that positron emission tomography (PET) scan can differentiate between lesions of toxoplasmosis and lymphoma. In the clinical setting described in this case, however, the most likely diagnosis is toxoplasmosis, based on the positive serology and the clinical presentation. Had the patient been taking trimethoprim-sulfamethoxazole prophylaxis for *Pneumocystis carinii* pneumonia (which also protects against toxoplasmosis) or had a negative serologic antibody test for *Toxoplasma gondii,* a PET scan may have been helpful; even then, however, the patient would likely have a brief trial of antitoxoplasmosis therapy or, more commonly, be referred for early brain biopsy instead of a PET scan.

Once a serologic test is positive for toxoplasmosis, it remains positive for life. Since most *Toxoplasma* disease is reactivation of previous infection, documentation of a rise in titer is not helpful in diagnosing active toxoplasmosis. Rather, it is the absence of a positive titer that is important in potentially ruling out *Toxoplasma* disease.

Bibliography

1. **Luft BJ, Hafner R, Korzun AH, Leport, Antoniskis D, Bosler EM, et al.** Toxoplasmic encephalitis in patients with the acquired immunodeficiency syndrome. Members of the ACTG 077p/ANRS 009 Study Team. N Engl J Med. 1993;329:995-1000.

2. **Dannemann B, McCutchan JA, Israelski D, Antoniskis D, Leport C, Luft B, et al.** Treatment of toxoplasmic encephalitis in patients with AIDS. A randomized trial comparing pyrimethamine plus clindamycin to pyrimethamine plus sulfadiazine. The California Collaborative Treatment Group. Ann Intern Med. 1993; 116:33-43.

HIV Disease Question 14
Answer: A

EDUCATIONAL OBJECTIVE: Select the proper screening test in a specific population.

This scenario meets the three criteria for selection of a screening test. Treatment of HIV-positive mothers is effective, and transmission of the infection to the child will cause a burden to society. The critical question is which test should be selected. PCR amplification is still not considered the screening test for diagnosis of an HIV infection in adults. Problems in the operating characteristics, especially the specificity due to the constant possibility of false-positive results, limit its applicability. However, it is important to screen pregnant women at risk for HIV infection, because antiretroviral treatment decreases the likelihood of transmission to the fetus and neonate. Testing of the newborn, if indicated because the mother did not receive any prenatal care, can be performed by detection of IgA antibodies (IgG antibodies may be transferred across the placenta from the HIV-positive mother and cause false-positive results). However, if the mother can be tested and counseled to receive treatment before delivery, she should.

ELISA testing for antibodies against HIV still remains the screening test of choice for HIV disease, supported by a positive Western blot. This combination of tests when used in a population with a high prevalence of disease has high positive and negative predictive values.

Bibliography

1. **Peckham C, Gibb D.** Mother-to-child transmission of the human immunodeficiency virus. N Engl J Med. 1995;333:298-302.

2. **Owens DK, Holodniy M, Garber AM, Scott J, Sonnad S, Moses L, et al.** Polymerase chain reaction for the diagnosis of HIV infection in adults. A meta-analysis with recommendations for clinical practice and study design. Ann Intern Med. 1996;124:803-15.

HYPERTENSION

Hypertension Question 1
Answer: C

EDUCATIONAL OBJECTIVE: Prescribe appropriate therapy for a pregnant woman with hypertension.

This 28-year-old woman's history establishes the diagnosis of chronic hypertension, rather than gestational hypertension or preeclampsia, because hypertension appeared before 20 weeks of gestation. Preexisting hypertension is often masked by the vasodilatation that occurs during pregnancy. The improbability of preeclampsia is supported by the absence of increased 24-hour urine protein excretion, renal insufficiency, or hyperuricemia. Although it is uncertain whether treatment of mild hypertension in pregnant women improves outcomes, it is generally agreed that severe hypertension should be treated. There is poorer fetal and maternal outcome when diastolic blood pressure is 110 mm Hg or greater in the first trimester. Methyldopa has been used extensively in the treatment of chronic hypertension in pregnant women and does not affect uteroplacental or fetal hemodynamics.

The use of atenolol in pregnant women has been associated with adverse effects on ureteroplacental and fetal hemodynamics. The use of diuretic agents is controversial during pregnancy because of the lack of prospective data, and it is uncertain whether these agents should be continued in patients in whom they had been started before the onset of pregnancy. A panel has suggested maintaining diuretic therapy in women with pre-existing treatment or in patients treated before 20 weeks of gestation. The usefulness of diuretic agents is greatest in patients with left ventricular hypertrophy or salt-sensitive hypertension. Diuretic agents should be discontinued if preeclampsia develops or in the presence of reduced fetal growth. Angiotensin-converting enzyme inhibitors such as enalapril have been associated with poor fetal outcome and should not be used, especially late in pregnancy.

Bibliography
1. **Sibai BM.** Treatment of hypertension in pregnant women. N Engl J Med. 1996;335:257-65.

Hypertension Questions 2-3
Answers: 2(D); 3(C)

EDUCATIONAL OBJECTIVE: Assess the risk of disease and probability of therapeutic benefit in a patient with level 1 hypertension.

At presentation, the patient's overall 10-year risk for the development of coronary heart disease (by far the predominant risk given her age and degree of hypertension) is less than 1%. If there were a 20% reduction in risk with successful antihypertensive treatment (a liberal estimate), the number of patients needed to treat to avoid one myocardial event is in excess of 500. In this setting, drug therapy is not indicated.

In contrast, the development of left ventricular hypertrophy represents a significant additional risk factor for coronary heart disease, and increases the patient's overall risk to approximately 12%. In this setting, the number needed to treat to avoid one myocardial infarction is approximately 40 and within the range that most clinicians would agree is appropriate for starting prophylactic treatment of minimal toxicity to avoid a major complication. In this setting, treatment would be for both hypertension and left ventricular hypertrophy. A direct vasodilator (for example, hydralazine) does not improve left ventricular hypertrophy. Diuretics may decrease left ventricular hypertrophy, primarily by decreasing ventricular dimensions but not by reducing ventricular wall thickness. ACE inhibitors (for example, captopril) are probably the most effective drugs for reducing blood pressure and left ventricular hypertrophy.

Bibliography
1. **Anderson KM, Wilson PW, Odell PM, Kannel WB.** An updated coronary risk profile. A statement for health professionals. Circulation. 1991;83:356-62.

Hypertension Question 4
Answer: B

EDUCATIONAL OBJECTIVE: Prescribe appropriate medications for the treatment of hypertension in pregnancy.

The use of methyldopa, hydralazine, propranolol, or labetalol is considered reasonable in the treatment of hypertension in the pregnant patient. The use of angiotensin-converting enzyme inhibitors is contraindicated because of evidence of abortion, stillbirths, and other severe complications of pregnancy that have been seen in humans and in animal studies.

Bibliography

1. **Carson JL, Elliot DL.** Care of the pregnant patient with medical illness. J Gen Intern Med. 1988;3:577-88.

Hypertension Question 5
Answer: B

EDUCATIONAL OBJECTIVE: Recognize the role of vasoconstricting nasal sprays in hypertension.

Lack of control of hypertension is commonly encountered in clinical practice. In this patient, the history of allergic rhinitis is consistent with the use of vasoconstricting nasal sprays, or systemic vasoconstricting medications, which typically produce habituation and are available without prescription. Allergic rhinitis is a common condition and is often self-treated by patients. Because of the tendency for rebound symptoms when a dose wears off, patients often continue treatment indefinitely, particularly because a prescription is unnecessary. This condition, referred to as *rhinitis medicamentosa,* may require a tapering course of systemic corticosteroids to reduce dependency.

Although noncompliance is a reasonable explanation, the presence of bilateral trace pitting edema suggests that the patient is receiving nifedipine, for which that physical finding is a fairly common side effect. Likewise, there is no evidence on physical examination of alternative explanations for edema. The patient is receiving a reasonable dosage of the drug, so dosage is unlikely to be responsible for treatment failure.

Although obesity is a risk factor for diastolic hypertension, it is described as mild in the patient's history. In any event, obesity would not be expected to produce this degree of diastolic hypertension. Secondary forms of hypertension, although always possible, are rare.

Bibliography

1. **Lake CR, Gallant S, Masson E, Miller P.** Adverse drug effects attributed to phenylpropanolamine: a review of 142 case reports. Am J Med. 1990;89:195-208.

Hypertension Question 6
Answer: C

EDUCATIONAL OBJECTIVE: Recognize the clinical presentation of aortic coarctation in an adult.

Coarctation of the aorta should be suspected in a young adult who has hypertension, leg claudication, and diminished or absent leg pulses. Supporting evidence would be a blood pressure difference between the arms and the legs. The diagnosis can be made by magnetic resonance angiography of the thoracic aorta, echocardiography, spiral computed tomography, or aortography. Surgical repair involves resection of the affected part of the aorta with subsequent end-to-end anastomosis. Percutaneous transluminal coronary angioplasty of the affected part of the aorta may also be used to treat the coarctation.

This patient's clinical features are not indicative of renal artery stenosis or suggestive of pheochromocytoma. Therefore, renal arteriography, captopril scintigraphy, and serum catecholamine testing are not indicated. Abdominal computed tomography will not diagnose the aortic coarctation, which typically occurs in the thoracic aorta near the insertion of the ductus ligamentosum.

Bibliography

1. **Hougen TJ, Sell JE.** Recent advances in the diagnosis and treatment of coarctation of the aorta. Curr Opin Cardiol. 1995;10:524-9.

Hypertension Question 7
Answer: A

EDUCATIONAL OBJECTIVE: Diagnose and manage acute aortic dissection.

The most appropriate response is to lower this woman's blood pressure immediately, using intravenous agents if necessary. Normally this would include use of a β-blocking agent to lower blood pressure, heart rate, and dp/dt, all of which are thought to promote extension of the aortic dissection. A second drug, frequently a vasodilating agent, is then added to the β-blocker.

Transthoracic echocardiography is relatively insensitive (31% to 55%) for distal aortic dissection, which is particularly likely in this patient. Its sensitivity is 78% to 100% for ascending dissection, but it is still less sensitive than transesophageal echocardiography. Therefore, some other imaging modality, including computed tomographic scanning or transesophageal echocardiography, would be preferred.

Calling a cardiovascular surgeon is less urgent than lowering the blood pressure. This patient has no clinical signs, such as aortic insufficiency, carotid or right arm pulse deficit, a neurologic syndrome, or anterior chest pain, that strongly suggest involvement of the ascending aorta. Ascending dissection is ordinarily a surgical emergency; descending dissection is not. As one simultaneously treats the hypertension and arranges for appropriate thoracic imaging, letting the on-call cardiovascular surgeon know about the patient is appropriate. However, rapid initial medical treatment and diagnosis are the first priority.

The option of ordering a series of spine radiographs addresses the possibility that a ruptured vertebral disc has caused such pain that the patient's hypertension is related to this rather than an aortic catastrophe. However, the first order of diagnostic strategy should be to rule out potentially life-threatening disease. Further work-up of less threatening possibilities would then follow.

Although aortic aneurysm with rupture is plausible, several features of the patient's presentation make the choice of abdominal ultrasonography less desirable than urgent lowering of blood pressure. First, there is no history of pre-existent aortic aneurysm. Second, the pain is interscapular, not in the flanks. Third, the patient presents with hypertension and a normal abdominal examination. Ordinarily, a ruptured abdominal aortic aneurysm is accompanied by abdominal tenderness and/or quiet bowel sounds, and frequently hypotension is present.

Bibliography

1. **Isselbacher EM, Eagle KA, DeSanctis RW.** Disease of the aorta. In: Braunwald E, ed. Heart Disease — A Textbook of Cardiovascular Medicine. Philadelphia: W.B. Saunders; 1996:1546-81.

2. **Cigarroa JE, Isselbacher EM, DeSanctis RW, Eagle KA.** Diagnostic imaging in the evaluation of suspected aortic dissection: old standards and new directions. N Engl J Med. 1993;328:35-43.

Hypertension Question 8
Answer: C

EDUCATIONAL OBJECTIVE: Diagnose white coat hypertension in a patient with elevated blood pressure in an office setting.

This 49-year-old woman has features suggesting so-called *white coat hypertension* with an elevated blood pressure noted only during her clinic visits and no evidence of end-organ effects. As many as 25% of all newly diagnosed cases of hypertension may be attributed to the transient rise in blood pressure some patients experience when being evaluated in the physician's office. Twenty-four hour ambulatory blood pressure monitoring (ABPM) is the most effective method of determining whether this observed elevation in blood pressure persists outside the office setting. Home blood pressure monitoring is an acceptable alternative approach. However, patients must be instructed on the use of the monitor and this method may not be as accurate as ABPM. Automated blood pressure devices are accurate if they are properly calibrated; however, many public devices are not properly maintained and therefore their results may not be reliable.

Repeated office visits to monitor the patient's blood pressure may not help clarify the problem. Documenting an elevated blood pressure outside the office setting is necessary to determine whether this patient has established hypertension. Furthermore, the expense of repeated office visits may exceed the cost of ABPM.

The clinical significance of white coat hypertension is controversial. Affected patients appear to represent a subgroup with an increased risk for developing hypertension. Transient elevation in blood pressure is not associated with an increase in cardiovascular events, and drug therapy is usually not warranted. However, most experts do recommend that these patients be counseled about lifestyle interventions to reduce the risk of cardiovascular disease.

Discontinuing the low-dose estrogen supplement is unlikely to lower the blood pressure, and starting antihypertensive therapy without excluding white coat hypertension would be premature.

Bibliography

1. **Appel LJ, Stason WB.** Ambulatory blood pressure monitoring and blood pressure self-measurement in the diagnosis and management of hypertension. Ann Intern Med. 1993;118:867-82.

2. **Pickering TG, Kaplan NM, Krakoff L, et al.** American Society of Hypertension Expert Panel: Conclusions and recommendations on the clinical use of home (self) and ambulatory blood pressure monitoring. Am J Hypertens. 1996;9:1.

Hypertension Question 9
Answer: A

EDUCATIONAL OBJECTIVE: Prescribe appropriate therapy for a black man with established hypertension.

This patient has established hypertension with evidence of early ventricular hypertrophy and type II diabetes mellitus. Lisinopril would be the most appropriate initial therapy. ACE inhibitor therapy in patients with diabetes mellitus and hypertension clearly prevents proteinuria and renal failure, and appears to prevent diabetic nephropathy, even in the absence of hypertension. Salt-sensitive hypertension is more common in blacks, and a diuretic or a calcium channel blocker is frequently the best initial choice for drug therapy. However ACE inhibitors are often effective in treating hypertension in blacks, and preventing diabetic nephropathy is the most important consideration in selecting the initial agent for this patient.

The different classes of calcium channel blockers appear to vary in their effect on proteinuria and renal function in diabetes. Diltiazem and nicardipine decrease glomerular pressure by increasing efferent arteriolar dilatation, thus decreasing proteinuria. By contrast, nifedipine, increases proteinuria by dilating both afferent and efferent arterioles and altering capillary permeability. Thiazide diuretics may exacerbate the hyperglycemia and hyperuricemia (though the effect is often trivial with low doses of the medication). α-Adrenergic blockers, such as doxazosin, offer no special advantages in this case. All of these agents can reduce left ventricular hypertrophy.

Bibliography

1. **Kasiske BL, Kalil RS, Ma JZ, Liao M, Keane WF.** Effect of antihypertensive therapy on the kidney in patients with diabetes: a meta-regression analysis. Ann Intern Med. 1993:118:129-38.

2. **Clark CM Jr, Lee DA.** Prevention and treatment of the complications of diabetes mellitus. N Engl J Med. 1995;332:1210-7.

Hypertension Question 10
Answer: B

EDUCATIONAL OBJECTIVE: Prescribe the appropriate therapy for a patient with diabetic nephropathy.

This patient has confirmed microalbuminuria, assuming that both urine specimens were obtained in the absence of menses or infection. The presence of retinopathy supports the interpretation that this is early diabetic nephropathy. A pathogenetic sequence in type 1 diabetes mellitus leads from microalbuminuria to clinical proteinuria and then, in most instances, to renal failure. Treatment with an angiotensin-converting enzyme inhibitor such as lisinopril at the earliest stage

(even before hypertension has appeared) decreases albumin excretion. This treatment also reduces the decline in glomerular filtration rate and the ultimate need for renal dialysis and is, therefore, the best currently available treatment of early nephropathy.

There is no strong evidence that losartan, an angiotensin-receptor blocker, has proven benefit for patients with early diabetic nephropathy, although it has been effective in hypertensive patients with other renal disease. A non-dihydropyridine calcium channel blocker such as verapamil can also decrease albumin excretion, but this drug class has not yet been definitively shown to decrease the long-term risk of renal insufficiency. Some evidence from animal and human studies implicates hyperlipidemia in the pathogenesis of nephropathy, but thus far lowering low-density lipoprotein (LDL) cholesterol has not been consistently shown to have long-term benefits in treatment of early nephropathy. However, if the patient has other risk factors or clinical evidence for coronary artery disease, simvastatin would be indicated to reduce LDL cholesterol to less than 130 mg/dL in the former case and to less than 100 mg/dL in the latter case. Hydrochlorothiazide and prazosin could both be useful later in this patient's course if she develops hypertension; however, they are not indicated for normotensive microalbuminuria.

Bibliography

1. **Gansevoort RT, de Zeeuw D, Shahinfar S, Redfield A, deJong PE.** Effects of the angiotensin II antagonist losartan in hypertensive patients with renal disease. J Hypertens. 1994;12(suppl 2):537-42.

2. **Lam KS, Cheng IK, Janus ED, Pang RW.** Cholesterol-lowering therapy may retard the progression of diabetic nephropathy. Diabetologia. 1995;38:604-9.

3. **Lewis EJ, Hunsicker LG, Bain RP, Rohde RD, the Collaborative Study Group.** The effect of angiotensin-converting-enzyme inhibition on diabetic nephropathy. N Engl J Med. 1993;329:1456-62.

4. Microalbuminuria Captopril Study Group. Captopril reduces the risk of nephropathy in IDDM patients with microalbuminuria. Diabetologia. 1996;39:587-93.

5. **Molitch ME.** ACE inhibitors and diabetic nephropathy. Diabetes Care.1994;17:756-60.

Hypertension Question 11
Answer: C

EDUCATIONAL OBJECTIVE: Prescribe the appropriate therapy for hypertension in a patient with type 2 diabetes mellitus.

This patient has essential hypertension based on family history, funduscopic findings, and absence of microalbuminuria. The hypertension has not responded adequately to weight reduction plus a large dose of enalapril. Black persons tend to have hypertension that is associated with an expanded extracellular fluid volume and a low plasma renin level. Therefore, addition of a diuretic agent such as hydrochlorothiazide is now appropriate. It should also improve the response to the angiotensin-converting enzyme (ACE) inhibitor. The patient's excellent glycemic control, current normal total cholesterol, and absence of family history of coronary artery disease suggest little risk from the diuretic agent, but he should be monitored for exacerbation of hyperglycemia or development of hyperlipidemia.

Adding or changing to another ACE inhibitor such as lisinopril is unlikely to be of any greater benefit than the first ACE inhibitor. A β-blocker is contraindicated by his asthma. As a house painter, he works at heights; therefore, α-adrenergic antagonists, which tend to cause orthostatic hypotension, should not be used unless they are essential to the control of hypertension. A hydroxymethylglutaryl coenzyme A (HMG-CoA) reductase inhibitor is not needed in a patient with a total cholesterol of 178 mg/dL unless the patient has remarkably low concentrations of both triglycerides and high-density lipoprotein cholesterol and, therefore, an elevated low-density lipoprotein cholesterol.

Bibliography

1. **Albu J, Konnarides C, Pi-Sunyer FX.** Weight control: metabolic and cardiovascular effects. Diab Rev. 1995;3:335-47.

2. **Bakris GL.** Pathogenesis of hypertension in diabetes. Diab Rev. 1995;3:460-76.

3. Consensus Development Conference. The treatment of hypertension in diabetes. Diabetes Care. 1993;16:1394-401.

4. **Elliott WJ, Stein PP, Black HR.** Drug treatment of hypertension in patients with diabetes. Diab Rev. 1995;3:477-509.

5. National High Blood Pressure Education Program Working Group. Report on hypertension in diabetes. Hypertension. 1994;23:145-58.

Hypertension Question 12
Answer: E

EDUCATIONAL OBJECTIVE: Diagnose fulminant preeclampsia and distinguish it from other diseases.

This woman has fulminant preeclampsia, a multisystem disease caused by widespread endothelial cell dysfunction resulting in fibrin deposits in the small vessels of the kidney, liver, and brain. Microangiopathic hemolytic anemia is present secondary to the widespread fibrin deposits.

Preeclampsia has many similarities to thrombotic thrombocytopenic purpura (TTP), but TTP causes damage to the endothelial cells by an immunologic mechanism. Fever virtually always is present in TTP, and hypertension is rare. This woman manifests the HELLP syndrome consisting of *h*emolysis, *e*levated *l*iver enzymes, and *l*ow *p*latelet count. The HELLP syndrome is always an indication for immediate delivery, which is the definitive treatment for preeclampsia.

Although hypertension occurs in preeclampsia, the pressure does not reach the levels seen in malignant hypertension, where diastolic pressure is usually above 120 mm Hg and hypertension itself causes endothelial cell damage. Thus, preeclampsia is not associated with retinal hemorrhages or exudates or papilledema, characteristically seen in malignant hypertension.

The hyperuricemia and proteinuria without microscopic hematuria or casts is typical of preeclampsia; with acute glomerulonephritis, however, microscopic hematuria accompanies proteinuria.

Liver involvement is common in preeclampsia, and fatty deposition in liver cells and fibrin deposits in the sinusoids have been found on percutaneous liver biopsy studies. Thrombocytopenia and elevated fibrin split products are consistent with widespread fibrin deposition, which can lead to a consumptive coagulopathy.

Bibliography

1. **Ferris TF.** Pre-eclampsia and hypertension in pregnancy. In: Burrow GN, Ferris TF, eds. Medical Complications During Pregnancy. 4th ed. Philadelphia, PA: WB Saunders Co; 1994.

2. **Martin JN, Blake PG Jr, Perry KG Jr, McCaul JF, Hess LW, Martin RW.** The natural history of HELLP syndrome: patterns of disease progression and regression. Am J Obstet Gynecol. 1991;164:1500-9.

Hypertension Question 13
Answer: B

EDUCATIONAL OBJECTIVE: Distinguish primary aldosteronism secondary to an adrenal adenoma from other complications in pregnancy.

This 28-year-old woman, who had hypertension preceding her pregnancy, is found to have hypokalemia accompanying severe hypertension in the 28th week of gestation. Although a renal artery stenosis could be present, the severe hypokalemia and high plasma aldosterone levels are more consistent with primary aldosteronism. Although plasma renin activity is usually undetectable with primary aldosteronism, the high plasma renin activity occurring with pregnancy is not completely suppressed. The high plasma aldosterone level at 8 AM followed by a decreased level after ambulation is most consistent with an adrenal adenoma.

Although malignant hypertension with secondary aldosteronism can occur in pregnancy, the normal funduscopic examination and the absence of significant proteinuria argue against this diagnosis.

The normal renal function, normal serum uric acid level, and minimal proteinuria argue against pre-eclampsia. When hyperaldosteronism is caused by adrenal hyperplasia, there is an exaggerated rise in plasma aldosterone levels with ambulation.

Bibliography

1. **Merrill RH, Dombroski RA, MacKenna M.** Primary hyperaldosteronism during pregnancy. Am J Obstet Gynecol. 1984;150:786-7.
2. **Neerhof MG, Shlossman PA, Poll DS, Ludmirsky A, Weiner S.** Idiopathic aldosteronism in pregnancy. Obstet Gynecol. 1991;78:489-91.

Hypertension Questions 14-18
Answers: 14(B); 15(D); 16(A); 17(D); 18(B)

EDUCATIONAL OBJECTIVE: Recognize co-existing conditions that help determine initial antihypertensive drug therapy in patients with high blood pressure.

The choice of first-line antihypertensive drug therapy is often determined by co-existing conditions.

In the 55-year-old man with diastolic dysfunction, there is no reason to select an antihypertensive drug on the basis of blood pressure reduction alone because each of these classes of drugs would be expected to lower blood pressure. However, some classes of drugs accentuate diastolic dysfunction by decreasing diastolic filling (for example, diuretics). In contrast, calcium channel blockers reduce contractility and increase time in diastole to enhance filling. Therefore, they would be the agent of choice in this patient.

In the 43-year-old woman with diabetes mellitus and high blood pressure, reductions in systemic pressure clearly have been shown to slow progression to end-stage renal disease. In addition, reductions in angiotensin II levels are also important. Angiotensin-converting enzyme (ACE) inhibitors are the agents of choice. They reduce resistance in efferent arteries more than in afferent arteries, thereby reducing glomerular pressure. Experimental studies have shown that this is associated with reductions in proteinuria and slower progression to end-stage renal disease. A recent study confirmed this hypothesis in patients with diabetes mellitus and serum creatinine in the 2.5 mg/dL range. ACE inhibitors were shown to reduce progression to end-stage renal disease, and ACE inhibitor therapy was associated with a 50% reduction in the risk of the combined end points of death, dialysis, and transplantation.

In the 72-year-old woman, several classes of antihypertensive therapy would be expected to reduce blood pressure. However, three recent trials (Systolic Hypertension in the Elderly Program, Swedish Trial in Old People, European Working Trial Party) have shown that thiazide diuretics reduce blood pressure as well as stroke and myocardial infarction in elderly hypertensive patients.

In the 53-year-old man with asymptomatic heart failure, all of the agents would be expected to reduce blood pressure. The choice of antihypertensive therapy is based on the results from the recent study of left-ventricular dysfunction trial (SOLVD). In this study, ACE inhibitors were compared with placebo in patients with chronic left ventricular dysfunction but without symptomatic heart failure. The results indicated that ACE inhibitors prevented clinical heart failure.

In the 65-year-old man with renal artery disease, this extent of stenosis is often associated with angiotensin II–dependent maintenance of the glomerular filtration rate. Although blood pressure would be expected to respond to ACE inhibitors, there is concern regarding reductions in efferent arteriolar tone in the presence of fixed up-stream stenosis. Therefore, although ACE inhibitors are the most effective therapy for non-bilateral renal artery stenosis, discontinuation of therapy due to worsening renal insufficiency occurs in up to 5% of treated patients, and calcium antagonists are an alternative therapy for these patients.

Bibliography

1. Effect of enalapril on mortality and the development of heart failure in asymptomatic patients with reduced left ventricular ejection fractions. The SOLVD Investigators. N Engl J Med. 1992;327:685-91.
2. **Frohlich ED, Apstein C, Chobanian AV, Devereux RB, Dustan HP, Dzau V, et al.** The heart in hypertension. N Engl J Med. 1992;327:998-1008.
3. **Lewis EJ, Hunsicker LG, Bain RP, Rohde RD.** The effect of angiotensin-converting-enzyme inhibitor on diabetic nephropathy. The Collaborative Study Group. N Engl J Med. 1993;329:1456-62.

4. Prevention of stroke by antihypertensive drug treatment in older persons with isolated systolic hypertension. Final results of the Systolic Hypertension in the Elderly Program (SHEP). SHEP Cooperative Research Group. JAMA. 1991;265:3255-64.

5. The fifth report of the Joint National Committee on Detection, Evaluation, and Treatment of High Blood Pressure. Arch Intern Med. 1993;153:154-83.

6. **Hollenberg NM.** Medical therapy for renovascular hypertension. Am J Hypertens. 1988;1:338S-343S.

Hypertension Question 19
Answer: D

EDUCATIONAL OBJECTIVE: Identify maneuvers proven to delay progression of end-stage renal disease.

The best management to slow progression of renal insufficiency is rigorous control of blood pressure. Several studies have also suggested that angiotensin-converting enzyme (ACE) inhibitors may have a particular advantage in slowing progression in both diabetic and nondiabetic causes of renal insufficiency, but hyperkalemia, as was present in this patient, may limit the utility of this agent. Lowering the labetalol dosage may relieve symptoms and thus ensure compliance, but the worsening of hypertension, which will likely ensue, will counteract this benefit. Results from a large United States multicenter trial (Klahr, 1994) have not confirmed a beneficial effect of protein restriction, although a meta-analysis of all studies examining protein restriction suggests that even moderate amounts of protein restriction may be of some benefit. However, the quantitative importance of protein restriction has not yet been defined and is not as well documented as the importance of blood pressure control. Although excess water ingestion may be useful in patients with recurrent nephrolithiasis, there is no evidence to suggest this has a beneficial effect in renal insufficiency.

Bibliography

1. **Walker WG.** Hypertension-related renal injury: a major contributor to end-stage renal disease. Am J Kidney Dis. 1993;22:164-73.

2. **Maschio G, Alberti D, Janin G Locatelli F, Mann JF, Motolese M, et al.** Effect of the angiotensin converting-enzyme inhibitor benazepril on the progression of chronic renal insufficiency. The Angiotensin-Converting-Enzyme Inhibition in Progressive Renal Insufficiency Study Group. N Engl J Med. 1996;334:939-45.

3. **Klahr S, Levey AS, Beck GJ, Caggiula AW, Hunsicker L, Kusek JW, et al.** The effects of dietary protein restriction and blood-pressure control on the progression of chronic renal disease. Modification of Diet in Renal Disease Study Group. N Engl J Med. 1994;330:877-84.

4. **Pedrini MT, Levey AS, Lau J, Chalmers TC, Wang PH.** The effects of dietary protein restriction on the progression of diabetic and nondiabetic renal diseases: a meta-analysis. Ann Intern Med. 1996;124:627-32.

JOINT DISEASE

Joint Disease Question 1
Answer: C

EDUCATIONAL OBJECTIVE: Obtain sufficient historical clues to diagnose a patient with *Neisseria gonorrhoeae*.

The patient presented with what she thought was a spider bite. However, the constitutional symptoms, joint pains, and presence of additional skin lesions suggest a systemic infection with *Neisseria gonorrhoeae*. The symptoms should clue the physician to inquire about a patient's sexual history. Repeated episodes of bacteremia with *Neisseria* species can be seen in patients with congenital or acquired complement deficiencies.

Spider bites can become secondarily infected but they usually spread locally. Certain spiders like the brown recluse and hobo spiders possess necrotizing toxins, but this is a localized phenomenon.

The skin lesions of varicella usually are vesicular in various stages of development and are more numerous. Most 24-year-old women have already been infected with varicella.

Larger vesicles in distribution of mouth, hands, and feet are consistent with hand, foot, and mouth disease caused by coxsackievirus. This infection can be acquired from young children in the home. The distribution of skin lesions does not suggest coxsackievirus infection.

Bibliography

1. **O'Brien JP, Goldenberg DL, Rice PA.** Disseminated gonococcal infection: a prospective analysis of 49 patients and a review of pathophysiology and immune mechanisms. Medicine. 1983;62:395-406.
2. Hobo spider bites in the Pacific Northwest. MMWR. 1996;45:433-6.

Joint Disease Question 2
Answer: E

EDUCATIONAL OBJECTIVE: Recognize, manage, and treat the signs and symptoms of an impingement syndrome of the shoulder with rotator cuff involvement.

The response to the subacromial injection (elimination of pain with elevation and strong and painless empty-can test) suggests that the patient's primary injury is impingement of the rotator cuff. The involvement is probably tendinitis rather than a tear. Imaging studies are not indicated at this time, and should be left to the discretion of an orthopedic surgeon if referral is considered. In addition, MRI examination of shoulders in asymptomatic patients in this age group often shows rotator cuff injury. The residual passive range of motion loss is problematic and indicates a stiffening ("frozen") shoulder. Subacromial corticosteroid injection can help decrease the inflammation in the subacromial space.

Specific shoulder exercises or referral to physical therapy can correct the reduced range of motion that resulted from several weeks of limited use of the shoulder, and will be more successful if the patient has increase in active ranges of motion after injection of the shoulder.

Bibliography

1. **Sher JS, Uribe JW, Posada A, Murphy BJ, Zlatkin MB.** Abnormal findings on magnetic resonance images of asymptomatic shoulders. J Bone Joint Surg. 1995;77:10-5.
2. **Melzer C, Wallny T, Wirth CJ, Hoffman S.** Frozen shoulder — treatment and results. Arch Orthop Trauma Surg. 1995;114:87-91
3. **Grubbs N.** Frozen shoulder syndrome: A review of the literature. J Orthop Sports Phys Ther. 1993;18:479-87.

Joint Disease Question 3
Answer: C

EDUCATIONAL OBJECTIVE: Select the most appropriate therapeutic regimen for a young patient who is disabled with rheumatoid arthritis.

Rheumatoid arthritis is an aggressive inflammatory disorder, and the therapeutic choices should be appropriate to the disease activity and severity. This 36-year-old woman has severe, active, seropositive, erosive disease. This disease profile demands the immediate institution of combination treatment, including a nonsteroidal anti-inflammatory drug (NSAID) to relieve pain and inflammation, a disease-controlling drug such as methotrexate, and physical therapy to improve function.

The choice of the disease-controlling drug may vary from physician to physician, but once the diagnosis of rheumatoid arthritis is confirmed, usually within 1 to 3 weeks after the first visit, disease-controlling drugs are mandatory. Physicians may consider using antimalarial drugs or sulfasalazine in patients with mild, nonerosive, seronegative disease with minimal functional limitation. In patients with more aggressive, seropositive, erosive disease, the institution of weekly methotrexate or parenteral gold would be more appropriate. Combination treatments, including antimalarial drugs and methotrexate, may be considered in patients with severe, progressive disease. Combination regimens, including both methotrexate and cyclosporine, may be helpful in patients with severe and progressive disease, but this combination has only been studied in a short-term, 6-month study.

NSAIDs are commonly used with disease-controlling drugs to rapidly control the inflammatory state and improve function. Short courses of corticosteroids (such as prednisone, 10 mg two times daily orally, with a complete taper over 5 days) may help to reset the level of inflammation. Tetracycline can inhibit metalloproteinases, the enzymes thought to contribute to cartilage and tissue damage in rheumatoid arthritis. For this reason, as well as the possibility that the triggering may in some way be related to *Mycoplasma* or other infectious agents, tetracycline drugs have been used in trials of affected patients. The clinical response has been moderate at best. Although some rheumatologists do add such medications to the treatment regimen, their use with NSAIDs as the sole agents would be inappropriate in this patient's aggressive disease.

Whatever the choice of medications, the physician must closely follow the disease course while the patient is following the recommended regimen. Results of functional tests such as the Health Assessment Questionnaire (HAQ) should be monitored along with the findings on clinical and laboratory assessments. If the patient's functional and inflammatory status is worsening while a specific regimen ids being followed, that treatment plan should be changed to avoid progressive joint damage.

Bibliography

1. **Cash JM, Klippel JH.** Second-line drug therapy for rheumatoid arthritis. N Engl J Med. 1995;330:1368-75.

Joint Disease Question 4
Answer: C

EDUCATIONAL OBJECTIVE: Recognize anserine bursitis.

Anserine bursitis is characterized by inflammation of a bursa beneath the insertion of the sartorius, gracilis, and semitendinosus muscles on the medial side of the proximal tibia. This is often confused with "pain in the knee." It frequently occurs in patients with osteoarthritis who seem predisposed to anserine bursitis, as in this example; it must be distinguished from an exacerbation of osteoarthritis, which would be characterized by symptoms and findings at the knee joint itself. The diagnosis is suggested by history and confirmed by localized tenderness and/or swelling. This condition is treated with local instillation of corticosteroids and/or local anesthetic, physical therapy, and administration of non-steroidal anti-inflammatory drugs (NSAIDs) or analgesics.

Prepatellar bursitis (housemaid's knee) is less common now than in the past. It is characterized by inflammation of the bursa anterior to the patella, and clinical diagnosis is usually obvious. Patellar tendinitis would reflect injury or irritation to this structure, at a different anatomic site and with a different pattern than this patient's symptoms. Nonarticular pain at the knee and calf may also be caused by arterial occlusive disease or referred neurologic pain. The new onset of localized extra-articular symptoms is not OA or an exacerbation of osteoarthritis, nor is it a presentation of osteonecrosis.

Bibliography

1. **Holtz HA, Kramer N, Paolino JS, Rosenstein ED, Panush RS.** Arthritis: it ain't necessarily so. Compr Ther. 1994;20:244-52.
2. **Larsson LG, Baum J.** The syndromes of bursitis. Bull Rheum Dis. 1986;36:1-8.

Joint Disease Question 5
Answer: C

EDUCATIONAL OBJECTIVE: Diagnose and manage fibromyalgia syndrome.

This patient has the clinical features generally accepted to constitute the fibromyalgia syndrome. Her laboratory tests are unremarkable. The history and physical examination documenting tender points make the clinical diagnosis of fibromyalgia syndrome. In this setting and without clinical information to raise suspicions for other or underlying disease, no additional testing is necessary. Although in the past, many clinicians had tested patients such as this for thyroid disease, dysproteinemia, other rheumatic disease, other systemic disease, or paraneoplastic syndromes, this approach is not cost effective and cannot be justified in the absence of any of the clinical clues suggesting that these would be reasonable possibilities.

Although many physicians utilize some of the selections suggested in managing patients with the fibromyalgia syndrome, there is scant convincing evidence available in the peer-reviewed literature to show consistent efficacy in long-term clinical trials for any of these. Nonsteroidal anti-inflammatory drugs and corticosteroids are rarely helpful. Plaquenil, methotrexate, antibiotics, or intravenous gamma globulin is inappropriate. Therapy with tricyclic agents and aerobic exercise programs, with supportive counseling interventions, are reasonable.

Bibliography

1. **Bennet RM.** Fibromyalgia and the facts. Sense or nonsense. Rheum Dis Clin. 1993;19:45-59.

2. **Block SR.** Fibromyalgia and the rheumatisms. Common sense and sensibility. Rheum Dis Clin North Am. 1993;19:61-77.

3. **Carette S, Bell MJ, Reynolds WJ, Haraoui B, McCain GA, Bykerk VP, et al.** Comparison of amitriptyline, cyclobenzaprine, and placebo in the treatment of fibromyalgia. A randomized, double-blind clinical trial. Arthritis Rheum. 1994;37:32-40.

4. **Wilke WS.** Treatment of "resistant" fibromyalgia. Rheum Dis Clin North Am. 1995;21:247-60.

5. **Goldenberg DL.** Management of fibromyalgia syndrome. Rheum Dis Clin North Am. 1989;15:499-512.

Joint Disease Question 6
Answer: B

EDUCATIONAL OBJECTIVE: Recognize the presence of seronegative rheumatoid arthritis using the American Rheumatism Association criteria.

The correct diagnosis in this patient is rheumatoid arthritis, which is seronegative. The patient satisfies a number of the important diagnostic American Rheumatism Association criteria for rheumatoid arthritis. She shows a symmetric polyarthritis that has lasted for over 3 months. She has swelling and synovial tissue increase in more than three joints, along with radiographic changes of periarticular osteopenia in the small joints of the hands and wrists. Although the serologic test for rheumatoid factor is negative and no bony or articular surface erosions are present on roentgenograms, the patient manifests definite prolonged

morning stiffness, which satisfies another criterion for the diagnosis of rheumatoid arthritis.

Examination of synovial fluid provides no evidence for crystalline-induced arthropathy, such as gout or chondrocalcinosis. There is nothing in the history to suggest reactive arthritis or osteoarthritis. A septic arthritis would be unlikely in a patient whose joint symptoms have persisted now for 6 to 8 months. Generally, after several months when a low-grade synovial space infection is present *(Mycobacterium tuberculosis)*, the cell differential in synovial fluid will show a predominance of mononuclear cells or lymphocytes.

Bibliography

1. **Gabriel SE, Luthra HS.** Rheumatoid arthritis: can the long-term outcome be altered? Mayo Clin Proc. 1988;63:58-68.

2. **Aho K, Palosuo T, Raunio V, Puska P, Aromaa A, Salonen JT.** When does rheumatoid arthritis start? Arthritis Rheum. 1985; 28:485-9.

3. **Aho K, Heliovaara M, Maatela J, Tuomi T, Palosuo T.** Rheumatoid factors antedating clinical rheumatoid arthritis. J Rheumatol. 1991;18:1282-4.

4. **Sharp JT.** Radiologic assessment as an outcome measure in rheumatoid arthritis. Arthritis Rheum. 1989;32:221-9.

5. **Wolfe F, Cathey MA, Roberts FK.** The latex test revisited. Rheumatoid factor testing in 8,287 rheumatic disease patients. Arthritis Rheum. 1991;34:951-60.

Joint Disease Question 7
Answer: D

EDUCATIONAL OBJECTIVE: Recognize trochanteric bursitis.

Nonarticular rheumatologic disorders at the hip and thigh include muscular disorders, vascular insufficiency (Leriche's syndrome), osteonecrosis, transient osteoporosis (regional migratory osteoporosis or osteolysis), herniated nucleus pulposus, spinal stenosis, meralgia paresthetica (lateral femoral cutaneous nerve entrapment), and tendinitis-bursitis. It is not uncommon for elderly patients to have pain at the knee, hip, or back without significant abnormalities in these joints. The physician may erroneously attribute the symptoms to these joints on the basis of minor degenerative changes on radiographs. The symptoms of claudication may be misleading. If an intact peripheral arterial system is found, attention should be focused on a detailed neurologic examination assessing the motor, sensory, and reflex functions of the legs. Often there will be minimal neurologic abnormalities, but clinical features will be sufficiently suggestive of spinal stenosis (pseudoclaudication) to justify doing an MRI or CT scan.

Two types of bursitis commonly occur at the hip and thigh. In ischial bursitis (weaver's bottom) the bursa overlying the ischial tuberosity is inflamed. This may cause pain in the buttocks, exacerbated by sitting and by flexion of the hip. With trochanteric bursitis, a bursal sac over the greater trochanter is inflamed. Pain is exacerbated by external rotation and standing. These entities, both common causes of hip pain, are managed with local injection of corticosteroids and/or analgesics, physical therapy, and administration of nonsteroidal anti-inflammatory drugs or analgesics.

Bibliography

1. **Holtz HA, Kramer N, Paolino JS, Rosenstein ED, Panush RS.** Arthritis: it ain't necessarily so. Compr Ther. 1994;20:244-52.
2. **Larsson LG, Baum J.** The syndromes of bursitis. Bull Rheum Dis. 1986;36:1-8.
3. **Shbeeb MI, Matteson EL.** Trochanteric bursitis (greater trochanter pain syndrome). Mayo Clin Proc. 1996;71:565-9.

Joint Disease Question 8
Answer: B

EDUCATIONAL OBJECTIVE: Recognize sausage digit of psoriatic arthritis.

This patient has tenosynovitis of two entire digits; these are classic symptoms of seronegative spondyloarthropathies and psoriatic arthritis in particular. The seronegative spondyloarthropathies differ from rheumatoid arthritis, which tends to cause symmetric inflammation of metacarpophalangeal joints or proximal interphalangeal joints but not inflammation along an entire digit in an asymmetric pattern. For reasons that are unknown, the seronegative spondyloarthropathies often appear to respond better to nonsalicylate-based nonsteroidal anti-inflammatory drugs than to aspirin. The best choice of therapy would be high-dose indomethacin rather than low-dose aspirin.

The history does not suggest infection, and therefore, antibiotic therapy would be inappropriate. Methotrexate is not indicated because of the limited nature of the arthritis, but methotrexate has been shown to be effective therapy for extensive psoriasis and psoriatic arthritis. A short course of methylprednisolone has no role in the management of the dactylitis of psoriatic arthritis.

Psoriatic arthritis is generally categorized according to clinical pattern. Inflammation of the small joints of the hands, including the distal interphalangeal joints is unique to the seronegative spondyloarthropathies,

but it is one of the less common patterns when present alone. More often, other joints are affected in an asymmetric pattern with or without spinal involvement. Therapy must be individualized and tailored to each patient's pattern and severity of arthritis.

Bibliography

1. **Gladman DD, Shuckett R, Russell ML, Thorne JC, Schacter RK.** Psoriatic arthritis (PSA) — an analysis of 220 patients. Q J Med. 1987;62:127-41.

Joint Disease Question 9
Answer: E

EDUCATIONAL OBJECTIVE: Identify appropriate management of medial compartment osteoarthritis of the knee.

This 75-year-old woman's history, physical examination, and radiographic findings confirm the diagnosis of medial compartment osteoarthritis of the knee. Acetaminophen is as effective as nonsteroidal anti-inflammatory drugs such as indomethacin for many patients and is safer in elderly patients. Reducing loading forces across the knee by having the patient lose weight, use a cane, and alter activities may be all that is necessary. Fitness walking and quadriceps strengthening reduces pain and improves function. Providing an instep orthotic to patients with pronated feet and medial compartment disease may realign the forces more equally across the joint space and reduce strain on the medial collateral ligament and other soft tissue structures.

The effectiveness of transcutaneous electrical stimulation and knee braces is unproved. Limiting activity is unnecessary and may be counterproductive.

Bibliography

1. **Hochberg MC, Altman RD, Brandt KD, Clark BM, Dieppe PA, Griffin MR, et al.** Guidelines for the medical management of osteoarthritis. Part II. Osteoarthritis of the knee. American College of Rheumatology. Arthritis Rheum. 1995;38:1541-6.

Joint Disease Question 10
Answer: D

EDUCATIONAL OBJECTIVE: Diagnose reflex sympathetic dystrophy syndrome.

This is a classic example of the reflex sympathetic dystrophy syndrome, previously known as the *shoulder–*

hand syndrome. The pathogenesis is not known, but a similar clinical presentation can be seen following peripheral nerve injury (sympathetic causalgia). Bone scans show increased uptake over the affected region, and radiographs show mottled osteoporosis. Treatment regimens include corticosteroids, physical therapy for the shoulder, cervical sympathetic block, and pain medications. Permanent contractures are not uncommon.

Lymphangitis, usually with cellulitis, may occur after axillary node dissection, but impressive fever, chills, and other clinical features of serious bacterial infection would be expected. Bland obstruction of the subclavian vein should not cause severe pain and tenderness in the hand. Pulmonary osteoarthropathy can produce focal tenderness resulting from periostitis, but it is associated with clubbing and arthritis, not diffuse swelling and tenderness.

Bibliography

1. **Veldman PH, Reynen HM, Arntz IE, Goris RJ.** Signs and symptoms of reflex sympathetic dystrophy: prospective study of 820 patients. Lancet. 1993;342:1012-6.

Joint Disease Question 11
Answer: A

EDUCATIONAL OBJECTIVE: Diagnose pseudogout.

The synovial fluid analysis immediately confirms that this is a pseudogout attack, although superimposed infection must be excluded by culture and Gram stain. Calcium pyrophosphate dihydrate deposition disease can manifest as chondrocalcinosis, pseudogout, osteoarthritis, rheumatoid-like arthritis, and neuropathic-like destructive arthritis. This patient had a typical pseudogout attack. All forms of calcium pyrophosphate dihydrate deposition disease tend to occur in elderly patients and are characterized by the presence of weakly positively birefringent, rod-shaped and rhomboidal crystals in synovial fluid. This patient should be evaluated for the causes of pyrophosphate dihydrate deposition disease, including hypercalcemia.

Calcium oxalate deposition disease occurs in primary and secondary oxalosis and is characterized by the presence of strongly positively birefringent bipyramidal crystals. Renal insufficiency and renal failure are the most common causes of this disease in adults, and this patient had normal renal function.

Basic calcium phosphate deposition disease, which tends to cause chronic bursitis and other joint

syndromes, is not characterized by positively birefringent crystals but rather by clumps and globules of nonrefringent aggregates. The identity of these crystals can be confirmed with electron microscopy.

Gout is characterized by needle-shaped, strongly negatively birefringent crystals. A gout attack can be initiated by starvation, trauma, surgery, or other stress and could occur in a patient like the one in this question.

Septic joints should always be suspected and can be superimposed on gout or calcium pyrophosphate dihydrate deposition arthritis. Thus, if the suspicion is high, antibiotic therapy should be initiated until the results of the synovial and blood cultures are available.

Bibliography

1. **Ryan LM.** Calcium pyrophosphate dihydrate crystal deposition and other crystal deposition diseases. Curr Opin Rheumatol. 1993;5:517-21.
2. **Hoffman GS.** Arthritis due to deposition of calcium crystals. In: Wilson JD, Braunwald E, Isselbacher KJ, Petersdorf RG, Martin JB, Fauci AS, et al. Harrison's Principles of Internal Medicine, 12th ed. New York: McGraw-Hill; 1992:1479-82.

Joint Disease Question 12
Answer: B

EDUCATIONAL OBJECTIVE: Identify the clinical presentation of gouty arthritis.

This patient has undergone renal transplantation, is taking cyclosporine (which may cause hyperuricemia), and develops an acute, febrile arthritis. The most likely explanation for the arthritis in this clinical setting is gout, which is characterized by needle-shaped, birefringent crystals. Synovial fluid must be examined to establish a diagnosis of gouty arthritis. Although gout typically affects metatarsophalangeal joints, it is not uncommon in the ankle.

All of the other responses suggest possible causes for acute arthritis, but they are less common than acute gouty arthritis in this setting. Infectious arthritis, caused either by gram-negative or gram-positive organisms, is a consideration in an immunosuppressed person. Acute pseudogout arthritis may also occur in such patients, but less often than gout, and acute pseudogout arthritis more typically involves the knee. Although lupus erythematosus cells may be seen in joint effusions of patients with systemic lupus erythematosus, this does not occur frequently; monoarticular lupus arthritis would not be likely in this patient.

Bibliography

1. **Lin HY, Rocher LL, McQuillan MA, Schmaltz S, Pallella TD, Fox IH.** Cyclosporine-induced hyperuricemia and gout. N Engl J Med. 1989;321:287-92.

2. **George T, Mandell BF.** Gout in the transplant patient. J Clin Rheumatol. 1995;1:328-34.

Joint Disease Question 13
Answer: B

EDUCATIONAL OBJECTIVE: Recognize the signs and symptoms of disseminated gonococcal infection and prescribe appropriate treatment.

Pain overlying the dorsum of the foot or ankle (or both) and accentuated by passive flexion of the toes is characteristic of tenosynovitis involving the extensor tendons of the foot. Tenosynovitis is often an initial manifestation of disseminated gonococcal infection. In this case, the presence of tenosynovitis in association with other acute articular findings in a young adult should prompt consideration of disseminated gonococcal infection. Particularly in women, these symptoms may present in the absence of antecedent signs or symptoms or vaginitis, pharyngitis, or urethritis. Arthrocentesis of affected joints in early disseminated gonococcal infection commonly fails to yield organisms on Gram stain; accordingly, treatment for disseminated gonococcal infection should be initiated even when the Gram stain is negative. The current treatment recommendations for disseminated gonococcal infection are to initiate treatment with ceftriaxone sodium until symptoms resolve, then (providing the organism is penicillinase negative) continue treatment with an oral course of cefuroxime, ciprofloxacin hydrochloride, or clavulanic acid/amoxicillin for a minimum of 7 days.

Given the prevalence of penicillinase-producing *Neisseria gonorrhoeae,* a regimen of ampicillin and probenecid is not recommended for the initial treatment of disseminated gonococcal infection. In the absence of other physical findings characteristic of disseminated gonococcal infection, institution of nafcillin sodium as initial empiric therapy for possible acute monarticular staphylococcal infection might also be appropriate. However, gonococcal infection is a frequent cause of acute monarticular arthritis in young adults, and use of nafcillin sodium alone in this setting would be inappropriate.

Tenosynovitis over the dorsum of the foot is commonly caused by overuse syndrome following activities such as hiking; it will usually respond to a short course of a nonsteroidal anti-inflammatory drug such as indomethacin.

Tenosynovitis in association with acute arthritis may also occur in patients with acute rheumatic fever, for which appropriate treatment is salicylates and penicillin. However, the absence of fever and polyarticular symptoms in this patient renders acute rheumatic fever unlikely. The acute onset of tenosynovitis in a teenager or sexually active adult in association with other articular symptoms or papular or pustular skin lesions should be treated as disseminated gonococcal infection unless proven otherwise. Although uncommon, primary infection of tendon sheaths has also been reported to occur with a variety of organisms, including *Yersinia enterocolitica* and *Mycobacterium tuberculosis.*

Bibliography

1. **Ho G Jr.** Bacterial arthritis. Curr Opin Rheumatol. 1991;3:603-9.

2. **Smith JW.** Infectious arthritis. Infect Dis Clin North Am. 1990; 4:523-38.

LIPID DISORDERS

Lipid Disorders Question 1
Answer: D

EDUCATIONAL OBJECTIVE: Determine serum lipid concentrations.

Total serum cholesterol is divided among the very low-density lipoprotein (VLDL), low-density lipoprotein (LDL), and high-density lipoprotein (HDL) cholesterol. Total cholesterol and HDL are generally directly measured, whereas, in the fasting state, VLDL cholesterol can be estimated as triglycerides/5. This approximation is only true for triglycerides less than approximately 400 mg/dL. Therefore, LDL cholesterol, which is generally not directly measured, is calculated as: total cholesterol − HDL cholesterol − triglycerides/5.

Bibliography

1. Report of the National Cholesterol Education Program Expert Panel on Detection, Evaluation and Treatment of High Blood Cholesterol in Adults. The Expert Panel. Arch Intern Med. 1988;148:36-69.
2. **Ryder RE, Hayes TM, Mulligan IP, Kingswood JC, Williams S, Owens DR.** How soon after myocardial infarction should plasma lipid values be assessed? BMJ. 1984;289:1651-3.
3. **Ronnemaa T, Viikari J, Irajala K, et al.** Marked decrease in serum HDL cholesterol level during acute myocardial infarction. Acta Med Scand. 1988;207:161.

Lipid Disorders Question 2
Answer: A

EDUCATIONAL OBJECTIVE: Recognize appropriate primary prevention in postmenopausal women with a high-risk lipid profile.

Diet and exercise are the first step in prevention. The benefits of weight loss, exercise, and fat restriction on lipid parameters and blood pressure have been shown in men and women of all ages. In this patient, a 1200-calorie American Heart Association step I diet (≤ 30% fat and < 10% saturated fat) and exercise for 30 minutes three to four times weekly may be expected to provide the following at 6 months: weight, 67 kg (148 lb); blood pressure, 138/86 mm Hg; fasting cholesterol, 238 mg/dL; triglycerides, 200 mg/dL; high-density lipoprotein (HDL) cholesterol, 38 mg/dL; and calculated low-density lipoprotein (LDL) cholesterol, 140 mg/dL.

Although evidence is not available from controlled trials, it is reasonable to place high-risk, postmenopausal, or posthysterectomy women on estrogens. Estrogen replacement therapy should be delayed until the cause and treatment of the increased triglycerides is resolved. Estrogens usually result in a mild increase in triglycerides, which may be marked in women with preexisting mild to moderate elevation.

The cost-to-benefit ratio of lipid-lowering for primary prevention of coronary artery disease in women is not clear. It is prudent to treat women at high risk, based on postmyocardial infarction secondary prevention trials of lipid lowering. This 53-year-old woman has two major risk factors: a family history of premature coronary disease and low HDL cholesterol. Additionally, her triglyceride level above the 95th percentile combined with a low HDL cholesterol and cholesterol/HDL cholesterol ratio greater than 5 markedly increase coronary risk. Hypertension, the third risk factor may be resolved with diet and exercise. The decision for lipid-lowering treatment must await the response to diet and exercise. Treatment with niacin would be an inexpensive method of normalizing the level of triglycerides, raising the HDL cholesterol, reducing the number of small LDL particles, and lowering the LDL cholesterol to less than 130 mg/dL as recommended in the ATP II guidelines. Gemfibrozil would be an alternative but is more expensive and may increase LDL cholesterol. The statin class of drugs would effectively lower LDL cholesterol but have only mild impact on HDL cholesterol and triglycerides, and the cost would be considerably more than that of niacin.

Bibliography

1. **Austin MA, King MC, Vranizan KM, Krauss RM.** Atherogenic lipoprotein phenotype. A proposed genetic marker for coronary heart disease risk. Circulation. 1990;82:495-506.
2. **Assmann G, Schulte H.** Relation of high density lipoprotein cholesterol and triglycerides to the incidence of atherosclerotic coronary artery disease (the PROCAM experience). Prospective Cardiovascular Munster study. Am J Cardiol. 1992;70:733-7.

3. **Superko HR, Krauss RM.** Differential effects of nicotinic acid in subjects with different LDL subclass patterns. Atherosclerosis. 1992;95:69-76.

4. **Frick MH, Elo O, Haapa K, Heinonen OP, Heinsalmi P, Helo P, et al.** Helsinki Heart Study: primary prevention trial with gemfibrozil in middle-aged men with dyslipidemia. Safety of treatment, changes in risk factors, and incidence of coronary heart disease. N Engl J Med. 1987;317:1237-45.

5. **Bradford RH, Shear CL, Chremos AN, Dujovne C, Dounton M, Franklin FA, et al.** Expanded clinical evaluation of Lovastatin (EXCEL) study results. I. Efficacy in modifying plasma lipoproteins and adverse event profile in 8245 patients with moderate hypercholesterolemia. Arch Intern Med. 1991;151:43-9.

Lipid Disorders Question 3
Answer: B

EDUCATIONAL OBJECTIVE: Select the most appropriate lipid treatment in a patient following myocardial infarction.

There is clear clinical trial–based evidence that HMG-CoA reductase inhibitors can be of benefit in men and women following myocardial infarction. Benefits, including decreases in mortality, recurrent myocardial infarction, and need for revascularization, are independent of age, gender, and left ventricular function. However, in the 4S trial (simvastatin versus placebo), the entry criterion was a low-density lipoprotein cholesterol (LDL) greater than 170 mg/dL; and in CARE (pravastatin versus placebo), where entry LDL cholesterol ranged from 100 to 169 mg/dL, there was no shown benefit when the LDL cholesterol was less than 125 mg/dL. CARE was not powered to detect benefits with LDL cholesterol less than 125 mg/dL, but in this patient the LDL cholesterol is only 118 mg/dL. This patient has two other lipid parameters associated with an increase in cardiac events and death in coronary artery disease particularly in women aged over 65 years: level of triglycerides greater than 200 mg/dL and a low level of high-density lipoprotein cholesterol (HDL). Moderate doses of niacin can both decrease triglycerides (15% to 30%) and increase the HDL cholesterol (10% to 20%). Although no trial data support specifically targeting the triglycerides and HDL cholesterol, niacin was the first lipid-lowering agent to reduce mortality following MI. Remarkably, in the Coronary Drug Project long-term follow-up, patients randomized to niacin had a reduced mortality at 14 years after myocardial infarction even if they discontinued niacin. Decreasing triglycerides and increasing HDL cholesterol has been shown to reduce new lesion formation, a finding which may explain the latter effect.

The Helsinki Heart Study, in which gemfibrozil reduced the 5-year coronary event rate by over 40%, was conducted only in men with no evidence of coronary artery disease. Although gemfibrozil has lipid-altering affects similar to those of niacin, there is no evidence of value in established coronary artery disease and no reduction has been shown in overall mortality. Bile resins should be reserved for lowering LDL cholesterol alone or in supplement to the HMG-CoA reductase inhibitors. The β-blocker metoprolol may be in part responsible for the increase in triglycerides and decrease in HDL cholesterol, but the benefit of β-blockade following myocardial infarction is well established.

Bibliography

1. National Cholesterol Education Program. Second Report of the Expert Panel on Detection, Evaluation, and Treatment of High Blood Cholesterol in Adults (Adult Treatment Panel II). Circulation. 1994;89:1333-445.

2. **Sacks FM, Pfeffer MA, Moye LA, Rouleau JL, Rutherford JD, Cole TG, et al.** The effect of pravastatin on coronary events after myocardial infarction in patients with average cholesterol levels. Cholesterol Recurrent Events Trial Investigators. N Engl J Med. 1996;335:1001-9.

3. **Canner PL, Berge KG, Wenger NK, Stamler J, Friedman L, Prineas RJ, et al.** Fifteen year mortality in the Coronary Drug Project patients: long term benefit with niacin. J Am Coll Cardiol. 1986;8:1245-55.

4. **Frick MH, Heinonen OP, Huttunen JK, Koskinen P, Manttari M, Manninen V.** Efficacy of gemfibrozil in dyslipidemic subjects with suspected heart disease. An ancillary study in the Helsinki Heart Study frame population. Ann Med. 1993;25:41-5.

Lipid Disorders Question 4
Answer: E

EDUCATIONAL OBJECTIVE: Recognize the role of antioxidant therapy in primary prevention for middle-aged men.

This man's lipid profile is normal other than the increased lipoprotein(a), which does not increase risk of coronary artery disease (CAD) in black persons. Antioxidants for primary prevention are attractive based on epidemiologic and experimental data, but there is no evidence that supplements are effective, particularly in the absence of CAD. High-dose vitamin A is hepatotoxic and should be avoided. β-carotene had no benefit on CAD and increased cancer mortality in asbestos workers who were at risk for CAD, and vitamin E was of no value for reducing cancer risk or CAD in smokers. Neither β-carotene nor vitamin E had a significant impact on preventing the development of clinical angina in smokers.

The epidemiologic studies concluding a benefit for supplemental vitamins E and C in women and men suffer from serious selection bias. Persons who take vitamin supplements are more likely to eat a low-fat diet, exercise, and adhere to other hygienic measures associated with decrease in CAD risk. Taking antioxidant supplements cannot be justified in healthy men and women. Secondary prevention has more support but not convincing evidence. In CLAS, a trial of the benefit of lipid-lowering therapy with coronary angiographic end points, increased dietary and supplemental vitamin E was associated with less progression of CAD, independent of lipids. These results must be interpreted with caution. The impact of vitamin E was not an a priori hypothesis. In CHAOS (a post-myocardial infarction trial of Vitamin E 400–800 IU versus placebo), vitamin E reduced subsequent ischemic events but with a slight (not significant) increase in overall mortality. CHAOS randomized only 2000 subjects. Much larger trials will be necessary to test the value of antioxidants following myocardial infarction.

Bibliography

1. **Mehra MR, Lavie CJ, Ventura HO, Milani RV.** Prevention of atherosclerosis. The potential role of antioxidants. Postgrad Med. 1995;98:175-6, 179-84.

2. **Stephens NG, Parsons A, Schofield PM, Kelly F, Cheeseman K, Mitchinson MJ.** Randomised controlled trial of vitamin E in patients with coronary disease: Cambridge Heart Antioxidant Study (CHAOS). Lancet. 1996;347:781-6.

3. **Hodis HN, Mack WJ, LaBree L, Cashin-Hemphill L, Sevanian A, Johnson R, et al.** Serial coronary arteriographic evidence that antioxidant vitamin intake reduces progression of coronary artery atherosclerosis. JAMA 1995;273:1849-54.

4. **Omenn GS, Goodman GE, Thornquist MD, Balmes J, Cullen MR, Glass A, et al.** Effects of a combination of beta carotene and vitamin A on lung cancer and cardiovascular disease. N Engl J Med. 1996;334:1150-5.

5. **Rapola JM, Virtamo J, Haukka JK, Heinonen OP, Albains D, Taylor PR, et al.** Effect of vitamin E and beta carotene on the incidence of angina pectoris. A randomized, double-blind, controlled trial. JAMA. 1996;275:693-8.

Lipid Disorders Question 5
Answer: B

EDUCATIONAL OBJECTIVE: Identify the clinical presentation of critical limb ischemia and select the most appropriate diagnostic test.

Leg discomfort with walking defines claudication, which is a typical symptom of a patient with peripheral arterial occlusive disease caused by atherosclerosis. Tobacco use and diabetes mellitus are the two most common causes of peripheral arterial disease. Disease progression may cause critical limb ischemia, resulting in persistent foot pain. Patients frequently sit with the foot dependent for pain relief. Rest pain is an indication for revascularization. Arteriography is done to see the nature and extent of the atherosclerotic lesions so that the appropriate revascularization procedure can be planned.

Acute arterial embolism from a cardiac source is a potential cause of acute limb ischemia. However, this patient's problem is a chronic one. Both legs are affected by peripheral atherosclerosis, as reflected in the pulse examination. Therefore, echocardiography is not indicated to plan revascularization. Pulse volume recordings will be abnormal, consistent with peripheral arterial disease. However, these data will provide little incremental information over that obtained by physical examination of this patient.

Venous ultrasonography is indicated if one suspects deep venous thrombosis. This patient's foot swelling is most likely secondary to prolonged dependency, because he spends most nights sitting up in a chair for relief. Patients with diabetes mellitus often have peripheral neuropathy that causes pain or paresthesias. This patient has evidence of peripheral neuropathy by physical examination, and this would most certainly be confirmed by a nerve conduction study. However, the findings on nerve conduction study will not affect the plan for revascularization.

Bibliography

1. Second European consensus document on chronic critical leg ischemia. Circulation. 1991;84:IV1-26.

Lipid Disorders Question 6
Answer: A

EDUCATIONAL OBJECTIVE: Select the best strategy for primary prevention of coronary artery disease in elderly women.

The general benefits of diet and exercise extend to elderly men and women who are often the most motivated and compliant group. The American Heart Association Step I diet consists of less than 30% fat and less than 10% saturated fat. The standard Western diet in the United States that avoids butter and eggs provides about 34% to 38% of calories from fat and 12% to 15% from saturated fat. With appropriate dietary counseling by the physician, nurse, or dietitian, the average lowering of total and low-density lipoprotein (LDL) cholesterol is about 10% and 7% respectively, but may be 25% to 40% depending on previous dietary fat and genetic factors.

Although age should not be a basis for excluding elderly patients from drug treatment, there is no proven benefit of cholesterol lowering in healthy women of any age without coronary risk factors, such as diabetes and low high-density lipoprotein (HDL). LDL cholesterol is a major risk factor in middle age, but there is minimal attributable effect in elderly women. Furthermore, in this patient the ratio of total cholesterol to HDL cholesterol ratio is optimal. It is estimated (without risk stratification) that only 6.5 coronary deaths would be prevented per 1000 treated by lowering cholesterol from 285 to 200 mg/dL in women aged 75 to 84 years.

Aspirin and estrogen should be considered in elderly women with established vascular disease or in the presence of factors suggesting a high probability of coronary artery disease, such as diabetes or low HDL cholesterol. Although regular use of one to six aspirin weekly (but not more) was associated with fewer coronary events in nurses aged over 50 years, this does not support beginning treatment in elderly persons where risk is not known. Age does influence the risk of regular aspirin use. Until evidence of benefit is available, estrogen and progestins should not "forced upon" women of any age.

Bibliography

1. **Gordon DJ, Rifkind BM.** Treating high blood cholesterol in the older patient. Am J Cardiol. 1989;63:48H-52H.

2. **Silagy CA, McNeil JJ, Donnan GA, Tonkin AM, Worsam B, Campion K.** Adverse effects of low-dose aspirin in a healthy elderly population. Clin Pharmacol Ther. 1993;54:84-9.

3. **Manson JE, Stampfer MJ, Colditz GA, Willett WC, Rosner B, Speizer FE, et al.** A prospective study of aspirin use and primary prevention of cardiovascular disease in women. JAMA. 1991;266:521-7.

4. **Bush TL, Barrett-Conner E, Cowan LD, Criqui MH, Wallace RB, Suchindran CM, et al.** Cardiovascular mortality and noncontraceptive use of estrogen in women: results from the Lipid Research Clinic Program Follow-up Study. Circulation. 1987;75:1102-9.

Lipid Disorders Question 7
Answer: B

EDUCATIONAL OBJECTIVE: Manage lipid levels in patients with coronary artery disease.

In patients with established coronary artery disease, the frequency of subsequent infarctions and mortality is closely related to total cholesterol and low-density lipoprotein (LDL) cholesterol. Prospective randomized trials have demonstrated that cholesterol lowering in patients with established coronary disease significantly reduces cardiovascular events, such as acute myocardial infarction, and total mortality. These findings have led the National Cholesterol Education Program (NCEP) to recommend the most aggressive lipid modification to be undertaken in patients with known coronary artery disease. Currently, recommendations are to lower LDL cholesterol to 100 mg/dL and raise high-density lipoprotein (HDL) cholesterol to 35 mg/dL.

Bibliography

1. Summary of the second report of the National Cholesterol Education Program (NCEP) Expert Panel on Detection, Evaluation, and Treatment of High Blood Cholesterol in Adults (Adult Treatment Panel II). JAMA. 1993; 269:3015-23.

2. **LaRosa JC, Cleeman JI.** Cholesterol lowering as a treatment for established coronary heart disease. Circulation. 1992;85:1229-35.

3. **Hunninghake DB, Stein EA, Dujovne CA, Harris WS, Feldman EB, Miller VT, et al.** The efficacy of intensive dietary therapy alone or combined with lovastatin in outpatients with hypercholesterolemia. N Engl J Med. 1993;328:1213-9.

4. **LaRosa JC.** Cholesterol lowering, low cholesterol, and mortality. Am J Cardiol. 1993;72:776-86.

Lipid Disorders Question 8
Answer: A

EDUCATIONAL OBJECTIVE: Manage hypertriglyceridemia in a patient with both type 2 diabetes mellitus and familial hypertriglyceridemia.

This 51-year-old man presented with uncontrolled type 2 diabetes mellitus, and his initial hypertriglyceridemia and hypercholesterolemia could have been solely a result of the diabetes. It was not possible to calculate his initial plasma low-density lipoprotein (LDL) cholesterol because his serum triglycerides were too high (> 400 mg/dL). Following marked improvement in diabetic control, his serum triglyceride level remains significantly elevated and along with his still low plasma high-density lipoprotein (HDL) cholesterol is a risk factor for coronary disease in type 2 diabetes mellitus. Given the family history, he is likely to have familial hypertriglyceridemia in addition to diabetic dyslipidemia. His calculated plasma LDL cholesterol is now 108 mg/dL (212-34-350/5).

Because it is unlikely that his serum triglycerides will normalize by further improvement in glycemic control, the appropriate treatment is gemfibrozil, which can lower serum triglycerides 40% and increase plasma HDL cholesterol 10%.

Changing his regimen from glyburide to metformin may further slightly decrease serum triglycerides and increase plasma HDL, but he has already reached normal weight and it is not worth the chance that his diabetic control will worsen. Nicotinic acid will lower triglycerides but may worsen plasma glucose control. Because his plasma LDL cholesterol is normal, neither an HMG-CoA reductase inhibitor nor a bile-acid resin is specifically indicated. If he develops coronary artery disease, one of these should be added to bring plasma LDL to less than 100 mg/dL.

Bibliography

1. **Frick MH, Elo O, Haapa K, Heinonen OP, Heinsalmi P, Helo P, et al.** Helsinki Heart Study: primary-prevention trial with gemfibrozil in middle-aged men with dyslipidemia. Safety of treatment, changes in risk factors, and incidence of coronary heart disease. N Engl J Med. 1987;317:1237-45.
2. **Garg A, Grundy SM.** Treatment of dyslipidemia in patients with NIDDM. Diab Rev. 1995;3:433-45.
3. **Howard BV.** Pathogenesis of diabetic dyslipidemia. Diab Rev. 1995;3:423-32.
4. **Laakso M.** Epidemiology of diabetic dyslipidemia. Diab Rev. 1995;3:408-22.
5. **Manninen V, Tenkanen L, Koskinen P, Huttunen JK, Mänttäri, Heinonen OP, Frick MH.** Joint effects of serum triglyceride and LDL cholesterol and HDL cholesterol concentrations on coronary heart disease risk in the Helsinki Heart Study. Circulation. 1992;85:37-45.

Lipid Disorders Question 9
Answer: B

EDUCATIONAL OBJECTIVE: Recognize proper management of a patient with elevated fasting total serum cholesterol level.

The National Cholesterol Education Project recommends that all adults be screened for nonfasting total cholesterol level. Patients with cholesterol levels below 200 mg/dL require reassessment at 5-year intervals. Values between 200 mg/dL and 239 mg/dL (borderline elevated) in the absence of established coronary heart disease, or two risk factors (one of which is male sex) should prompt dietary instruction and annual reassessment.

The presence of risk factors, established coronary heart disease, or a cholesterol level of 240 mg/dL or higher is an indication for fasting lipoprotein analysis. Additional fasting past 12 hours is unlikely to lower cholesterol levels further. Exercise or family testing may be appropriate parts of a risk modification program, but specific recommendations are not indicated until after a fasting lipoprotein analysis reveals abnormal cholesterol subfractions.

Bibliography

1. Report of the National Cholesterol Education Program Expert Panel on Detection, Evaluation and Treatment of High Blood Cholesterol in Adults. The Expert Panel. Arch Intern Med. 1988;148:36-69.

Lipid Disorders Question 10
Answer: B

EDUCATIONAL OBJECTIVE: Distinguish the patterns of hyperlipidemia seen in the nephrotic syndrome and identify their treatments.

There is no current evidence that treatment lowers the risk of cardiovascular disease in patients with the nephrotic syndrome. Nevertheless, reduction of the abnormal lipids is generally recommended based on data derived from studies in non-nephrotic populations. Debate remains about the mechanism for the hyperlipidemia, but reduction of proteinuria and elevation of serum albumin concentration towards normal will lead to reduction of the high concentrations of plasma cholesterol. This may be done by specific methods of using immunosuppressive medications, inducing remissions of the nephrotic syndrome, or by using ACE inhibitors, which often reduce proteinuria as long as the ACE inhibition is continued. HMG-CoA reductase inhibitors have been used in many short-term and several long-term studies in nephrotic patients. In general, they have been proved effective at lowering total cholesterol and LDL cholesterol concentrations without significant side effects.

Hyperlipidemia is common in the nephrotic syndrome. Most patients have elevated concentrations of total cholesterol, LDL cholesterol, and often very low LDL (VLDL) cholesterol with variable concentrations of high-density lipoprotein cholesterol. Although patients with the nephrotic syndrome have been shown to have an increased risk of cardiovascular mortality, this risk has not necessarily been related to the elevated cholesterol concentrations.

Bibliography

1. **Appel G.** Nephrology Forum. Lipid abnormalities in renal diseases. Kidney Int. 1991;39:169-83.

2. **Ordonez JD, Hiatt RA, Killebrew EJ, Fireman BH.** The increased risk of coronary heart disease associated with the nephrotic syndrome. Kidney Int. 1993;44:638-42.

3. **Radhakrishnan J, Appel AS, Valeri A, Appel GB.** The nephrotic syndrome, lipids, and risk factors for cardiovascular disease. Am J Kidney Dis. 1993;22:135-42.

4. **Spitalewitz S, Porush JG, Cattran D, Wright N.** Treatment of hyperlipidemia in the nephrotic syndrome: the effects of pravastatin therapy. Am J Kidney Dis. 1993;22:143-50.

LIVER DISORDERS

Liver Disorders Question 1
Answer: B

EDUCATIONAL OBJECTIVE: Distinguish between the use of laboratory tests to make a diagnosis or monitor the course of therapy.

The detection of serum antibodies against hepatitis C is a relatively inexpensive diagnostic tool and is widely used for the diagnosis of an infection. However, the titer of the antibody does not accurately reflect disease activity. The hepatitis C virus is extremely difficult to study in vitro, and the two most widely accepted methods to measure disease activity are either liver biopsy or quantification of serum viral RNA levels. Nucleic acid amplification techniques, when performed under rigorous control, are probably less expensive than a liver biopsy and also not as invasive. Therapy for chronic hepatitis C is still not very effective, and many patients have persistent hepatic inflammation after a 6-month course of interferon therapy. Tests that detect viral RNA in the serum, especially with more widespread implementation of the amplification methodologies, are used both to assess treatment success and to determine the need for more therapy. The goal of therapy is to eliminate viral RNA from the serum.

Bibliography

1. **Hoofnagle JH, Lau D.** Chronic viral hepatitis—benefits of current therapies. N Engl J Med. 1996;334:1470-1.

2. **Poynard T, Bedossa P, Chevallier M, Mathurin P, Lemonnier C, Trepo C, et al.** A comparison of three interferon alfa-2b regimens for the long-term treatment of chronic non-A, non-B hepatitis. Multicenter Study Group. N Engl J Med. 1995;332:1457-62.

3. **Shindo M, Di Bisceglie AM, Cheung L, Shih JW, Christiano K, Feinstone SM, et al.** Decrease in serum hepatitis C viral RNA during alpha-interferon therapy for chronic hepatitis C. Ann Intern Med. 1991;115:700-4.

Liver Disorders Question 2
Answer: B

EDUCATIONAL OBJECTIVE: Diagnose autoimmune hepatitis.

This 36-year-old woman has recent onset of nonspecific symptoms, physical findings suggestive of chronic liver disease, and historical and laboratory features consistent with autoimmune hepatitis. A third of patients with autoimmune hepatitis present with a clinical picture suggestive of acute hepatitis, although complete evaluation shows evidence of chronic liver disease in most patients, including the physical findings indicative of cirrhosis as described in this patient (palmar erythema, spider angiomata, palpable left lobe in the subxiphoid area).

Approximately 4% of patients with autoimmune hepatitis have false-positive results for anti-HCV by second-generation ELISA, a much lower false-positive rate than found with the first-generation assay. Approximately 28% of patients with chronic viral hepatitis have seropositivity of ANA at low titer ($\leq$1:40). Patients with autoimmune hepatitis typically have ANA at high titer ($\geq$1:320). Additional findings in this patient supporting the diagnosis of autoimmune hepatitis include the high total globulin of 4.5 g/dL, an associated autoimmune disease (hypothyroidism), and an aggressive chronic inflammation in the liver biopsy specimen. The differentiation of autoimmune hepatitis from chronic viral hepatitis with positive autoimmune markers is important because of treatment implications: mistakenly treating autoimmune hepatitis with interferon can intensify immune-mediated hepatocellular inflammation of autoimmune hepatitis, whereas corticosteroid therapy for chronic viral hepatitis will increase the viral burden.

Acetaminophen toxicity is a major cause of acute liver injury and can occur at doses as low as 3 g/d in the setting of chronic alcohol use. However, chronic hepatitis and cirrhosis are not in the spectrum of acetaminophen liver injury, and acetaminophen at the dosage taken by this patient would not contribute to liver injury. Fatty liver is the most common cause of minor aminotransferase elevations and can, in a minority of patients, progress to cirrhosis in the setting of nonalcoholic steatohepatitis (NASH), but NASH typically occurs in persons with obesity or other risk factors for fatty liver and has a histologic appearance distinct from that of chronic hepatitis. However, in approximately 40% of patients with NASH, such risk factors are absent.

Bibliography

1. **Czaja AJ.** Autoimmune hepatitis. Evolving concepts and treatment strategies. Dig Dis Sci. 1995;40:435-56.
2. **Czaja AJ.** Autoimmune hepatitis and viral infection. Gastroenterol Clin North Am. 1994;23:547-66.
3. **Krawitt EL.** Autoimmune hepatitis. N Engl J Med. 1996;334:897-903.
4. **Bacon BR, Farahvash MJ, Janney CG, Neuschwander-Tetri BA.** Nonalcoholic steatohepatitis: an expanded clinical entity. Gastroenterology. 1994;107:1103-9.

Liver Disorders Question 3
Answer: C

EDUCATIONAL OBJECTIVE: Distinguish acute hepatotoxicity caused by acetaminophen in an alcoholic patient from other causes of liver injury.

The values of the liver enzymes in this patient suggest acute hepatocellular injury. These findings are typical of a "therapeutic misadventure" with acetaminophen in a chronic alcohol user. Such toxicity typically develops in patients who drink more than 80 g of alcohol per day. The characteristic feature of the syndrome is very large elevations of aspartate aminotransferase (AST) concentration, ranging from 3000 to 48,000 U/L in more than 90% of cases, and typically lower alanine aminotransferase (ALT) levels. The mortality rate based on cases reported in the literature is 20%. Alcohol appears to lower the threshold for acetaminophen hepatotoxicity not only by inducing the cytochrome P-450 system, which enhances formation of the reactive intermediary metabolite, but also by depleting glutathione, which is essential for detoxification of the metabolite. In alcoholic hepatitis, the pattern is typically a modest increase of aminotransferases (AST of approximately 150 to 250 U/L). Acute cholecystitis may have a presentation similar to that of acute alcoholic hepatitis, with fever, right upper quadrant pain, and jaundice. However, the aminotransferase values are typically more modestly elevated than in this case. This case is more typical of acute hepatocellular injury. Although acute hepatitis B could result in aminotransferase levels like those in this patient, she has no recent history of hepatitis exposure. A presentation as acute hepatitis C is uncommon. The most likely diag-

nosis is acetaminophen hepatotoxicity because the elevation of aminotransferases is marked. Alcoholics, whether or not they have alcohol-related liver disease, should be advised to avoid or limit the use of acetaminophen. In alcoholics with suspected acetaminophen-induced liver injury, *N*-acetylcysteine should be administered.

Bibliography

1. **Maddrey WC.** Hepatic effects of acetaminophen. Enhanced toxicity in alcoholics. J Clin Gastroenterol. 1987;9:180-5.
2. **Zimmerman HJ, Maddrey WC.** Acetaminophen (paracetamol) hepatotoxicity with regular intake of alcohol: analysis of instances of therapeutic misadventure. Hepatology. 1995;22:767-73.
3. **Lee WM.** Drug-induced hepatotoxicity. N Engl J Med. 1995;333:1118-27.

Liver Disorders Question 4
Answer: C

EDUCATIONAL OBJECTIVE: Recognize the clinical characteristics of nonalcoholic steatohepatitis

This patient has the characteristic clinical presentation of nonalcoholic steatohepatitis. This disorder is commonly seen in moderately obese patients with hyperlipidemia. Diabetes mellitus has also been suggested as a predisposing condition. Affected patients are usually asymptomatic, and often have only mild aminotransferase elevations noted on routine screening. The liver biopsy findings are similar to those seen with alcoholic liver disease, with large-droplet steatosis and mild inflammation. The course of the illness is usually benign, but it can progress to fibrosis and cirrhosis. The best therapeutic approach is to treat the underlying obesity, hyperlipidemia, and diabetes, if present.

Hepatitis B and C are unlikely in the absence of antibodies to the virus. Interferon therapy, therefore, would be inappropriate. Interferon therapy even in the presence of non-B, non-C hepatitis is controversial. The biopsy findings alone are not pathognomonic of ethanol-induced liver disease. The clinical, laboratory, and biopsy findings are not suggestive of biliary disease. Endoscopic retrograde cholangiopancreatography (ERCP) is not needed for the diagnosis. Corticosteroid therapy would be indicated for autoimmune hepatitis, but such therapy has no role in nonalcoholic steatohepatitis.

Bibliography

1. **Bacon BR, Farahvash MJ, Janney CG, Neuschwander-Tetri BA.** Nonalcoholic steatohepatitis: an expanded clinical entity. Gastroenterology. 1994;107:1103-9.

2. **Sheth SG, Gordon FD, Chopra S.** Nonalcoholic steatohepatitis. Ann Intern Med. 1997;126:137-45.

Liver Disorders Question 5
Answer: E

EDUCATIONAL OBJECTIVE: Manage a patient with asymptomatic cholelithiasis.

The majority of gallstones are asymptomatic and require no therapy. Multiple studies have demonstrated that significant complications rarely occur in the absence of preceding symptoms. The risk for developing symptoms of cholelithiasis is 1% to 2% per year. In this patient who has no symptoms of cholecystitis or choledocholithiasis, there is no reason to use any of the listed therapies. The presence of comorbid illnesses, such as diabetes mellitus, does not increase the risk for biliary tract complications and does not warrant therapy. Ursodeoxycholic acid therapy dissolves 30% to 50% of cholesterol stones less than 2 cm in diameter. The recurrence rate, however, is more than 50%. Endoscopic retrograde cholangiopancreatography (ERCP) is indicated only when choledocholithiasis is suspected. When stones are symptomatic, cholecystectomy is appropriate. Laparoscopic surgery has less morbidity than the open approach.

Bibliography

1. **Ransohoff DF, Gracie WA.** Treatment of gallstones. Ann Intern Med. 1993;119:606-19.

Liver Disorders Question 6
Answer: C

EDUCATIONAL OBJECTIVE: Counsel a patient concerning treatment for chronic hepatitis C.

Interferon therapy for persons with chronic hepatitis C using the Food and Drug Administration (FDA)-approved regimen of interferon alfa, 3 million IU three times per week for 6 months, results in normalization of elevated alanine aminotransferase (ALT), usually accompanied by disappearance of hepatitis C virus (HCV) RNA from the serum, in 40% of patients. However, after cessation of 6 months of treatment, the ALT concentration again becomes elevated and HCV RNA reappears in the serum in approximately 60% of responders. Consequently, 15% to 20% of patients demonstrate sustained response to standard interferon therapy. The FDA recently approved interferon therapy for 12 months based on the results of trials that showed that prolonging treatment for patients who show an initial response to interferon reduces by half their chance of relapse (recurrent ALT elevation and reappearance of virus in the serum) after cessation of treatment. Patients whose serum ALT fails to normalize or who do not lose serum HCV RNA after 3 months of interferon therapy have very low sustained loss of HCV after treatment. Therefore, a National Institutes of Health (NIH) consensus conference (reference 4 below) recommended that interferon therapy in such patients be discontinued.

Characteristics associated with favorable response to interferon therapy include shorter duration of infection, absence of fibrosis on liver biopsy, and low viral load by quantitative testing. Definitive evidence is not yet available that successful treatment, defined as sustained clearance of the virus, as indicated by loss of HCV RNA from the serum, reduces the rate of progression to cirrhosis or risk for hepatocellular carcinoma, although preliminary evidence suggests that this may be the case.

Bibliography

1. **Hoofnagle JH.** Therapy of acute and chronic viral hepatitis. Adv Intern Med. 1994;39:241-75.

2. **Conjeevaram HS, Everhart JE, Hoofnagle JH.** Predictors of a sustained response to interferon alfa therapy in chronic hepatitis C. Hepatology. 1995;22:1326-9.

3. **Poynard T, Bedossa P, Chevallier M, Mathurin P, Lemonnier C, Trepo C, et al.** A comparison of three interferon alfa-2b regimens for the long-term treatment of chronic non-A, non-B hepatitis. N Engl J Med. 1996;332:1457-62.

4. The National Institutes of Health Consensus Development Conference. Management of hepatitis C. Hepatology. 1997;26:1S-155S. (also available via the Internet at http://odp.od.nih.gov/consensus/statements/cdc/105/105/stmt.html)

Liver Disorders Question 7
Answer: A

EDUCATIONAL OBJECTIVE: Counsel a patient concerning diagnosis and family screening for hemochromatosis.

Alcoholic liver injury can result in an increased serum ferritin and transferrin saturation. To confirm a suspected diagnosis of genetic hemochromatosis, a liver biopsy should be done to determine the level of hepatic iron and to calculate the hepatic iron index (hepatic iron [(mol)/dry weight of liver [g]/patients age [y]), which is diagnostic if >2.0. If a liver biopsy is not practicable, serial phlebotomy should be initiated, and the amount of drawn blood required to precipitate anemia will indicate if the diagnosis is correct. When the diagnosis of this autosomal recessive disorder is confirmed, the family members most at risk, the proband's siblings, who have a one in four chance of being homozygous, should be screened. When a proband has been identified, HLA typing can be useful. Because the probability of homozygosity in either the parents or the children is in the range of 100 to 200, the gene frequency in the population, it is not necessary that they be screened.

With the identification of the genetic defect responsible for most cases of genetic hemochromatosis, blood tests capable of identifying affected patients are anticipated for clinical use in the near future. Because the finding of fibrosis and cirrhosis puts the patient at risk for hepatoma despite adequate iron depletion with phlebotomy, the biopsy should still be performed both for definitive diagnosis and to determine the need for future screening for hepatoma.

Bibliography

1. **Adams PC, Dertesz AE, Valberg LS.** Clinical presentation of hemochromatosis: a changing scene. Am J Med. 1991;90:445-9.
2. **Deugnier YM, Turlin B, Powell LW, Summers KM, Moirand R, Fletcher L, et al.** Differentiation between heterozygotes and homozygotes in genetic hemochromatosis by means of a histologic hepatic iron index: a study of 192 cases. Hepatology. 1993;17:30-4.

Liver Disorders Question 8
Answer: D

EDUCATIONAL OBJECTIVE: Counsel a patient with chronic hepatitis B concerning viral hepatitis vaccination and treatment.

Hepatitis A vaccine is recommended for all susceptible persons with chronic liver disease because of their limited hepatic reserve, which predisposes them to more severe acute hepatitis virus infection. Specifically, the mortality rate of acute hepatitis A among adults with chronic hepatitis B has been found to be considerably increased.

Active vaccination with hepatitis B vaccine for household contacts of persons with chronic hepatitis B is recommended; however, passive vaccination with hepatitis immune globulin is not necessary. This is to be distinguished from recommendations for acute exposure to persons with acute hepatitis B in the home or prevention of transmission of hepatitis B from an infected mother to an infant, which would include both the hepatitis B vaccine and the hepatitis B immune globulin.

Persons infected with hepatitis B virus (HBV) in the replicative phase have hepatitis B e antigen (HBeAg) in the serum, which correlates with high levels of circulating HBV DNA. Such patients are candidates for interferon therapy with the intent of eliminating HBeAg and eventually clearing the infection. The patients who are most likely to respond to interferon therapy are those with evidence of ongoing immune-mediated necroinflammatory activity in the liver, as suggested by an alanine aminotransferase (ALT) concentration greater than 100 U/L, but relatively modest levels of circulating virus, as indicated by HBV DNA levels <200 pg/mL. This patient meets these criteria and would be expected to respond to interferon therapy, with response defined as loss of the HBeAg within 6 months after completion of treatment, of at least 40%. Most patients who respond to interferon therapy with clearance of HBeAg from the serum demonstrate a transient rise in serum aminotransferases, which is presumably associated with interferon-mediated specific immune attack by activated T lymphocytes on infected hepatocytes. Among patients with evidence of decompensated cirrhosis due to hepatitis B, as indicated by a history of portosystemic encephalopathy, ascites, or variceal hemorrhage, interferon therapy can present considerable risk of infectious complications or hepatic decompensation precipitated by an immune-mediated flare. Consequently, interferon therapy for patients with hepatitis B and decompensated cirrhosis should be considered only at specialized centers where expertise in liver disease and liver transplantation is available.

Bibliography

1. **Dusheiko GM.** Rolling review—the pathogenesis, diagnosis and management of viral hepatitis. Aliment Pharmacolol Ther. 1994;8:229-53.
2. **Perillo RP.** Interferon in the management of chronic viral hepatitis B. Dig Dis Sci. 1993;38:577-93.
3. **Wong DK, Cheung AM, O'Rourke K, Naylor CD, Detsky AS, Heathcote J, et al.** Effect of alpha-interferon treatment in patients with hepatitis B e antigen–positive chronic hepatitis B. A meta-analysis. Ann Intern Med. 1993;119:312-23.
4. **Perrillo R, Tamburro C, Regenstein F, Balart L, Bodenheimer H, Silva M, et al.** Low-dose, titratable interferon alfa in decompensated liver disease caused by chronic infection with hepatitis B virus. Gastroenterology. 1995;109:908-16.

Liver Disorders Questions 9-12
Answers: 9(C); 10(B); 11(D); 12(A)

Educational Objective: Distinguish the serologic patterns of chronic viral hepatitis B, C, and D.

The 53-year-old man has chronic hepatitis C due to remote injection drug use, as is indicated by persistent anti–hepatitis C virus (HCV) positivity, which almost invariably denotes persistent viremia in persons with previous parenteral blood exposure. The IgM component of anti-HBc indicates acute hepatitis B virus (HBV) infection and drops below detectable levels after 4 to 6 months after resolution of the acute infection. However, persistence of total anti-HBc indicates past exposure to HBV. Resolution of acute HBV infection is indicated by loss of HBsAg and development of anti-HBs.

The 32-year-old nurse was vaccinated for HBV as indicated by persistent anti-HBs, but because she has had no exposure to the HBV virion, she is negative for anti-HBc. Since her exposure to HCV by needlestick, newly developed alanine aminotransferase (ALT) elevation suggests she is in the minority of recipients of occupation-related needlestick exposure to HCV (<10%) to acquire HCV infection. Consequently, she is anti-HCV positive.

In the 45-year-old male injection drug user, chronic HBV infection is indicated by the presence of HBsAg and total anti-HBc, and the absence of IgM anti-HBc indicates that this is not acute hepatitis B. Hepatitis D virus (HDV) infection develops either as coinfection or superinfection. Coinfection is indicated by evidence of acute HDV and HBV infection (positive IgM anti-HBc). HDV superinfection is indicated by development of anti-HDV superimposed on chronic HBV serologic markers. Typically, HDV infection suppresses HBV replication and is accompanied by negative HBeAg.

In the 59-year-old man who is chronically infected with HBV, the presence of HBsAg indicates persistent infection. Because this patient has been exposed to HBV, anti-HBc is present in the serum, but the IgM subclass of anti-HBc is negative, indicating that this is not a recently acquired infection. The presence of circulating HBeAg is associated with ongoing viral replication, relatively high levels of circulating virus (as indicated by high levels of HBV DNA in the serum), and usually the presence of active necroinflammatory activity in the liver.

Bibliography

1. **Hoofnagel JH.** Therapy of acute and chronic viral hepatitis. Adv Intern Med. 1994;39:241-5.

2. **Herrera JL.** Serologic diagnosis of viral hepatitis. South Med J. 1994;87:677-84.

3. **Hoofnagle JH, Di Bisceglie AM.** The treatment of chronic viral hepatitis. N Engl J Med. 1997;336:347-56.

Liver Disorders Questions 13-16
Answers: 13(D); 14(B); 15(A); 16(C)

Educational Objective: Distinguish between the clinical presentations of different cholestatic diseases.

Various disorders may produce a similar picture of cholestasis, with nearly identical laboratory values. Visualization of the biliary tree is often required to identify the underlying cause. Patients with AIDS may develop a cholangiopathy of the extrahepatic biliary tree that radiographically resembles sclerosing cholangitis. The cause of this disorder is probably infectious, rather than autoimmune. *Cryptosporidium, Microsporidia,* cytomegalovirus, and HIV have all been suggested to cause the characteristic picture of ductal irregularity and narrowing. Patients with idiopathic inflammatory bowel disease, particularly ulcerative colitis, are at an increased risk for sclerosing cholangitis. This can occur in the setting of quiescent bowel disease or it may even precede the diagnosis of colitis. Patients usually develop progressive cholestasis, with intermittent fevers from bacterial infection of the obstructed portions of the biliary tree. Diagnosis requires cholangiography. No medical therapy has been proven effective in this disorder, and most patients ultimately require liver transplantation.

Primary biliary cirrhosis often has a subtle presentation of pruritus or asymptomatic cholestasis. It occurs most frequently in women. Antimitochondrial antibodies are present in over 90% of affected patients. Cholangiography is normal, but the disease is progressive, with advancing pruritus and osteopenia. A syndrome of cholestasis, normal bile ducts on cholangiography, and a paucity of bile ducts on liver biopsy specimen has been called "the vanishing bile duct syndrome." The pathophysiology of this disorder is unknown, but it has been associated with some medications, including chlorpromazine.

Bibliography

1. **Beaugerie L, Teilhac MF, Deluol AM, Fritsch J, Girard PM, Rozenbaum W, et al.** Cholangiopathy associated with Microsporidia infection of the common bile duct mucosa in a patient with HIV infection. Ann Intern Med. 1992;117:401-2.

2. **Lee YM, Kaplan MM.** Primary sclerosing cholangitis. N Engl J Med. 1995;332:924-33.

3. **Kaplan MM.** Primary biliary cirrhosis. N Engl J Med. 1996;335:1570-80.

Liver Disorders Question 17
Answer: B

EDUCATIONAL OBJECTIVE: Recognize acute gallstone-induced pancreatitis and the most appropriate treatment for this serious illness.

This patient clearly has acute ascending cholangitis and gallstone pancreatitis. Recent prospective controlled trials have shown that endoscopic retrograde pancreatography (ERCP) with papillotomy and either removal of a common duct stone or placement of a stent are more effective therapy than emergency surgery. The morbidity and mortality rates are lower and the success rates higher with emergency endoscopic treatment than with surgery. Similar controlled trials have shown that emergency endoscopy in the critically ill patient with gallstone pancreatitis is better than conservative therapy, such as antibiotics and supportive care. Lithotripsy is rarely done now, even for removal of gallbladder gallstones, and is at best experimental and rarely done in bile duct stones. Laparoscopic cholecystectomy is typically done electively in asymptomatic patients and should not be done in critically ill patients with gallstone pancreatitis.

Bibliography

1. **Johnston DE, Kaplan MM.** Pathogenesis and treatment of gallstones. N Engl J Med. 1993;328:412-21.
2. **Lai EC, Mok FP, Tan ES, Lo CM, Fan ST, You KT, et al.** Endoscopic biliary drainage for severe acute cholangitis. N Engl J Med. 1992;326:1582-6.
3. **Carr-Locke DL.** Acute gallstone pancreatitis and endoscopic therapy. Endoscopy. 1990;22:180-3.

Liver Disorders Question 18
Answer: C

EDUCATIONAL OBJECTIVE: Recognize primary biliary cirrhosis and the most efficacious way of diagnosing it.

This is the classic description of primary biliary cirrhosis. Itching is the most common specific symptom of early primary biliary cirrhosis. Approximately 70% of affected patients have enlarged livers. The best screening test for suspected primary biliary cirrhosis is the antimitochondrial antibody study. It is positive in 95% of affected patients and has a 98% specificity if newer ELISA tests are used. Serum protein electro-

phoresis might show a diffuse increase in immunoglobulins; however, this finding is nonspecific and may be found in many chronic liver diseases. Anti–smooth-muscle antibody tests are positive in some patients with autoimmune chronic hepatitis; however, the test is nonspecific and not terribly useful. The sulfur colloid technetium liver-spleen scan is useful for detecting portal hypertension and hypersplenism; however, it is not specific and would not be helpful in diagnosing primary biliary cirrhosis. Endoscopic retrograde cholangiopancreatography (ERCP) is typically normal in patients with primary biliary cirrhosis. Its only role in the diagnosis of primary biliary cirrhosis is in the patient who presents with a similar syndrome but who has a negative antimitochondrial antibody test. ERCP would then be used to look for other causes of disease such as primary sclerosing cholangitis.

Bibliography

1. **Kaplan MM.** Primary biliary cirrhosis. N Engl J Med. 1987;316:521-8.
2. **Kaplan MM.** Primary biliary cirrhosis. In: Schiff L, Schiff ER, eds. Diseases of the Liver. 7th ed. Philadelphia: J.B. Lippincott Co.; 1993:377-410.
3. **Van de Water J, Cooper A, Surh CD, Coppel R, Danner D, Ansari A, et al.** Detection of autoantibodies to recombinant mitochondrial proteins in patients with primary biliary cirrhosis. N Engl J Med. 1989;320:1377-80.

Liver Disorders Questions 19-22
Answers: 19(A); 20(D); 21(C); 22(B)

EDUCATIONAL OBJECTIVE: Distinguish the causes of jaundice in pregnancy.

Jaundice during pregnancy can occur from a variety of causes. The most common cause is acute viral hepatitis, which can occur at any time during pregnancy, with the characteristic elevations in aminotransferases and history of appropriate exposure, as in the 24-year-old woman with the history of injection drug abuse. Acute fatty liver of pregnancy occurs late and presents with evidence of liver failure, including encephalopathy, coagulopathy, and jaundice, as in the 35-year-old woman in her eighth month of pregnancy. Liver biopsy shows characteristic small-droplet steatosis. This often fatal disease requires vigorous support and immediate delivery of the child.

Intrahepatic cholestasis of pregnancy is a usually benign disease for the mother, but it does slightly increase the risk for fetal death. Patients often present with pruritus, cholestasis, and mild elevation of aminotransferases, as in the 23-year-old woman in her eighth month of pregnancy. The disorder may recur with subsequent pregnancies and with the use of oral contraceptives. Patients with preeclampsia can develop a syndrome of hemolysis, elevated liver enzymes, and low platelet count called the HELLP syndrome, as in the 25-year-old woman in her seventh month of pregnancy. Jaundice is usually mild. The abnormalities resolve after delivery, but hepatic infarction and even hepatic rupture can occur.

Bibliography

1. **Reyes H, Sandoval L, Wainstein A, Ribalta J, Donoso S, Smok G, et al.** Acute fatty liver of pregnancy: a clinical study of 12 episodes in 11 patients. Gut. 1994;35:101-6.

2. **Sjogren MH.** Hepatic emergencies in pregnancy. Med Clin North Am. 1993;77:1115-27.

3. **Reyes H.** The spectrum of liver and gastrointestinal disease seen in cholestasis of pregnancy. Gastroenterol Clin North Am. 1992;21:905-21.

Liver Disorders Question 23
Answer: C

EDUCATIONAL OBJECTIVE: Diagnose the cause of ascites from the laboratory test results, specifically the serum-to-ascites albumin gradient, the leukocyte count, and the aspartate aminotransferase (AST)–alanine aminotransferase (ALT) ratio.

This patient clearly has chronic liver disease complicated by ascites. The paracentesis demonstrates that the serum-ascites albumin gradient is 2. A value greater than 1.1 suggests that the ascites is due to por-

tal hypertension. Although both alanine aminotransferase (ALT) and aspartate aminotransferase (AST) are elevated, the AST-ALT ratio is greater than 3, a finding common in alcoholic liver disease but not in any of the other diseases listed. The pattern of the aminotransferases, the elevated bilirubin, and the serum-ascites albumin gradient greater than 1.1 make ovarian carcinoma and tuberculous peritonitis unlikely diagnoses. The serum-ascites albumin gradient in this patient is consistent with Budd-Chiari syndrome, although the ascitic fluid albumin concentration is frequently higher. However, the AST-ALT ratio makes Budd-Chiari syndrome unlikely. The presentation, AST-ALT ratio, and slight elevation of alkaline phosphatase make primary biliary cirrhosis unlikely. Therefore, the combination of the serum-ascites albumin pattern and the AST-ALT ratio make alcoholic cirrhosis the most likely diagnosis. The characteristic ratio of AST to ALT in alcoholic liver disease is due to a relative deficiency of pyridoxal phosphate in alcoholic patients. Many such patients have nutritionally deficient diets and therefore ingest low amounts of vitamin B_6. Equally important, alcoholism itself increases the turnover of pyridoxal phosphate concentration even in patients with a normal diet.

Bibliography

1. **Runyon BA, Montano AA, Akriviadis EA, Antillon MR, Irving MA, McHutchison JG.** The serum-ascites albumin gradient is superior to the exudate-transudate concept in the differential diagnosis of ascites. Ann Intern Med. 1992;117:215-20.

2. **Kaplan MM.** Laboratory tests. In: Schiff L, Schiff ER, eds. Diseases of the Liver. 7th ed. Philadelphia: JB Lippincott Co; 1993:108-44.

3. **Runyon BA.** Care of patients with ascites. N Engl J Med. 1994;330:337-42.

MYOCARDIAL INFARCTION

Myocardial Infarction Question 1
Answer: E

EDUCATIONAL OBJECTIVE: Diagnose cardiogenic shock and select appropriate treatment based on clinical and hemodynamic findings.

This patient has both clinical and hemodynamic findings of cardiogenic shock. This is manifest by hypotension and tachycardia with signs of peripheral hypoperfusion (metabolic acidosis, cool skin, and low urine output). The presence of adequate volume is suggested by the patient's rales on physical examination. However, once diuretics are given, the patient may in fact be normovolemic with slow clearing of the pulmonary edema fluid. In this situation it is beneficial to place a Swan-Ganz catheter to determine precisely the patient's volume status. This patient appears to be adequately hydrated on the basis of a wedge pressure of 25 mm Hg. In addition, he has signs of a low cardiac output and a high systemic vascular resistance, all consistent with cardiogenic shock.

Intra-aortic balloon pumping has been found to be a useful adjunct in patients with ongoing ischemia and severe left ventricular dysfunction. It has been shown to reduce the systemic vascular resistance, improve cardiac output, reduce pulmonary capillary wedge pressures, as well as improve the perfusion of the coronary arteries. Therefore, balloon pumping should reduce the myocardial oxygen demand while improving the supply. Improving coronary perfusion of the infarct as well as non-infarct zones may reduce global myocardial ischemia. Patients with cardiogenic shock generally have infarcted at least 40% of the left ventricle. Use of thrombolytic therapy in shock patients is associated with low rates of coronary reperfusion as well as high mortality rates (70% to 80%). These critically ill patients should have their coronary anatomy defined by emergency cardiac catheterization, even if interhospital transfer is required. The use of emergency coronary angioplasty or bypass surgery may reduce the mortality rate to 50%.

Digoxin therapy is not effective at acutely augmenting left ventricular function. Intravenous diuretics may lower the pulmonary capillary wedge pressure further; however, this treatment will not result in an increase in blood pressure. Diuretics are not necessary at this point, as long as the patient is oxygenating well. In addition, this patient may need a higher left ventricular filling pressure in order to maintain blood pressure, given his degree of left ventricular dysfunction. It is better to intubate the patient if necessary rather than over-diurese a patient who is already hypotensive; however, given the arterial blood gases, intubation is not necessary.

Dopamine therapy may be useful as a temporary strategy to raise the blood pressure; however, in the setting of an elevated systemic vascular resistance, dopamine will cause further vasoconstriction and tachycardia, with a subsequent increase in the myocardial oxygen demand. Dobutamine may be useful in temporarily augmenting cardiac output and reducing wedge pressure; however, inotropic agents have not altered the mortality of patients with cardiogenic shock.

Bibliography

1. **Forrester JS, Diamond G, Chatterjee K, Swan HJ.** Medical therapy of acute myocardial infarction by application of hemodynamic subsets. N Engl J Med. 1976;295:1404-13.
2. **DeWood MA, Notske RN, Hensley GR, Shields JP, O'Grady WP, Spores J, et al.** Intraaortic balloon counterpulsation with and without reperfusion for myocardial infarction shock. Circulation. 1980;61:1105-12.
3. **Bates ER, Topol EJ.** Limitations of thrombolytic therapy for acute myocardial infarction complicated by congestive heart failure and cardiogenic shock. J Am Coll Cardiol. 1991;18:1077-84.
4. **O'Neill WW.** Angioplasty therapy of cardiogenic shock: are randomized trials necessary? J Am Coll Cardiol. 1992;19:915-7.
5. **Maekawa K, Liang CS, Hood WB Jr.** Comparison of dobutamine and dopamine in acute myocardial infarction. Effects of systemic hemodynamics, plasma catecholamines, blood flows and infarct size. Circulation. 1983;67:750-9.

Myocardial Infarction Question 2
Answer: A

EDUCATIONAL OBJECTIVE: Determine the appropriate role for catheterization and angioplasty following acute myocardial infarction.

This patient is in an exceedingly low-risk category following myocardial infarction. He is young, has no prior cardiac problems, has sustained an inferior myocardial infarction, and has well-preserved ventricular function. Discharge on medical therapy is the appropriate management.

Although the exercise thallium scan is somewhat equivocal, given his low risk (less than 1% mortality per year), it is unlikely that any diagnostic or therapeutic procedure would be of benefit. Therefore, additional exercise testing is not warranted. Furthermore, most of the data regarding the predictive value of exercise testing were derived in an era when reperfusion therapy was not applied. More recent data suggest that it is very difficult to predict which patients may have subsequent recurrent ischemia and infarction after thrombolysis, and the very expensive noninvasive evaluation that this patient had may not be warranted. In this low-risk patient, risk stratification should include an estimate of ejection fraction and exercise treadmill testing. Conversely, some have advocated early cardiac catheterization with *no* noninvasive testing as a means to determine patients' risk stratification and expedite hospital discharge.

Although catheterization may obviate the need for multiple, expensive noninvasive testing, catheterization is not indicated at this time, because this patient has already had a battery of tests that placed him in a low-risk category. Conventionally, catheterization is done either to eliminate need for noninvasive testing or in patients who are at higher risk of having a subsequent cardiac event (signs of left ventricular dysfunction, recurrent ischemia, or evidence of prior myocardial infarction).

A patient who is clinically stable following thrombolysis generally does not benefit from routine coronary angioplasty. However, if the patient has had a history of prior myocardial infarction, evidence of hemodynamic compromise, or recurrent ischemia, catheterization with revascularization has been shown to be beneficial.

Bibliography

1. SWIFT trial of delayed elective interventional conservative treatment after thrombolysis with anistreplase in acute myocardial infarction. SWIFT (Should We Intervene Following Thrombolysis?) Trial Study Group. BMJ. 1991;302:555-60.

2. Comparison of invasive and conservative strategies after treatment with intravenous tissue plasminogen activator in acute myocardial infarction. Results of the Thrombolysis in Myocardial Infarction (TIMI) phase II trial. The TIMI Study Group. N Engl J Med. 1989;320:618-27.

3. **Mueller HS, Cohen LS, Braunwald E, Forman S, Feit F, Ross A, et al.** Predictors of early morbidity and mortality after thrombolytic therapy of acute myocardial infarction. Analysis of patient subgroups in the Thrombolysis In Myocardial Infarction (TIMI) phase II trial. Circulation. 1992;85:1254-64.

Myocardial Infarction Questions 3-5
Answers: 3(B); 4(D); 5(C)

EDUCATIONAL OBJECTIVE: Differentiate adjunctive medical therapy in patients with acute myocardial infarction.

Several classes of drugs have been found to alter significantly the outcome of patients experiencing acute myocardial infarction. In addition to thrombolytic therapy, early administration of aspirin and beta-blockers has been shown to reduce subsequent mortality. Early administration of an angiotensin-converting enzyme (ACE) inhibitor was not associated with mortality reduction in the Consensus II trial. Late administration (after about 1 week) of ACE inhibitors does reduce subsequent mortality and cardiovascular events, as do aspirin and beta-blockers. Moreover, ventricular dilatation (infarct expansion) is also reduced. Several studies have shown that beta-blocker therapy reduces subsequent sudden death as well as overall mortality. Calcium channel blocker therapy increases mortality in patients with acute myocardial infarction in the presence of clinical congestive heart failure or depressed left ventricular function.

Bibliography

1. **Swedberg K, Held P, Kjebshus J, Rasmussen K, Ryden L, Wedel H.** Effects of the early administration of enalapril on mortality in patients with acute myocardial infarction. Results of the Cooperative New Scandinavian Enalapril Survival Study II (Consensus II). N Engl J Med. 1992;327:678-84.

2. **Woods KL, Fletcher S, Roffe C, Haider Y.** Intravenous magnesium sulfate in suspected acute myocardial infarction: results of the second Leicester Intravenous Magnesium Intervention Trial (LIMT-II). Lancet. 1992;339:1553-8.

3. **Yusuf S, Sleight P, Held P, McMahon S.** Routine medical management of acute myocardial infarction. Lessons from overviews of recent randomized controlled trials. Circulation. 1990;82:II117-34.

4. **Pfeffer MA, Braunwald E, Moyel A, Basta L, Brown EJ Jr, Cuddy JE, et al.** Effect of captopril on mortality and morbidity in patients with left ventricular dysfunction after myocardial infarction. Results of the Survival and Ventricular Enlargement trial. The SAVE Investigators. N Engl J Med. 1992;327:669-77.

5. The effect of diltiazem on mortality and reinfarction after myocardial infarction. The Multicenter Diltiazem Postinfarction Trial Research Group. N Engl J Med. 1988;319:385-92.

Myocardial Infarction Question 6
Answer: D

EDUCATIONAL OBJECTIVE: Identify the cause of hypotension in the setting of acute myocardial infarction.

Although the precordial ST-segment depressions may suggest the presence of anterior ischemia, a more unifying diagnosis is provided by an inferior posterior myocardial infarction with right ventricular involvement. This hemodynamic complication of an inferior myocardial infarction is associated with a significantly higher mortality rate and identifies a high-risk subgroup for whom acute reperfusion therapy is especially considered. Most patients show a return of normal right ventricular systolic function over a period of several days to weeks, which is partly related to a concomitant improvement in left ventricular dysfunction and reduction of right ventricular afterload. Any factor that reduces preload (such as nitrates), interferes with normal atrioventricular synchrony (atrial fibrillation), or increases right ventricular afterload (for example, left ventricular failure) will predictably worsen hemodynamic function.

Despite the history of antacid use, the elevated jugular venous pressure and negative test for occult blood in the stool argue against hypovolemia. Cardiogenic shock from primary left ventricular pump failure would be unusual in the setting of an inferior posterior myocardial infarction without evidence of an antecedent event in another coronary territory. A murmur of mitral regurgitation may be absent in as many as 50% of patients with acute papillary muscle dysfunction and/or rupture. Myocardial rupture, however, most commonly occurs 3 to 7 days after the initial injury. Radiographic pulmonary edema is the rule rather than the exception with acute mitral regurgitation.

The clinical findings of hypotension with elevated venous pressure and clear lung fields are suggestive of right ventricular involvement. Although not done in this case, electrocardiography with right precordial leads should be obtained in any patient with an inferior ST-segment elevation myocardial infarction. Demonstration of 1-mm ST-segment elevation in lead V_4R allows the diagnosis of right ventricular infarction with 88% sensitivity and 78% specificity.

The concomitant finding of ST-segment depression in leads V_1 and V_2 is problematic. The differential diagnosis includes true posterior infarction, anteroseptal subendocardial ischemia (ischemia at a distance), or reciprocal change. It is distinctly unusual for ST-segment depressions to be observed in lead V_1 in the setting of either anteroseptal subendocardial ischemia or reciprocal change. An echocardiogram can often identify acute right ventricular dilatation and free wall hypokinesis to aid in the differential diagnosis.

Bibliography

1. **Berger PB, Ryan TJ.** Inferior myocardial infarction. High-risk subgroups. Circulation. 1990;81:401-11.

2. **Dell'Italia LJ, Starling MR, Crawford MH, Boros BL, Chadhuri TK, O'Rourke RA.** Right ventricular infarction: identification by hemodynamic measurements before and after volume loading and correlation with noninvasive techniques. J Am Coll Cardiol. 1984;4:931-9.

3. **Zehender M, Kasper W, Kauder E, Schonthaler M, Geibel A, Olschewski M, et al.** Right ventricular infarction as an independent predictor of prognosis after acute inferior myocardial infarction. N Engl J Med. 1993;328:981-8.

Myocardial Infarction Question 7
Answer: B

EDUCATIONAL OBJECTIVE: Recognize the role of β-blocking drugs in patients with stable coronary artery disease with impaired ventricular function.

β-blocking drugs are indicated in this patient. Benefits will include antihypertensive and anti-ischemic effects and reduced probability of sudden death. With the exclusion of an implantable defibrillator, β-blocking drugs are the most effective agents for reducing sudden death in high-risk patients. This woman has an impaired left ventricle with an ejection fraction less than 35%. Diltiazem should be discontinued because of its adverse effect on left ventricular function and its potential to induce congestive heart failure (CHF). Amlodipine can be given safely to patients with an impaired left ventricle and a history of CHF, but in the absence of angina it offers no additional benefit over angiotensin-converting enzyme (ACE) inhibitors. The benefit of β-blockade is highest in persons with an impaired left ventricle, and precipitation of congestive heart failure is very uncommon. Long-acting nitrates have no role in coronary artery disease with an impaired left ventricle in the absence of angina or heart failure. Diuretic agents should be avoided because of their adverse effects on neurohumoral response, unless there is evidence of pulmonary congestion or edema. In the absence of CHF there is no indication for digoxin. The Digoxin Investigator Group (DIG) trial sponsored by the National Heart, Lung, and Blood Institute showed that digoxin decreased CHF symptoms and reduced the need for hospitalization, but there was no survival benefit.

Bibliography

1. **Kendall MJ, Lynch KP, Hjalmarson A, Kjekshus J.** Beta-blockers and sudden cardiac death. Ann Intern Med. 1995;123:358-67.

2. **Kennedy HL, Rosenson RS.** Physician use of beta-adrenergic blocking therapy: a changing perspective. J Am Coll Cardiol. 1995;26:547-52.

3. **Packer M, O'Connor CM, Ghali JK, Pressler ML, Carson PE, Belkin RN, et al.** Effect of amlodipine on morbidity and mortality in severe chronic heart failure. Prospective Randomized Amlodipine Survival Evaluation Study Group. N Engl J Med. 1996;335:1107-14.

4. The effect of digoxin on mortality and morbidity in patients with heart failure. The Digitalis Investigation Group. N Engl J Med. 1997;336:525-33.

Myocardial Infarction Question 8
Answer: E

EDUCATIONAL OBJECTIVE: Assess coronary risk factors following a myocardial infarction.

Lowering low-density lipoprotein (LDL) cholesterol following an acute myocardial infarction has proven efficacy, and dietary and drug treatment should begin early. The concentrations of cholesterol, triglycerides, high-density lipoprotein (HDL) cholesterol, and calculated LDL cholesterol obtained within 24 hours of onset of symptoms fairly reflect the pre-event lipid profile, but after 24 hours the cholesterol concentrations decrease significantly, the triglycerides may increase markedly, and HDL cholesterol is not predictable. This patient may not be a candidate for lipid-lowering drugs based on the predischarge values, but the concentrations measured at 4 weeks following thrombolytic therapy reflect the preinfarction values and those measured at 3 months the postinfarction values.

The most common lipid abnormality in persons with premature coronary artery disease is an increase in lipoprotein(a) concentration, but laboratory standards are not available and treatment is limited. The most important parameters are fasting cholesterol, triglycerides, and HDL cholesterol, which allow calculation of LDL cholesterol and estimation of LDL particle size. Based on laboratory variability and the effects of the myocardial infarction, the 4-week cholesterol concentration could range from 200 to 240 mg/dL and HDL cholesterol from 33 to 45 mg/dL. Each of the lipid

parameters helps to determine treatment goals, diet, and drug therapy. The concentration of apolipoprotein B would be of interest but would not change treatment strategy. An increase in fibrinogen and platelets is found in persons with premature coronary disease, but there is no treatment and routine measurement is not advised. Although homocysteine is an important risk factor and measurement in persons with premature coronary artery disease is appropriate, the value of treatment is not established.

Bibliography

1. **Sacks FM, Pfeffer MA, Moye LA, Rouleau JL, Rutherford JD, Cole TG, et al.** The effect of pravastatin on coronary events after myocardial infarction in patients with average cholesterol levels. Cholesterol and Recurrent Events Trial Investigators. N Engl J Med. 1996;335:1001-9.

2. **Durrington PN, Ishola M, Hunt L, Arrol S, Bhatnagar D.** Apolipoproteins (a), AI, and B and parental history in men with early onset ischemic heart disease. Lancet. 1988;1:1070-3.

3. **Kannel WB, Wolf PA, Castelli WP, D'Agostino RB.** Fibrinogen and risk of cardiovascular disease. The Framingham Study. JAMA. 1987;258:1183-6.

4. **Genest JJ Jr, McNamara JR, Upson B, Salem DN, Ordovas JM, Schaefer EF, et al.** Prevalence of familial hyperhomocysteinemia in men with premature coronary artery disease. Arterioscler Thromb. 1991;11:1129-36.

5. **Carlsson R, Lindberg G, Westin L, Israelsson B.** Serum lipids four weeks after acute myocardial infarction are a valid basis for lipid lowering intervention in patients receiving thrombolysis. Br Heart J. 1995;74:18-20.

Myocardial Infarction Question 9
Answer: D

EDUCATIONAL OBJECTIVE: Select the optimal management of ventricular fibrillation occurring within the early phases of an acute transmural myocardial infarction.

The mortality rate of patients who develop ventricular fibrillation within 48 hours of an acute myocardial infarction depends on the presence or absence of heart failure. In the absence of significant left ventricular dysfunction, the 1-year mortality rate is extremely low. In these patients, treatment with β-blockade alone is recommended. In contrast, patients who have sustained a large infarction have a lower rate of survival. At most centers, treatment of these higher-risk patients is limited to standard care following myocardial infarction, including β-blockers, angiotensin-converting enzyme inhibitors, and revascularization, if required. According to published guidelines, an electrophysiologic study is not indicated in patients with sudden death occurring within the first 48 hours of an acute myocardial infarction.

The routine treatment of patients following myocardial infarction with amiodarone is also not routinely recommended. The EMIAT and CAMIAT studies evaluated the role of empiric treatment of high-risk postinfarction patients with amiodarone (identified based on an ejection fraction of less than 40%, non-sustained ventricular tachycardia, or frequent ventricular ectopy). Although amiodarone lowered the incidence of arrhythmic deaths in both studies, there was no difference in overall mortality.

Treatment with atenolol would therefore represent the optimal approach to management of this patient at the present time. No data exist to suggest that treatment with a class I antiarrhythmic agent such as procainamide will have any survival benefit. Neither an electrophysiologic study nor placement of an implantable defibrillator is indicated. Although amiodarone could be considered in this setting, this approach is controversial and currently undergoing further investigation.

Bibliography

1. **O'Nunain S, Ruskin J.** Cardiac arrest. Lancet. 1993;341:1641-7.

2. **Zipes DP, DiMarco JP, Gillette PC, Jackman WM, Myerberg RJ, Rahmintoola SH, et al.** Guidelines for clinical intracardiac electrophysiological and catheter ablation procedures. A report of the American College of Cardiology/American Heart Association Task Force on Practice Guidelines (Committee on Clinical Intracardiac Electrophysiologic and Catheter Ablation Procedures), developed in collaboration with the North American Society of Pacing and Electrophysiology. J Am Coll Cardiol. 1995;26:555-73.

3. **Tofler GH, Stone PH, Muller JE, Rutherford JD, Willich SN, Gustafson NF, et al.** Prognosis after cardiac arrest due to ventricular tachycardia or ventricular fibrillation associated with acute myocardial infarction (the MILIS study). Multicenter Investigation of the Limitation of Infarct Size. Am J Cardiol. 1987;60:755-61.

Myocardial Infarction Question 10
Answer: C

EDUCATIONAL OBJECTIVE: Anticipate recurrent ischemic events in patients with stable coronary disease.

Rupture of a plaque with a superimposed thrombus is responsible for most acute coronary ischemic events (myocardial infarction [MI] or unstable angina) in patients with silent or known coronary artery disease. Gradual progression to occlusion without a thrombus is usually silent and not often the cause of acute MI. Severe (> 75% to 90%) chronic MI-associated lesions have increased fibrous tissue, which stabilizes the plaque. Most MI-associated lesions seen at coronary angiography or postmortem examination are mild to moderate (40% to 70%) and not heavily calcified. In this patient, the multiple circumflex lesions typify lesions that are prone to rupture. Coronary arteriography is not a good predictor of site of future infarction. Reversible defects on thallium-201 stress imaging increase the probability of future acute events but do not effectively predict the site. Sites of previous percutaneous transluminal coronary angioplasty (PCTA) do not have a predilection for plaque instability, and plaque rupture in the left main coronary artery occurs but is relatively uncommon.

Bibliography

1. **Falk E, Shah PK, Fuster V.** Pathogenesis of plaque disruption. In: Fuster V, Ross R, Topol E, eds. Atherosclerosis and Coronary Artery Disease. Philadelphia: Lippincott-Raven; 1996:491-507.

2. **Fuster V, Badimon L, Badimon JJ, Chesebro JH.** The pathogenesis of coronary artery disease and the acute coronary syndromes (2). N Engl J Med. 1992;326:310-8.

3. **Little WC, Constantinescu M, Applegate RJ, Kutcher MA, Burrows MT, Kahl FR, et al.** Can coronary arteriography predict the site of subsequent myocardial infarction in patients with mild-to-moderate coronary artery disease? Circulation. 1988;78:1157-66.

4. **Naqvi T, Hachamovitch R, Berman D, Buchbinder N, Kiat H, Shah PK.** Does the presence and site of myocardial ischemia on perfusion scintigraphy predict the occurrence and site of future myocardial infarction in patients with stable coronary artery disease? Am J Cardiol. 1997;79:1521-4.

5. **Waller BF, Pinkerton CA, Orr CM, Slack JD, VanTassel, JW, Peters T.** Restenosis 1 to 24 months after clinically successful coronary balloon angioplasty: a necropsy study of 20 patients. J Am Coll Cardiol. 1991;17:58B-70B.

Myocardial Infarction Question 11
Answer: B

EDUCATIONAL OBJECTIVE: Recognize the correct role of angiotensin-converting enzyme inhibitor therapy in the treatment of asymptomatic left ventricular dysfunction following an extensive anterior myocardial infarction.

The proper treatment of this patient should be guided by the results of recent clinical trials. A growing number of controlled trials have examined the role of angiotensin-converting enzyme (ACE) inhibitor therapy following acute myocardial infarction. The goals of such treatment include a decrease in short- and long-term mortality and a reduction in the risk of developing overt heart failure, reinfarction, and progressive left ventricular dilatation. Some debate continues regarding the optimal timing and duration of ACE inhibitor treatment in patients who receive concomitant treatment with aspirin and β-blockers. The SAVE (captopril), AIRE (ramipril), and TRACE (trandolapril) trials all selected high-risk populations as identified by clinical evidence of overt heart failure or marked left ventricular dysfunction (left ventricular ejection fraction below 40%) following myocardial infarction (MI). Treatment with an oral ACE inhibitor was initiated between days 3 and 16 post-MI, and all three trials showed a substantial (19% to 27%) reduction in all-cause mortality. Conversely, the CATS (captopril), CAPTIN (captopril), and CONSENSUS-II (intravenous enalaprilat followed by oral enalapril) trials all initiated therapy within the first 6 hours. All three studies showed a high incidence of hypotension and a trend toward increased early mortality. A third treatment strategy was adopted in the GISSI-3 (lisinopril), ISIS-4 (captopril), and SMILE (zofenopril) trials. Oral treatment was initiated early (within 24 hours) but continued for only 4 to 6 weeks. The aim of these studies was to treat a broad spectrum of patients with varied degrees of left ventricular dysfunction rather than limit ACE inhibitor treatment to high-risk populations. The treatment interval was limited to the period of time when the risk of reinfarction or abnormal left ventricular remodeling was thought to be greatest. All three trials showed a small but significant benefit of short-term therapy on 6- to 12-month mortality.

For this patient, the best choice is to begin oral enalapril within 48 hours. Well-conducted controlled trials have shown that ACE inhibitor therapy should be initiated within 48 hours and continued indefinitely in post-MI patients with left ventricular ejection fractions below 40% and in those individuals who have had an episode of overt heart failure beyond the initial 24 hours of presentation. Initiation of an oral ACE inhibitor should be delayed for 24 to 72 hours, until hemodynamic stability has been established.

There are less convincing arguments for long-term treatment of patients with transient post-MI heart failure in whom recovery of left ventricular function occurs. For small myocardial infarctions, the greatest benefit of ACE inhibitor treatment may be achieved by decreasing the extent of early left ventricular remodeling, which occurs during the first 4 to 6 weeks. In such patients, the drug might be safely discontinued at 6 weeks. However, if the ongoing QUIET (quinapril) trial

shows a substantial reduction in reinfarction, a stronger case may be made for treating all post-MI patients with an ACE inhibitor indefinitely. This approach cannot be recommended for all patients at this time.

Bibliography

1. **Latini R, Maggioni AP, Flather M, Sleight P, Tognoni G.** ACE inhibitor use in patients with myocardial infarction. Summary of evidence from clinical trials. Circulation. 1995;92:3132-7.

2. **Swedberg K, Held P, Kjeksus J, Rasmussen K, Ryden L, Wedel H, et al.** Effects of the early administration of enalapril on mortality in patients with acute myocardial infarction. Results of the cooperative new Scandinavian enalapril survival study II (CONSENSUS II). N Engl J Med. 1992;327:678-84.

3. Six-month effects of early treatment with lisinopril and transdermal glyceryl trinitrate singly and together withdrawn six weeks after acute myocardial infarction: the GISSI-3 trial. Gruppo Italiano per lo Studio della Sopravvivenza Nell'Infarcto Miocardico. J Am Coll Cardiol. 1996;27:337-44.

4. ISIS-4: A randomized factorial trial assessing early oral captopril, oral mononitrate, and intravenous magnesium sulphate in 58,050 patients with suspected acute myocardial infarction. ISIS-4 (Fourth International Study of Infarct Survival) Collaboration Group. Lancet. 1995;345:669-85.

5. **Ryan TJ, Anderson JL, Antman EM, Braniff BA, Brooks NH, Califf RM, et al.** ACC/AHA guidelines for the management of patients with acute myocardial infarction: executive summary. A report of the American College of Cardiology/ American Heart Association Task Force on Practice Guideline (Committee on Management of Acute Myocardial Infarction). Circulation. 1996;94:2341-50.

Myocardial Infarction Question 12
Answer: A

EDUCATIONAL OBJECTIVE: Recognize and treat post-infarction pericarditis.

This patient has developed symptoms and electrocardiographic signs to suggest postinfarction pericarditis, the incidence of which has declined in the thrombolytic era. The absence of a pericardial friction rub does not exclude the diagnosis, especially given the rather compelling features of the history (positional pain) and the PR-segment depression. The expression of pericarditis generally implies transmural myocardial necrosis with irritation of the overlying pericardial surfaces. It is imperative to distinguish the pain of pericarditis from that of recurrent ischemia. Pericardial effusions are detected by echocardiography in up to 40% of patients but are by no means as specific as they are noted in most patients with myocardial infarction.

Salicylate is the treatment of choice (class I recommendation of the American College of Cardiology/American Heart Association guidelines). Medications that interfere with wound healing, such as nonsteroidal anti-inflammatory agents and corticosteroids are contraindicated, given case reports that these drugs are associated with a relatively higher incidence of thinning, aneurysm formation, and myocardial rupture. Colchicine is reserved for the treatment of recurrent, idiopathic pericarditis.

Bibliography

1. **Ryan TJ, Anderson JL, Antman EM, Braniff BA, Brooks NH, Califf RM, et al.** ACC/AHA guidelines for the management of patients with acute myocardial infarction: a report of the American College of Cardiology/American Heart Association Task Force on Practice Guidelines (Committee on Management of Acute Myocardial Infarction). J Am Coll Cardiol. 1996;28:1328-428.

2. **Becker RC, Gore JM, Lambrew C, Weaver WD, Rubison RM, French WJ, et al.** A composite view of cardiac rupture in the United States National Registry of Myocardial Infarction. J Am Coll Cardiol. 1996;27:1321-6.

3. **Oliva PB, Hammill SC.** The clinical distinction between regional postinfarction pericarditis and other causes of postinfarction chest pain: ancillary observations regarding the effect of lytic therapy upon the frequency of postinfarction pericarditis, postinfarction angina, and reinfarction. Clin Cardiol. 1994;17:471-8.

4. **Berman J, Haffajee CI, Alpert JS.** Therapy of symptomatic pericarditis after myocardial infarction: retrospective and prospective studies of aspirin, indomethacin, prednisone, and spontaneous resolution. Am Heart J. 1981;101:750-3.

5. **Adler Y, Zandman-Goddard G, Ravid M, Avidan B, Zemer D, Ehrenfeld M, et al.** Usefulness of colchicine in preventing recurrences of pericarditis. Am J Cardiol. 1994;73:916-7.

Myocardial Infarction Question 13
Answer: C

EDUCATIONAL OBJECTIVE: Identify the absolute and relative contraindications to the use of thrombolytic therapy for the treatment of acute myocardial infarction.

The American Heart Association/American College of Cardiology Guidelines for the Management of Acute Myocardial Infarction list the following as absolute contraindications to the use of thrombolytic therapy:

1. Previous hemorrhagic stroke at any time; other strokes or cerebrovascular events within the past year
2. Known intracranial neoplasm (or arteriovenous malformation)
3. Active internal bleeding
4. Suspected aortic dissection

There are several relative contraindications or cautions, which include:

1. Severe and uncontrolled hypertension at time of presentation (blood pressure greater than 180/100 mm Hg)
2. Any history of a previous cerebrovascular accident or known intracerebral pathology
3. Current use of anticoagulants in therapeutic doses and/or a known bleeding diathesis
4. Recent trauma (within the past 2 to 4 weeks) or a traumatic or prolonged cardiopulmonary resuscitation (greater than 10 minutes) or major surgery within the past 3 weeks
5. Noncompressible vascular punctures (for example, at the subclavian vein)
6. Recent internal bleeding (within the past 2 to 4 weeks)
7. Pregnancy
8. Active peptic ulcer disease
9. History of chronic severe hypertension
10. Previous exposure (within the past 5 days to 2 years) or history of previous allergic reaction to streptokinase or anistreplase

The chronic use of warfarin to a therapeutic international normalized ratio would clearly make the use of thrombolytic therapy unnecessarily hazardous in this octogenarian. Age alone is not a contraindication to the use of thrombolytic therapy. The Fibrinolytic Therapy Trialists' overview suggested that the absolute survival benefit at 5 weeks with the use of fibrinolytic therapy was similar for young and old patients (for example, 15 lives saved per 1000 treated patients less than 55 years of age, 13 lives saved per 1000 treated patients 75 years of age or older). Indeed, advanced age (greater than 70 years) is an indicator of increased risk and should usually engender an aggressive strategy unless strong contraindications exist. This patient's stroke 4 years before her presentation is a relative contraindication to the use of thrombolytic therapy. The small but increased risk of intracranial hemorrhage needs to be balanced against the much higher risk of cardiac mortality predicated on her age, the location of the infarction, presentation with atrial fibrillation, and the presence of heart failure. Philosophical judgments regarding the propriety of aggressive reperfusion strategies in such patients are difficult to render in an emergency room environment.

Although the beneficial effects of thrombolytic therapy are greatest for those patients with ST-segment elevation infarctions treated within 12 hours of the onset of symptoms, individual patients of this type with clear evidence of persistent injury and hemodynamic embarrassment of uncertain temporal duration are also likely to benefit from such a reperfusion strategy.

This patient's blood pressure at the time of presentation was not high enough to provide a contraindication to thrombolytic therapy. The presence of left ventricular hypertrophy on the electrocardiogram would imply that hypertension has been a chronic issue. Yet, like her age and gender, her chronic hypertension is but a relative risk factor for thrombolytic-related hemorrhage, all of which must be balanced against the magnitude and severity of her presenting infarction.

Bibliography

1. Fibrinolytic Therapy Trialists' (FTT) Collaborative Group. Indications for fibrinolytic therapy in suspected acute myocardial infarction: collaborative overview of early mortality and major morbidity results from all randomized trials of more than 1000 patients. Lancet. 1994;343:311-22.

2. **Maggioni AP, Maseri A, Fresco C, Franzosi MG, Mauri F, Santoro E, et al.** Age-related increase in mortality among patients with first myocardial infarctions treated with thrombolysis: The Investigators of the Gruppo Italiano per lo Studio della Sopravvivenza nell'Infarto Miocardico (GISSI-2). N Engl J Med. 1993;329:1442-8.

3. **Collins R, Peto R, Baigent C, Sleight P.** Aspirin, heparin, and fibrinolytic therapy in suspected myocardial infarction. N Engl J Med. 1997;336:847-60.

4. **Maggioni AP, Franzosi MG, Santoro E, White H, Van de Werf F, Tognoni G.** The risk of stroke in patients with acute myocardial infarction after thrombolytic and antithrombotic treatment. Gruppo Italiano per lo Studio della Sopravvivenza nell'Infarto Miocardico II (GISSI-2), and The International Study Group. N Engl J Med. 1992;327:1-6.

5. **Ryan T, Anderson JL, Antman EM, Braniff BA, Brooks NH, Califf RM, et al.** ACC/AHA guidelines for the management of patients with acute myocardial infarction. A report of the American College of Cardiology/American Heart Association Task Force on Practice Guidelines (Committee on Management of Acute Myocardial Infarction). J Am Coll Cardiol. 1996;1328-428.

Myocardial Infarction Questions 14-18 Answers: 14(C); 15(D); 16(B); 17(A); 18(B)

EDUCATIONAL OBJECTIVE: Choose the appropriate reperfusion strategy for acute myocardial infarction as specified by the patient's clinical condition.

The 64-year-old man has had a recent inferior-posterior myocardial infarction complicated by ventricular septal rupture. Although this complication can sometimes be difficult to distinguish from papillary muscle rupture with mitral regurgitation on clinical grounds alone, a bedside transthoracic echocardiogram with Doppler interrogation should be diagnostic. Both ventricular septal rupture and papillary muscle rupture tend to occur 3 to 5 days after the index event. A murmur (loudest at the lower left sternal border) is present in as many as 90% of patients with ventricular septal defect, but only 50% of patients with mitral regurgitation (heard between the lower left sternal border and apex). Patients with acute mitral regurgitation tend to have more impressive signs of pulmonary edema. Survival with medical therapy alone for either of these two mechanical complications is quite poor. Catheterization with oximetry and coronary angiography are urgently indicated. Temporary stability can be achieved with intra-aortic balloon counterpulsation. Prompt surgery is mandated unless severe comorbidities exist. Coronary revascularization is routinely done at the time of mechanical repair.

The 55-year-old man appears to have had an apical lateral posterior myocardial infarction within the past 48 hours and now arrives pain-free without signs of persistent injury by electrocardiographic criteria or hemodynamic embarrassment. At this stage in the evolution of his infarction there would be no predictable benefit from the initiation of an acute reperfusion strategy. It would be appropriate to institute conservative medical therapy, including aspirin, a β-blocker, and an angiotensin-converting enzyme inhibitor, and then to assess his residual left ventricular function and ischemic potential, unless recurrent injury were to intervene.

The 81-year-old woman presents with clear indications for and no apparent contraindications to thrombolytic therapy. Within the time frame of her arrival less than 1 hour from symptom onset, tissue plasminogen activator and streptokinase should provide essentially equal survival and functional benefit. Age alone is not a contraindication to thrombolytic therapy. Streptokinase is less expensive (by a factor of 11) and may be associated with a lower risk of intracranial hemorrhage. In the GUSTO I trial of 41,021 patients, there was a significant excess of hemorrhagic stroke with accelerated tissue plasminogen activator ($P = 0.03$) and with the strategy of combination tissue plasminogen activator and streptokinase ($P < 0.001$) compared with streptokinase alone.

The 60-year-old man with type 1 diabetes mellitus and a defective anginal warning system arrives in cardiogenic shock owing to primary left ventricular pump failure in the setting of his acute anterolateral myocardial infarction superimposed on his previous inferior event. Conservative management, even if it were to include inotropic therapy and intra-aortic balloon counterpulsation, would still be associated with a near 80% hospital mortality rate. Several nonrandomized and retrospective studies done over the past two decades have suggested that successful mechanical revascularization with either percutaneous transluminal coronary angioplasty (of the culprit vessel only) or coronary artery bypass graft surgery is associated with hospital survival rates that may approach 50%. Important determinants of survival include age and the time to revascularization. Aggressive strategies of this type may not be appropriate for patients over 80 years of age. The few data that do exist from the thrombolytic literature would suggest that pharmacologic reperfusion strategies may be less effective. This may, in turn, reflect the extent of intracoronary thrombus burden or the difficulties in achieving reflow in states of significant coronary hypoperfusion.

The 52-year-old man presents with an anterior ST-segment elevation myocardial infarction, perhaps complicated by new right bundle branch block. There are no contraindications to thrombolytic therapy, including the small right knee effusion 6 months after arthroscopic surgery. Subgroup analysis from the GUSTO I trial suggests that accelerated-dose tissue plasminogen activator is most beneficial in men of this age group with anterior infarctions. In the overall GUSTO I trial, accelerated-dose tissue plasminogen activator was associated with a 14% mortality rate reduction when compared with the combined streptokinase groups. The mechanism of this improved benefit was related to a higher rate of infarct vessel patency with normal flow (TIMI grade 3).

Bibliography

1. **Bengtson JR, Kaplan AJ, Pieper KS, Wildermann NM, Mark DB, Pryor DB, et al.** Prognosis in cardiogenic shock after acute myocardial infarction in the interventional era. J Am Coll Cardiol. 1992;20:1482-9.

2. The GUSTO investigators. An international randomized trial comparing four thrombolytic strategies for acute myocardial infarction. N Engl J Med. 1993;329:673-82.

3. **Hochman JS, Boland J, Sleeper LA, Porway M, Brinker J, Coe J, et al.** Current spectrum of cardiogenic shock and effect of early revascularization on mortality. Results of an International Registry. SHOCK Registry Investigators. Circulation. 1995;91:873-81.

4. **Michels KB, Yusuf S.** Does PTCA in acute myocardial infarction affect mortality and reinfarction rates? A quantitative overview (meta-analysis) of the randomized clinical trials. Circulation. 1995;91:476-85.

5. **Simoons ML, Maggioni AP, Knatterud G, Leimberger JD, de Joegere P, van Domburg R, et al.** Individual risk assessment for intracranial hemorrhage during thrombolytic therapy. Lancet. 1993;342:1523-8.

NOSOCOMIAL INFECTION

Nosocomial Infection Question 1
Answer: D

EDUCATIONAL OBJECTIVE: Define current therapy and infection control measures for isolation patients.

Because there has been documented spread via fomites and medical equipment such as thermometers and blood pressure cuffs, the use of dedicated, non-essential medical equipment is encouraged for vancomycin-resistant enterococci (VRE) patient isolation. The patient has two separate organisms—methicillin-resistant *Staphylococcus aureus* (MRSA) and VRE—which require enforcement of isolation guidelines. The patient therefore may not be placed in the same room as another MRSA patient unless that patient also has VRE. All patient contact requires adherence to standard precautions even if there is no active infection due to the presence of MRSA in the sputum. Vancomycin should not be used when there is colonization of the sputum with MRSA in the absence of an infiltrate on chest radiography or physical examination findings consistent with pneumonia. Ciprofloxacin would not be indicated for MRSA treatment for the same reason; in addition, there has been development of ciprofloxacin resistance when it is used to attempt eradication of colonization. Ciprofloxacin would also be ineffective against vancomycin-resistant *Enterococcus faecium*. Laminar flow rooms have never been proven useful in the isolation of patients with nosocomial colonization or infection.

The patient's fever may be the result of autonomic dysregulation owing to the stroke or more likely to an undiagnosed infection. It would be prudent to search for other sites of infection before starting empiric antibiotic therapy, especially because of the presence of multidrug-resistant organisms. The work-up might include computed tomography (CT) of the chest (for aspiration pneumonia), CT of the sinuses, urinalysis and culture, and possibly lumbar puncture and blood culture for possible line infection.

Bibliography

1. **Livornese LL Jr, Dias S, Samel C, Romanowski B, Taylor S, May P, et al.** Hospital-acquired infection with vancomycin-resistant *Enterococcus faecium* transmitted by electronic thermometers. Ann Intern Med. 1992;117:112-6.

2. Centers for Disease Control and Prevention. Recommendations for preventing the spread of vancomycin resistance. Recommendations of the Hospital Infection Control Practices Advisory Committee. MMWR. 1995;44(RR-12):1-13.

3. **Tablan OC, Anderson LJ, Arden NH, Breiman RF, Butler JC, McNeil MM.** Guideline for prevention of nosocomial pneumonia. The Hospital Infection Control Practices Advisory Committee, Centers for Disease Control and Prevention. Am J Infect Control. 1994;22:247-92.

4. **Slaughter S, Hayden MK, Nathan C, Hu TC, Rice T, Van Voorhis J, et al.** A comparison of the effect of universal use of gloves and gowns with that of glove use alone on acquisition of vancomycin-resistant enterococci in a medical intensive care unit. Ann Intern Med. 1996;125:448-56.

5. **Mulligan ME, Ruane PJ, Johnston L, Wong P, Wheelock JP, MacDonald K, et al.** Ciprofloxacin for eradication of methicillin-resistant *Staphylococcus aureus* colonization. Am J Med. 1987;82:215-9.

Nosocomial Infection Question 2
Answer: D

EDUCATIONAL OBJECTIVE: Recognize disseminated fungal infection in a patient with prolonged granulocytopenia.

The development of nodular or hemorrhagic skin lesions along with pulmonary infiltrates in an immunocompromised host should always trigger strong consideration of disseminated fungal infection or nocardiosis. Patients with hematologic malignancies and prolonged granulocytopenia are at particular risk for disseminated infection with *Aspergillus (A. fumigatus* or *A. flavus)* or *Fusarium* species. Both may present with nodular or hemorrhagic skin lesions, pulmonary nodules, and/or sinusitis. As was the case in this patient, biopsy specimens of skin nodules frequently reveal branching, acutely angular, septate hyphae invading dermal blood vessels. Culture of the biopsy material is typically useful for identification of both *Aspergillus* and *Fusarium* species. As opposed to *Aspergillus, Fusarium* species can be grown readily from blood cultures using the lysis-centrifugation technique. Cultures of both blood and biopsy material from this patient grew *Fusarium solani.*

Disseminated aspergillosis and fusariosis require treatment with high-dose amphotericin B (1.0 to 1.5 mg/kg per day). Survival depends most upon the prompt resolution of granulocytopenia. Liposomal preparations of amphotericin B offer important potential advantages in therapy, but controlled treatment trials of disseminated aspergillosis and fusariosis in patients with granulocytopenia have yet to be published. Oral itraconazole, although potentially useful in the prevention of *Aspergillus* infection in granulocytopenic patients, cannot be relied upon for treatment of established, disseminated infection in these patients. Fluconazole, used for prophylaxis against *Candida albicans* infections in this patient, has limited activity against *Aspergillus* and *Fusarium* species. Disseminated infections with non-albicans candidal species, such as *C. glabrata* and *C. kruseii,* may also occur in granulocytopenic patients given fluconazole prophylaxis.

The addition of vancomycin to empiric antibiotic regimens targeting aerobic gram-negative rods in granulocytopenic patients with persistent fever can be important, especially because mucositis and central venous catheters predispose such patients to infections with *Staphylococcus* species and *Streptococcus mitis.* However, these infections do not typically present with subcutaneous and pulmonary nodules. Concern about an allergic reaction to ceftazidime might prompt the substitution of aztreonam or imipenem-cilastatin therapy in the presence of a skin rash more suggestive of an allergic reaction. In any case, a skin biopsy is often useful in distinguishing between disseminated infection and allergic response. Bronchoscopy and transbronchial biopsy are frequently instrumental in the diagnosis of pulmonary infiltrates in granulocytopenic patients. In this patient, skin biopsy was a far more benign procedure and was likely to be of higher yield because the two small (1 cm in diameter) peripheral pulmonary nodules in the right upper lobe were not particularly accessible to transbronchial biopsy.

Bibliography

1. **Pizzo PA.** Management of fever in patients with cancer and treatment-induced neutropenia. N Engl J Med. 1993;328:1323-32.

2. **Rabodonirina M, Piens MA, Monier MF, Gueho E, Fiere D, Mojon M.** Fusarium infections in immunocompromised patients: case reports and literature review. Eur J Clin Microbiol Infect Dis. 1994;13:152-61.

3. **Walsh TJ, Hiemenz JW, Anaissie E.** Recent progress and current problems in treatment of invasive fungal infections in neutropenic patients. Infect Dis Clin North Am. 1996;10:365-400.

Nosocomial Infection Question 3
Answer: B

EDUCATIONAL OBJECTIVE: Select the best antibiotic regimen for a granulocytopenic patient with fever, severe mucositis, and a possible Hickman catheter exit-site infection.

The combination of vancomycin and ceftazidime is the most appropriate listed choice for this patient. Based on data from the 1970s and 1980s indicating the frequency and severity of gram-negative infections, the empiric therapy recommended for patients with granulocytopenic fever has consisted of an antipseudomonal β-lactam antibiotic—such as ceftazidime, imipenem-cilastatin, piperacillin-tazobactam, or ticarcillin-clavulanic acid—combined with an aminoglycoside. Several recent studies suggest that ceftazidime or imipenem-cilastatin monotherapy is equivalent to combination therapy in neutropenic, febrile patients who have no readily identifiable focus of infection. With the onset of fluoroquinolone prophylaxis in the 1990s, most septicemias suffered by febrile granulocytopenic patients are gram-positive rather than gram-negative in origin. Nonetheless, the routine empiric use of vancomycin has been discouraged by many authors who fear the emergence of vancomycin resistance in enterococci and staphylococci and argue that vancomycin therapy for possible gram-positive infections can be safely delayed in many instances until organisms are detected in the blood.

Empiric antibiotic therapy must be individualized for each patient. The empiric use of vancomycin is justified in this patient because she has an exit-site infection of her Hickman catheter that may be associated with bacteremia, as suggested by her shaking chill. Most of these infections are caused by coagulase-negative staphylococci (up to 80% of which are resistant to methicillin and other β-lactam antibiotics) or *Staphylococcus aureus.* This patient, by virtue of the severe mucositis of the upper gastrointestinal tract, is also at risk for life-threatening infection with streptococci, such as *Streptococcus mitis,* that are relatively resistant to penicillin and respond poorly to β-lactam antibiotic treatment. In this particular patient, concern about promoting the development of vancomycin-resistant organisms is outweighed by the risks of failing to treat a likely gram-positive infection.

Bibliography

1. **Greene JN.** Catheter-related complications of cancer chemotherapy. Infect Dis Clin North Am. 1996;10:255-95.

2. **De Pauw BE, Deresinski SC, Feld R, Lane-Allman EF, Donnelly JP.** Ceftazidime compared with piperacillin and tobramycin for the empiric treatment of fever in neutropenic patients with cancer. A multicenter randomized trial. The Intercontinental Antimicrobial Study Group. Ann Intern Med. 1994;120:834-44.

3. **Winston DJ, Ho WG, Bruckner DA, Champlin RE.** Beta-lactam antibiotic therapy in febrile granulocytopenic patients. A randomized trial comparing cefoperazone plus piperacillin, ceftazidime plus piperacillin, and imipenem alone. Ann Intern Med. 1991;115: 849-59.

4. **Jansen J, Cromer M, Akard L, Black JR, Wheat LJ, Allen SD.** Infection prevention in severely myelosuppressed patients: a comparison between ciprofloxacin and a regimen of selective antibiotic modulation of the intestinal flora. Am J Med. 1994;96:335-41.

5. **Bochud PY, Eggiman P, Calandra T, Van Melle G, Saghafi L, Francioli P.** Bacteremia due to viridans streptococcus in neutropenic patients with cancer: clinical spectrum and risk factors. Clin Infect Dis. 1994;18:25-31.

6. **Shlaes DM, Gerding DN, John JF Jr, Craig WA, Bornstein DL, Duncan RA, et al.** Society for Healthcare Epidemiology of America and Infectious Diseases Society of America Joint Committee on the Prevention of Antimicrobial Resistance: Guidelines for the prevention of antimicrobial resistance in hospitals. Clin Infect Dis. 1997;25:584-99.

Nosocomial Infection Question 4
Answer: E

EDUCATIONAL OBJECTIVE: Recognize the appropriate use of vancomycin in light of the spread of vancomycin-resistant enterococci.

A spread of vancomycin-resistant enterococci (VRE) has become an important public health and hospital infection control problem. Unfortunately, enterococci resistant to vancomycin are usually resistant to other antibiotics. These organisms in hospitals can cause infections with high mortality. In addition, once these isolates appear in hospitals, they may continue to cause infections in other patients. Because of these problems, guidelines have been published to reduce the spread of these highly resistant organisms. Fundamental to the control of VRE is reduction in the use of vancomycin, except for certain indications.

In addition to restriction of the use of vancomycin, a crucial aspect of controlling the spread of VRE is recognition by the microbiology laboratory of an isolate with prompt reporting to hospital infection control authorities and prompt dissemination of the information. It is recognized that such patients need to be placed under strict barrier precautions, because they are reservoirs of rapid spread to other patients through contamination of the environment and person-to-person transmission. In addition, once the colonized or infected patient has appeared in the hospital, it is prudent to search for other colonized patients who may continue to contaminate the environment and cause further spread of infection.

Many common uses of vancomycin are not recommended. Patients with neutropenia should not receive vancomycin until cultures are available and unless they have clinical clues suggesting a gram-positive infection, such as an infected intravenous line. However, in some locations, resistant *Streptococcus mitis* causes infections in neutropenic patients, justifying empiric use of vancomycin. Because oral use of vancomycin is particularly important in encouraging the selection of resistant enterococci, initial vancomycin use in the treatment of antibiotic colitis is discouraged.

Vancomycin should not be used to treat isolates of staphylococci that are likely contaminates, such as only one positive blood culture of multiple cultures obtained. Phlebotomists should be trained to properly obtain blood cultures to minimize contamination.

Vancomycin is also not routinely recommended for surgical prophylaxis, unless there is evidence in the hospital of very frequent resistance to β-lactam antibiotics among staphylococci causing wound infections. As usual in surgical wound prophylaxis, only one dose is recommended in a 2-hour window before the surgical incision.

Bibliography

1. Recommendations for preventing the spread of vancomycin resistance. Recommendations of the Hospital Infection Control Practice Advisory Committee (HICPAC). MMWR. 1995;44(RR-12):1-13.

2. **Morris JG Jr, Shay DK, Hebden JN, McCarter RJ Jr, Perdue BE, Jarvis W, et al.** Enterococci resistant to multiple antimicrobial agents, including vancomycin. Establishment of endemicity in a university medical center. Ann Intern Med. 1995;123:250-9.

Nosocomial Infection Question 5
Answer: B

EDUCATIONAL OBJECTIVE: Manage tunneled central venous catheter infections.

Infection ultimately occurs in about 25% of patients with central venous access devices. In general, catheter-related infections can be categorized as exit-site infections, tunnel infections, catheter-related bacteremias or fungemias, septic thrombophlebitis, and infusate-related bacteremias or fungemias. Most catheter-associated bacteremias are caused by gram-positive organisms, especially coagulase-negative staphylococci, and can be treated successfully without removal of the catheter, unless blood cultures remain positive after 48 hours of treatment. Immediate catheter removal should be considered when bacteremia is caused by *Pseudomonas aeruginosa,* vancomycin-resistant enterococci, *Corynebacterium* JK, *Bacillus* species, or *Lactobacillus* species. Almost all authors recommend catheter removal for fungemia.

Candida albicans is the most common offender, although the incidence of infections caused by non-albicans candidal species has increased dramatically, in part as a result of fluconazole prophylaxis in neutropenic patients. Risk factors for catheter-associated candidemias include the number of antibiotics used previously, parenteral hyperalimentation, visible colonization of mucosal sites such as the perineum or oropharynx, recent abdominal surgery, corticosteroid therapy, and diabetes mellitus. In one large study, removal of all intravascular catheters was associated with a reduction of candidemia from 5 or 6 days to 2 or 3 days. In other studies, mortality has been closely related to the duration of candidemia. Authors of a study involving 155 patients with candidemia associated with central venous catheters concluded that prompt catheter removal was indicated because the mortality rate of patients treated with antifungal therapy alone was 82%.

Catheter exit-site infections due to bacteria (defined by inflammation confined to an area less than 2 cm from the exit site) can usually be cured with antibiotic treatment alone. For example, in one study, 55 of 65 exit-site infections were managed effectively with antibiotic treatment alone. However, exit-site infections caused by *Pseudomonas aeruginosa* frequently require catheter removal. Tunnel infections typically occur much earlier after catheter placement than other types of infection and almost always require catheter removal (20 of 29 patients in one study).

Neutropenia is not an indication for catheter removal during bacteremia, because 90% to 95% of patients can be managed successfully with antibiotic treatment alone. Catheters should not be removed routinely in patients with unexplained and persistent neutropenic fevers. *Staphylococcus epidermidis* is the most common cause of catheter-related infections. Up to 80% of these organisms are resistant to methicillin and thus do not respond to nafcillin or cefazolin. Vancomycin should be used in empiric treatment regimens rather than nafcillin or cefazolin.

Bibliography

1. **Greene JN.** Catheter-related complications of cancer therapy. Infect Dis Clin North Am. 1996;10:255-95.

2. **Rex JH, Bennett JE, Sugar AM, Pappas PG, Serody J, Edwards JE, et al.** Intravascular catheter exchange and duration of candidemia. NIAID Mycoses Study Group and the Candidemia Study Group. Clin Infect Dis. 1995;21:994-6.

3. **Lecciones J, Lee JW, Navarro EE, Witebsky FG, Marshall D, Steinberg SM, et al.** Vascular catheter-associated fungemia in patients with cancer: analysis of 155 episodes. Clin Infect Dis. 1992;14:875-83.

4. **Raad II, Bodey GP.** Infectious complications of indwelling vascular catheters. Clin Infect Dis. 1992;15:197-208.

Nosocomial Infection Question 6
Answer: D

EDUCATIONAL OBJECTIVE: Recognize the importance of catheters in patients with candidemia and know the appropriate management of a transient candidemia.

Candidemia is most common in the setting of the patient with a complicated illness; the source of the *Candida* isolate is unclear. However, any blood isolate of a yeast should be regarded as clinically significant. Even if candidemia resolves, there is a risk of progressive retinal infection; all patients with candidemia should undergo a retinal examination by an ophthalmologist. Because the intravenous catheter is often the primary site, the catheter should be removed and the tip cultured. Failure to replace the intravenous catheter is associated with increased risk of clinical failure. Moreover, a new catheter site should be selected if possible, because replacement at the same site over a J wire may not cure fungemia as readily as a bacterial infection. Catheter replacement thus shortens the period of fungemia.

Transient candidemia (a positive blood culture followed by multiple negative cultures) is not benign. Some patients may have no further problem after a catheter is removed, but some remain candidemic, and there is no way at present to predict who will need antifungal therapy. Therefore, in addition to catheter replacement, antifungal therapy is warranted. Although amphotericin B is the standard therapy, large well-controlled studies have found that fluconazole, intravenously and then orally, is as effective as amphotericin B for primary treatment of fungemia. Of interest, this holds true for both albicans and non-albicans candidal species. The latter, especially *C. krusei* and *C. glabrata,* tend to be resistant to fluconazole in vitro and are associated with clinical fluconazole failures. In one large study the initiation of fluconazole treatment, at least until the fungus was identified as non-albicans, was not associated with clinical failure. However, in this study relatively few isolates were fluconazole-resistant.

Bibliography

1. **Lecciones JA, Lee JW, Navarro EE, Witebsky FG, Marshall D, Steinberg SM, et al.** Vascular catheter-associated fungemia in patients with cancer: analysis of 155 episodes. Clin Infect Dis. 1992;14:875-83.

2. **Phillips P, Shafran S, Garber G, Rotstein C, Smaill F, Fong I, et al.** Multicenter randomized trial of fluconazole versus amphotericin B for treatment of candidemia in nonneutropenic patients. Canadian Candidemia Study Group. Eur J Clin Microbiol Infect Dis. 1997;16:337-45.

3. **Rex JH, Rinaldi MG, Pfaller MA.** Resistance of *Candida* species to fluconazole. Antimicrob Agents Chemother. 1995;39:1-8.

Nosocomial Infection Questions 7-11
Answers: 7(B); 8(E); 9(C); 10(D); 11(A)

EDUCATIONAL OBJECTIVE: Distinguish the different types of isolation precautions required in various clinical settings.

The United States Public Health Service has published a document titled "Guidelines for Isolation Precautions in Hospitals" (standard precautions) to assist physicians, hospitals, and hospital infection control programs to understand the changing terminology and different categories of isolation. The guidelines, which are always evolving, contain changes from the original 1970s guidelines that were subsequently adapted. Universal precautions were instituted in the mid-1980s largely as a response to the HIV epidemic and hepatitis B infections. Universal precautions focused on avoidance of bloodborne exposure, such as needle-stick exposure, and contact with other potentially infected secretions. This area of precaution, also called "Blood and Body Fluid Precautions," became one element in addition to the other types of isolation such as disease-specific and category-specific systems (body substance isolation). The current guidelines merge elements of the other types of precautions into one document and collapse seven categories of isolation (contact isolation, strict isolation, respiratory isolation, tuberculosis isolation, enteric precautions, drainage/secretion precautions) and disease-specific isolations into three sets of precautions based on routes of transmission. All guidelines are suggestions that can be modified according to what is possible, practical, and prudent.

Standard precautions apply to all patients receiving hospital care, regardless of their diagnosis. These include hospital personnel use of gowns and gloves, handwashing, and guidelines pertaining to patient placement (cohorting), patient transportation, patient-care articles, personal protective equipment, and routine and terminal room cleaning. In addition to the standard precautions, three subcategories exist: airborne precautions, droplet precautions, and contact precautions.

All patients would require standard precautions to be observed in addition to the particular set of isolation precautions dictated by their diagnosis. A patient with disseminated varicella-zoster, which can be spread by both contact and airborne methods, requires both these types of isolation in addition to the standard precautions. A patient with measles requires airborne isolation but not contact isolation. A patient with meningococcemia and disseminated intravascular coagulation should be placed on droplet precautions. A patient with *Clostridium difficile*–associated diarrhea should be placed on contact isolation. An HIV-infected patient without other reason for isolation requires only standard precautions. The prevention of the spread of bloodborne pathogens should be practiced in all patient contacts, as is also appropriate for this patient.

Bibliography

1. **Slaughter S, Hayden MK, Nathan C, Hu TC, Rice J, Van Voorhis J, et al.** A comparison of the effect of universal use of gloves and gowns with that of glove use alone on acquisition of vancomycin-resistant enterococci in a medical intensive care unit. Ann Intern Med. 1996;125:448-56.

2. **Garner JS.** Guideline for Isolation Precautions in Hospitals. The Hospital Infection Control Practices Advisory Committee. Infect Control Hosp Epidemiol. 1996;17:53-80.

3. **Larson EL.** APIC guideline for handwashing and hand antisepsis in health care settings. Am J Infect Control. 1995;23:251-69.

Nosocomial Infection Question 12
Answer: A

EDUCATIONAL OBJECTIVE: Manage a febrile intubated patient, recognizing essential diagnostic testing.

The patient described has fever and a new lung infiltrate, a clinical picture suggesting the possibility of ventilator-associated pneumonia. The clinical features are not specific, and critically ill patients can have multiple causes of fever and a variety of reasons for lung infiltrates. Fever can be the result of infection at other sites (urine, central venous line), the result of a drug reaction, the consequence of atelectasis or pulmonary embolus, or the result of antibiotic complications such as *Clostridium difficile* colitis. In addition, patients in the intensive care unit may develop radiographic evidence of maxillary sinusitis, which is often infectious and may coexist with nosocomial pneumonia. The incidence of nosocomial sinusitis is increased if gastric or tracheal tubes are inserted through the nose and can be markedly reduced by oral insertion of tubes.

The patient described is likely to have early-onset (before day 5 of mechanical ventilation) ventilator-associated pneumonia, an entity that is likely caused by *Staphylococcus aureus*, pneumococcus, *Haemophilus influenzae*, and non-pseudomonal enteric gram-negative organisms. The diagnosis is made clinically, and the patient should be started on empiric antibiotic therapy directed at the aforementioned organisms. Because initial therapy is likely to be broad spectrum, it can be focused once culture results of endotracheal aspiration become available. Although endotracheal aspiration cultures are not diagnostic of pneumonia (and thus not specific), they are likely to contain any of the pathogenic organisms and thus are as sensitive for finding these organisms as a procedure such as bronchoscopy; hence, these cultures should be obtained. It is unnecessary to do a bronchoscopy or nonbronchoscopic bronchoalveolar lavage in order to obtain quantitative cultures in this setting, and delaying antibiotic therapy in order to do so may be harmful. Although the patient has a risk factor for sinusitis because of the presence of a nasogastric tube, aspiration of the sinuses should not even be considered until a radiograph, preferably a computed tomographic (CT) scan, shows findings of sinusitis.

Bibliography

1. **Bonten MJ, Gaillard CA, Wouters EF, van Tiel FH, Stobberingh EE, van der Geest S.** Problems in diagnosing nosocomial pneumonia in mechanically ventilated patients. A review. Crit Care Med. 1994;22:1683-91.

2. **Rouby JJ, Laurent P, Gosnach M, Cambau E, Lamas G, Zouaoui A, et al.** Risk factors and clinical relevance of nosocomial maxillary sinusitis in the critically ill. Am J Respir Crit Care Med. 1994;150:776-83.

3. **Rumba MJ, Bass RL.** Tracheal aspirate correlates with protected specimen brush in long-term ventilated patients who have clinical pneumonia. Chest. 1994;106:531-4.

4. **Antonelli M, Moro ML, Capelli O, De Blasi RA, D'Errico RR, Conti G, et al.** Risk factors for early onset pneumonia in trauma patients. Chest. 1994;105:224-8.

Nosocomial Infection Question 13
Answer: C

EDUCATIONAL OBJECTIVE: Select the preferred treatment approach for a patient with neutropenia and fever.

In the 1960s and 1970s fever in a patient neutropenic from cytotoxic therapy was reportedly due to defined infection (bacterial, fungal, or viral) 60% to 70% of the time. With improved prophylactic approaches, fever can be ascribed to infection in a lower percentage of patients (30% to 40% in published series). Nevertheless, prompt initiation of broad-spectrum antibiotics and early use of antifungal therapy in persistently febrile neutropenic patients are recommended. The latter has been shown to reduce morbidity and mortality from opportunistic mycoses, such as aspergillosis. Controversy has surrounded the issue of how long to continue antimicrobial therapy in persistently neutropenic patients. Because of relapses of severe infections in some patients when antimicrobial therapy was discontinued in the face of persistent neutropenia, consensus now favors continuation of treatment until the neutropenia has resolved.

Because this patient is no longer febrile and her general condition appears stable, addition of amphotericin B or other antifungal therapy would not be warranted at this time. Empiric vancomycin treatment is recommended to cover *Staphylococcus epidermidis* or *S. aureus* (rarely diphtheroids), causing intravenous catheter-related infections in nosocomial settings. Staphylococci are easily recovered from blood cultures if present and would be less likely to respond to treatment with ceftazidime and tobramycin than gram-negative rods. In this improving patient, addition of vancomycin would not be appropriate at this time. Neutropenic patients do not generally have immunoglobulin deficiency, and no benefit can be expected from intravenous immune globulin given therapeutically. Use of granulocyte colony-stimulating factor may hasten the resolution of neutropenia and could be a good adjunct to antibiotic therapy in this patient.

Bibliography

1. **Pizzo PA.** Drug therapy: management of fever in patients with cancer and treatment-induced neutropenia. N Engl J Med. 1993;328:1323-32.

2. **EORTC International Antimicrobial Therapy Group.** Empiric antifungal therapy in febrile granulocytopenic patients. Am J Med. 1989;86:668-72.

3. **Hughes WT, Armstrong D, Bodey GP, Feld R, Mandell G, Meyers JD, et al.** Guidelines for the use of antimicrobial agents in neutropenic patients with unexplained fever: a statement by the Infectious Diseases Society of America. J Infect Dis. 1990;161:381-96.

4. **Pizzo PA.** Fever in immunocompromised patients. N Engl J Med. 1999;341:893-900.

PNEUMONIA

Pneumonia Question 1
Answer: D

EDUCATIONAL OBJECTIVE: Manage a patient with possible multidrug-resistant tuberculosis.

A presumptive diagnosis of tuberculosis can be made in this patient and will be confirmed by culture of sputum. Because he is potentially infectious and because of his symptoms, therapy should be started immediately. Given his history of inadequate and erratic prior therapy and nonadherence, drug resistance should be suspected, and at least two new drugs that the patient has not previously received should be provided. Because the exact previous treatment is unknown, none of the two- or three-drug regimens listed would be satisfactory empiric therapy. In addition, because pyrazinamide primarily affects a limited population of intracellular tubercle bacilli, it should not be relied on to prevent the emergence of resistant organisms. The patient's likely nonadherence must be taken into account. Directly observed therapy given either from the start of therapy or after a brief period (for example, 2 to 4 weeks) of daily treatment is indicated. If intermittent therapy (twice weekly) is prescribed from the start, the addition of streptomycin will probably enhance the effectiveness of the regimen. The regimen of isoniazid, rifampin, ethambutol, pyrazinamide, and streptomycin (choice D) is likely to contain at least two active drugs and provide maximal efficacy. This regimen can be modified when drug susceptibility test results are available.

Bibliography

1. **Iseman MD.** Treatment of multidrug-resistant tuberculosis. N Engl J Med. 1993;329:784-91.
2. **Davidson PT.** Treating tuberculosis: what drugs, for how long? Ann Intern Med. 1990;112:393-5.
3. Centers for Disease Control. Initial therapy for tuberculosis in the era of multidrug resistance. Recommendations of the Advisory Council for the Elimination of Tuberculosis. MMWR. 1993;42(RR-7):1-8.
4. **Van Scoy RE, Wilkowske CJ.** Antituberculosis agents. Mayo Clin Proc. 1992;67:179-87.

Pneumonia Question 2
Answer: E

EDUCATIONAL OBJECTIVE: Prescribe the most appropriate therapy for a pregnant patient with community-acquired pneumonia.

Many antibiotics can be toxic, even in late pregnancy. However, there are sufficient data to indicate a cephalosporin would be safe for treating pregnant patients with community-acquired pneumonia. Physicians should consult the literature on any drug being given to the pregnant patient for its particular recommendation in pregnancy.

Choosing to use no antibiotic therapy would deny a patient useful therapy, particularly in the last trimester, when a relative state of immunosuppression exists. Ofloxacin or tetracycline would not be warranted. There are no data to support the use of ofloxacin in pregnant patients, and tetracycline could cause tooth enamel discoloration in the infant. Chloramphenicol could lead to an encephalopathic syndrome (gray syndrome) in the newborn when given late in the pregnancy.

Bibliography

1. Safety of antimicrobial agents in pregnancy. Med Let. 1987;29:61-3.
2. **Briggs GG, Freeman RK, Yaffe SJ, eds.** Drugs in Pregnancy and Lactation: A Guide to Fetal & Neonatal Risk. 4th ed. Baltimore, MD: Williams and Wilkins; 1994.

Pneumonia Question 3
Answer: C

EDUCATIONAL OBJECTIVE: Recognize and treat *Pneumocystis carinii* pneumonia in an immunocompromised patient without AIDS.

This patient, with the combination of severe dysfunction in cell-mediated and humoral immunity, has a diffuse pneumonia unresponsive to antibiotic therapy directed toward *Streptococcus pneumoniae*, *Haemophilus influenzae*, *Mycoplasma pneumoniae*, and *Legionella* species. The remaining differential diagnosis encompasses a wide array of viral, bacterial, fungal, and parasitic pathogens, including cytomegalovirus, herpes simplex virus, varicella-zoster virus, *Mycobacterium tuberculosis, Cryptococcus neoformans, Histoplasma capsulatum, Coccidioides immitis, Pneumocystis carinii,* and *Toxoplasma gondii.* Other considerations in patients with hematologic malignancies and pulmonary infiltrates include congestive heart failure, pulmonary hemorrhage, adult respiratory distress syndrome from a primary infectious process originating outside the lungs, and lung injury induced by previous radiation therapy or chemotherapeutic agents such as bleomycin, busulfan, or carmustine. Pursuit of a specific diagnosis is of paramount importance not only to ensure that the correct treatment is rendered, but also to limit toxicities caused by the multiple medications usually required to cover the most likely diagnostic possibilities.

The best diagnostic approach in such patients is influenced by the clinical presentation of pneumonia (whether, for example, it is lobar or diffuse), the rapidity of its progression, the response to empiric therapy, and specific expertise available (for example, bronchoscopy versus closed fine-needle aspiration). In this patient, bronchoscopy with transbronchial biopsy is the procedure that will most likely yield a specific diagnosis (or at least exclude some of the diagnostic possibilities with sufficient certainty to narrow empiric therapy). High-resolution computed tomographic chest scanning can be useful in distinguishing between congestive heart failure and diffuse pneumonitis and can aid the bronchoscopist in selecting a biopsy site for focal infiltrates. In this patient, congestive heart failure can be excluded on clinical grounds alone. Tuberculosis is but one diagnostic possibility of many; therefore, empiric therapy for this alone would be unwise. Bone marrow biopsy can be helpful in the diagnosis of disseminated mycobacterial and fungal infections, but would be less likely than bronchoscopy to be diagnostic in this patient with an active pneumonia.

The Giemsa stain from the bronchoalveolar lavage fluid shows numerous trophozoites of *Pneumocystis carinii,* and the Gomori's methenamine silver stain from the transbronchial biopsy shows cyst forms of the same organism. *Pneumocystis* pneumonia virtually always occurs in patients with compromised cell-mediated immunity. Examples include patients with AIDS, patients who have had radiation and/or cytotoxic chemotherapy for hematologic malignancies or autoimmune diseases, and patients with lymphocytic leukemia. Before the onset of AIDS, the conditions most closely associated with *Pneumocystis* pneumonia in

young adults were Hodgkin's disease and organ or bone marrow transplantation; in older adults, it was chronic lymphocytic leukemia. The number of episodes of rejection treatment (more than two) and posttransplant cytomegalovirus disease increase the risk for *Pneumocystis* pneumonia in patients with renal transplants, and probably in patients with other organ transplants as well. In immunocompromised patients who do not have AIDS, the clinical presentation of *Pneumocystis* pneumonia can be more accelerated, with severe dyspnea occurring within a few days of the onset of the first symptoms. The organism burden in these patients may not be as high as that in patients with AIDS, and this may lead to false-negative bronchoalveolar fluid examinations in some patients. Trimethoprim-sulfamethoxazole is the drug of choice for treatment, especially because it is generally well tolerated by non-AIDS patients.

Bibliography

1. **Dohn MN, Frame PT.** Clinical manifestations in adults. In: Walzer PD, ed. *Pneumocystis carinii* Pneumonia. 2nd ed. New York: Marcel Dekker, Inc; 1993:331-59.

2. **Arend SM, Westendorp RG, Kroon FP, van't Wout JW, Vandenbroucke JP, van Es LA, van der Woude FJ.** Rejection treatment and cytomegalovirus infection as risk factors for *Pneumocystis carinii* pneumonia in renal transplant patients. Clin Infect Dis. 1996;22:920-5.

3. **Schimpff SC.** Infections in the cancer patient—diagnosis, prevention, and treatment. In: Mandell GL, Bennet JE, Dolin R, eds. Principles and Practice of Infectious Diseases. 4th ed. New York: Churchill Livingstone;1994:2666-75.

4. **Bergen GA, Shelhamer JH.** Pulmonary infiltrates in the cancer patient. New approaches to an old problem. Infect Dis Clin North Am. 1996;10:297-325.

Pneumonia Question 4
Answer: E

EDUCATIONAL OBJECTIVE: Recognize that *Streptococcus pneumoniae* is the most common cause of overwhelming infection in a patient who has undergone splenectomy.

The spleen contributes to the immune response in a variety of complex ways. For example, it serves as a phagocytic filter that can remove poorly opsonized microbes, circulating antigenic complexes, and parasitized erythrocytes. IgM production and memory B-cell differentiation occur in the spleen. Patients who have undergone splenectomy, whether for treatment of hematologic malignancy or trauma, are at increased risk for overwhelming infections from encapsulated bacteria. The earlier in age the splenectomy is done and the more serious the underlying condition necessitating the splenectomy, the greater the risk. The risk is greatest within the first 2 years following splenectomy, but overwhelming infection, sepsis, and rapid death can occur decades later. *Streptococcus pneumoniae* accounts for about 70% of serious bacterial infections in these patients, and in fact, the pneumococcus was the cause of pneumonia, septicemia, and meningitis that proved fatal for this patient.

Most of the other serious infections related to splenectomy are caused by *Haemophilus influenzae, Neisseria meningitidis, Capnocytophaga canimorsus* (DF-2), and encapsulated gram-negative rods such as *Klebsiella* species. Rapidly administered empiric antibiotic coverage for these organisms is imperative, but even early diagnosis does not ensure survival. Prevention with vaccination with polyvalent pneumococcal and *H. influenzae* type B conjugate twice over a period of 2 to 3 years is recommended by some authors. Some authors recommend the meningococcal vaccine as well, although the vaccine does not prevent disease from type B meningococci, the most prevalent cause of disease in the United States and Western Europe. Daily oral penicillin prophylaxis has been effective in preventing pneumococcal infections in children and adults following splenectomy.

Although, as a farmer, this patient might be exposed to tick-borne illnesses such as Rocky Mountain spotted fever *(Rickettsia rickettsii)* or human ehrlichiosis, the time of year, the lack of prodromal symptoms, and the rapidity of onset of signs and symptoms of sepsis and meningitis make these illnesses less likely. Both *Pseudomonas aeruginosa* and *Staphylococcus aureus* can produce fulminant illness with purpuric skin lesions; however, nothing in the case history suggests a particular predilection for overwhelming infection with these organisms. An epidemic of the Hantavirus pulmonary syndrome occurred in the southwestern United States in 1993, and several cases have been described elsewhere in the United States. A febrile prodrome lasting 2 to 5 days is followed by a clinical picture and shock resembling adult respiratory distress syndrome. Disease from other Hantaviruses more typically produces thrombocytopenia and renal failure.

Bibliography

1. **Brozovic M.** Infection in non-malignant hematological disease and splenic dysfunction. Curr Opin Infect Dis. 1994;7:450-5.
2. **Breiman RF, Butler JC, Tenover FC, Elliott JA, Facklam RR.** Emergence of drug-resistant pneumococcal infections in the United States. JAMA. 1994;271:1831-5.

Pneumonia Question 5
Answer: D

EDUCATIONAL OBJECTIVE: Diagnose and treat a patient with community-acquired pneumonia.

The patient has a classic presentation and sputum Gram's stain for pneumococcal pneumonia. Patients with respiration rates greater than or equal to 30/min have an increased mortality rate and should be hospitalized. Ceftriaxone and cefotaxime are active against most *Streptococcus pneumoniae* isolates. The prevalence of penicillin- and multidrug-resistant pneumococci is increasing.

Ciprofloxacin has Food and Drug Administration (FDA)–approved indications for pneumococcal pneumonia but is not the first choice for the patient with pneumococcal pneumonia, because the minimal inhibitory concentrations for many pneumococcal pneumonia infections are close to the maximum serum concentrations of ciprofloxacin.

Vancomycin is active against pneumococci, including multidrug-resistant isolates. Recommendations from the Centers for Disease Control suggest restricting vancomycin use for patients in whom alternate therapy is not available to prevent further development of vancomycin-resistant organisms.

The effectiveness of trimethoprim-sulfamethoxazole against pneumococci is decreasing. This patient takes trimethoprim-sulfamethoxazole for prophylaxis and may be more likely to have colonization with a resistant *Streptococcus pneumoniae.*

Ceftazidime and ceftizoxime have poor in-vitro activity against many isolates (up to 25%) of *S. pneumoniae.*

Bibliography

1. **Emori TG, Gaynes RP.** An overview of nosocomial infections, including the role of the microbiology laboratory. Clin Microbiol Rev. 1993;6:428-42.

Pneumonia Question 6
Answer: B

EDUCATIONAL OBJECTIVE: Recognize an exacerbation of pulmonary infection in an adult patient with cystic fibrosis and select the most appropriate therapy.

The early recognition and treatment of exacerbations of pulmonary infection with effective antibiotics have played a major role in improved longevity in patients with cystic fibrosis. As in this patient, exacerbations of pulmonary infection may present subacutely with mild progressive dyspnea, decreased exercise tolerance, and anorexia and weight loss associated with worsening airflow obstruction on serial pulmonary function tests; changes in sputum production and appearance, fever, leukocytosis, or chest radiographic changes may not always be present.

Placebo-controlled studies have shown that prolonged, 14- to 21-day courses of intravenous antibiotics, guided by culture and susceptibility testing, are additive to but also substantially more effective than combined chest physiotherapy and bronchodilator treatment for restoring symptoms and pulmonary function to baseline levels. Most adult patients with cystic fibrosis have chronic infection with *Pseudomonas aeruginosa* and are treated with dual antibiotic therapy with an aminoglycoside and β-lactam antibiotic. Because of increased clearance and volume of distribution, larger-than-usual doses of both antibiotics are often required. Oral fluoroquinolone is an alternative regimen for milder exacerbations.

Meta-analyses suggest that long-term maintenance therapy with inhaled aminoglycosides may slightly improve pulmonary function and reduce the frequency of hospitalization, but inhaled antibiotics do not appear to be useful for treatment of acute infectious exacerbations. Inhaled recombinant deoxyribonuclease daily maintenance therapy may improve pulmonary function and reduce the frequency of acute infectious exacerbations but is not specifically useful during an acute exacerbation. Chest physiotherapy is useful both for acute infectious exacerbations and as chronic maintenance therapy, but as in this patient, compliance is often poor.

Bibliography

1. **Regelmann WE, Elliott GR, Warwick WJ, Clawson CC.** Reduction of sputum *Pseudomonas aeruginosa* density by antibiotics improves lung function in cystic fibrosis more than do bronchodilators and chest physiotherapy alone. Am Rev Respir Dis. 1990;141:914-21.

2. **Ramsey BW.** Management of pulmonary disease in patients with cystic fibrosis. N Engl J Med. 1996;335:179-88.

3. **Touw DJ, Brimicombe RW, Hodson ME, Heijerman HGM, Bakker W.** Inhalation of antibiotics in cystic fibrosis. Eur Respir J. 1995;8:1594-604.

4. **Davis PB, Drumm M, Konstan MW.** Cystic fibrosis. Am J Respir Crit Care Med. 1996;154:1229-56.

Pneumonia Question 7
Answer: A

EDUCATIONAL OBJECTIVE: Manage a patient with bronchiectasis and a positive acid-fast bacilli smear, and initiate appropriate management for both possible atypical mycobacterial infection and *Mycobacterium tuberculosis*.

The patient described has bronchiectasis as a consequence of childhood respiratory infection, with chronic cough and sputum production, in the absence of a history of cigarette smoking. Patients with bronchiectasis are prone to frequent episodes of acute airway infection, and these require antibiotic therapy. Now the patient has symptoms suggesting a new parenchymal lung infection, with blood streaking of the sputum and a cavitary infiltrate. The finding of acid-fast bacilli in the sputum is of concern, but patients with bronchiectasis can develop infection with either *Mycobacterium tuberculosis* or atypical mycobacteria.

With the finding of a positive acid-fast bacilli smear, it is necessary to assume the patient has *M. tuberculosis* and to remember that atypical mycobacterial infection is also a strong consideration. The clinician must manage the patient for both possibilities. Appropriate management would be to collect more sputum for culture, because the diagnosis of atypical mycobacterial infection is established by repeated isolation of the organism in association with a compatible cavitary chest radiographic pattern, and it is helpful for *M. tuberculosis* infection to have multiple samples sent for culture and sensitivity testing. Therapy should not be delayed until culture data are available, because this would put the patient at risk if *M. tuberculosis* were present. Thus, after sputum samples are collected, the patient should be started on multiple tuberculous medications directed at *M. tuberculosis* until final culture and sensitivity data become available. Appropriate therapy would be isoniazid, rifampin, and pyrazinamide for 2 months, followed by isoniazid and rifampin for 4 months, if the organism is drug-sensitive. The options to use a combination of isoniazid and ethambutol, or isoniazid and pyrazinamide, are not adequate for the possibility of *M. tuberculosis*.

If the final cultures show an atypical mycobacterial pathogen, therapy can be adjusted when more details about the organism's identity are known. Given the fact that the sputum smear is already positive for acid-fast organisms, the diagnosis of atypical mycobacterial infection can be established in this patient if repeated cultures are positive, because the patient has a compatible clinical course; therefore, there is no need to show tissue invasion with a transbronchial biopsy.

Although the final diagnosis can be established only by sputum culture results, there are several clinical clues that this patient has atypical mycobacterial infection. In comparing patients with atypical mycobacterial infection with those with tuberculosis, it is noteworthy that pre-existing lung disease and older age are more common in patients without tuberculosis.

Bibliography

1. **Al Jarad N, Demertzis P, Jones DJ, Barnes NC, Rudd RM, Gaya H, et al.** Comparison of characteristics of patients and treatment outcome for pulmonary non-tuberculous mycobacterial infection and pulmonary tuberculosis. Thorax. 1996;51:137-9.

Pneumonia Question 8
Answer: E

EDUCATIONAL OBJECTIVE: Distinguish the various testing approaches to the diagnosis of acute *Legionella* infection.

The patient described has severe community-acquired pneumonia with diastolic hypotension, a respiratory rate greater than 30/min, multilobar pneumonia, and severe hypoxemia. With these findings and with the epidemiologic data provided, *Legionella* pneumonia is an important concern, along with pneumococcus and gram-negative bacilli; broad-spectrum empiric therapy directed at this organism and other likely pathogens should be started immediately, without waiting for any further diagnostic confirmation of *Legionella* infection. A number of diagnostic tests are available for *Legionella*; however, in the absence of suspicion of serogroup I infection, there is no single test that is likely to be positive at the time of presentation with *Legionella* pneumonia.

If serogroup I infection were likely, urinary antigen testing has a yield of slightly greater than 50%. Acute titers for *Legionella* antibodies are rarely positive; the serologic diagnosis has a high yield only if both acute and convalescent immunofluorescent antibody titers to *Legionella* are examined for a fourfold increase. In one study of 68 patients with documented *Legionella* infection, most diagnoses were made in this manner; the collection of a single acute titer led to a diagnosis in less than 10% of cases, and false-positive results were almost as common as true-positive results when only acute titers were examined. Sputum staining with direct fluorescent antibody for *Legionella* has a highly variable yield, usually positive in less than 50% of cases.

Although sputum culture can also document *Legionella* infection, the yield is low, with only about 2% of nearly 1000 samples being positive in one laboratory's experience. In that study, sputum samples that were positive on culture generally did not have fewer than 10 squamous cells and more than 25 neutrophils per low-power field on a Gram's stain of sputum, the criteria used by most laboratories to screen sputum samples before culture. Urinary antigen testing is useful and is more likely to be positive at the time of acute infection than an acute immunofluorescent titer. However, the current urinary antigen test is specific for serogroup I infection and thus would probably not be valuable in this patient (the index case was known to be a non–serogroup I organism).

The data about *Legionella* diagnosis make it clear that serologic testing for organisms can have a high yield, but only if both acute and convalescent titers are collected, a process that requires a time period of 4 to 6 weeks. These test results are therefore of epidemiologic value but of no great help in the management of patients with acute infection. This has led to the suggestion that serologic testing not be used routinely in patients with community-acquired pneumonia because convalescent titers are rarely drawn, and if they are drawn, they give results too late to be of immediate clinical value.

Bibliography

1. **Ingram JG, Plouffe JF.** Danger of sputum purulence screens in culture of *Legionella* species. J Clin Microbiol. 1994;32:209-10.

2. **Plouffe JF, File TM Jr, Breiman RF, Hackman BA, Salstrom SJ, Marston BJ, et al.** Reevaluation of the definition of Legionnaires' disease: use of the urinary antigen assay. Community Based Pneumonia Incidence Study Group. Clin Infect Dis. 1995;20:1286-91.

3. **Bates JH, Campbell GD, Barron AL, McCracken GA, Morgan PN, Moses EB, et al.** Microbial etiology of acute pneumonia in hospitalized patients. Chest. 1992;101:1005-12.

Pneumonia Question 9
Answer: A

EDUCATIONAL OBJECTIVE: Manage an outpatient with mild community-acquired pneumonia and select appropriate therapy.

It is impossible to use a patient's clinical presentation, distinguishing between typical and atypical syndromes, to define the likely etiology and select the correct initial therapy. An algorithm for initial therapy—based on an assessment of severity of illness, place of therapy (requirement for hospitalization or intensive care unit), and the presence of comorbid illness and age greater than 60 years—has been proposed as a basis for selecting empiric therapy in patients with community-acquired pneumonia. The patient described has mild to moderate community-acquired pneumonia (not requiring hospitalization), is less than 60 years of age, and has no identified comorbid illness, suggesting that the most likely etiologic pathogens are pneumococci, *Mycoplasma pneumoniae*, viruses, and *Chlamydia pneumoniae*. Because the patient is a cigarette smoker, *Haemophilus influenzae* is a concern as well, even in the absence of proven chronic obstructive pulmonary disease. Therapy should be empiric, with all these organisms being considered and treated.

In order to determine the severity of pneumonia, it is important to assess respiratory rate to determine whether it is above 30/min, to determine whether the infiltrate is focal or multilobar, to define whether severe hypoxemia (Pao_2/Fio_2 ratio < 250) is present, and to determine whether severe sepsis (sepsis syndrome) or septic shock is present. This patient has no adverse prognostic findings, and therefore, his pneumonia can be characterized as mild and he can be treated out of the hospital.

Of the therapeutic options listed, azithromycin has activity against pneumococci, *H. influenzae,* and atypical pathogens such as *M. pneumoniae* and *C. pneumoniae.* Other macrolides, such as erythromycin, could be used, but erythromycin leads to more intestinal intolerance and is not active against *H. influenzae.* The cephalosporins listed as options, ceftriaxone and cefuroxime, are effective against pneumococcus and *H. influenzae* but have no activity against *M. pneumoniae* and *C. pneumoniae,* pathogens that should also be covered empirically in this 45-year-old patient. Although tetracycline is a reasonable choice for the treatment of pneumonia, it is not as active against pneumococcus as azithromycin and represents a second-choice therapeutic option. Although penicillin G is a form of highly focused therapy, it is not active against any of the likely pathogens except pneumococcus.

Bibliography

1. **Niederman MS, Bass JB Jr, Campbell GD, Fein AM, Grossman RF, Mandell LA, et al.** Guidelines for the initial management of adults with community-acquired pneumonia: diagnosis, assessment of severity, and initial antimicrobial therapy. American Thoracic Society. Am Rev Respir Dis. 1993;148:1418-26.

2. **Mandell LA.** Antibiotics for pneumonia therapy. Med Clin North Am. 1994;78:997-1014.

Pneumonia Question 10
Answer: C

EDUCATIONAL OBJECTIVE: Manage a patient with complicated *Streptococcus pneumoniae* infection.

Computed tomography of the patient's chest showed many loculated collections that were not seen on chest radiograph. After drainage of purulent pleural fluid, the patient had a complicated but gradually improving course. The second set of blood cultures still positive for penicillin-sensitive *Streptococcus pneumoniae* indicates uncontrolled bacterial infection, and penicillin rather than vancomycin or imipenem still remains the antibiotic of choice. The problem relating to lack of control of *S. pneumoniae* infections is need for drainage. And indium-labeled leukocyte scan would show increased uptake in the chest without localizing drainable pus.

Bibliography

1. **Bryant RE, Salmon CJ.** Pleural empyema. Clin Infect Dis. 1996;22:747-62.

Smoking

Smoking Question 1
Answer: A

EDUCATIONAL OBJECTIVE: Compare the value of reducing known coronary risk factors.

This patient has five risk factors and four are modifiable. Although each of the risk factors should be addressed, smoking cessation offers the greatest yield. After 1 or 2 years the risk of a coronary event attributable to smoking is reduced by 50% and at 5 years by nearly 100%. Exercise and a low-fat diet are excellent advice, but the benefits are difficult to measure. Depression, hostility and anger, and stress (particularly work-related) are associated with increased coronary event rates and should always be addressed. When personality traits are modified by an intense program, coronary disease progression may be reduced. In this patient the S_4 gallop, consistent with hypertensive heart disease, and retinal findings support the need to treat his high blood pressure, but the major impact of treating hypertension is reduction in strokes and congestive heart failure, not acute coronary ischemic events. Although his lipids should clearly be treated with diet and exercise, the attributable risk of his lipid profile is considerably less than that of smoking.

Bibliography

1. **Tsevat J, Weinstein MC, Williams LW, Tostesen AN, Goldman L.** Expected gains in life expectancy from various coronary heart disease risk factor modifications. Circulation. 1991;83:1194-201.

2. **Manson JE, Tosteson H, Ridker PM, Satterfield S, Herbert P, O'Connor GT, et al.** The primary prevention of myocardial infarction. N Engl J Med. 1992;326:1406-13.

3. **Collins R, Peto R, Macmahon S, Herbert P, Fiebach NH, Eberlein K, et al.** Blood pressure, stroke, and coronary heart disease. Part 2, Short term reductions in blood pressure: overview of randomized drug trials in their epidemiological context. Lancet. 1990;335:827-91.

4. **Theorell T.** The psychosocial environment, stress, and coronary heart disease. In: Marmot M, Elliot P, eds. Coronary Heart Disease Epidemiology: From Etiology to Public Health. New York: Oxford University Press; 1992:256-73.

Smoking Question 2
Answer: A

EDUCATIONAL OBJECTIVE: Diagnose and recommend treatment for thromboangiitis obliterans.

The clinical findings of critical limb ischemia, arterial occlusive disease involving distal blood vessels, and venulitis in a young man are most consistent with the diagnosis of thromboangiitis obliterans. Cigarette smoking has been linked closely to thromboangiitis obliterans, and smoking cessation may reduce progression.

Pentoxifylline is purported to improve limb blood flow by increasing red cell deformability and decreasing blood viscosity. However, its efficacy in treating critical limb ischemia secondary to thromboangiitis obliterans is not established. Neither calcium channel blockers, such as nifedipine, nor α-adrenergic receptor blockers have been shown to improve blood flow in patients with critical limb ischemia. Nifedipine and α-adrenergic blockers reduce symptoms of Raynaud's phenomenon, but this is not the patient's problem. Simvastatin, an hydroxymethylglutaryl coenzyme A (HMG-CoA) reductase inhibitor, reduces cardiovascular events in patients with atherosclerosis, but this agent has not been shown to have a role in patients with thromboangiitis obliterans. The affected blood vessels in this patient, as is typical for many patients with thromboangiitis obliterans, are distal and located in the foot and digits. More proximal revascularization procedures are usually not effective, because they do not correct downstream lesions. Moreover, percutaneous transluminal angioplasty of the tibioperoneal trunk is associated with a high restenosis rate and would not be effective in the long-term management of this patient.

Bibliography

1. **Olin JW.** Thromboangiitis obliterans. Curr Opin Rheumatol. 1994;6:44-9.

2. **Olin JW, Young JR, Graor RA, Ruschhaupt WF, Bartholomew JR.** The changing clinical spectrum of thromboangiitis obliterans (Buerger's disease). Circulation. 1990;82:IV3-8.

Smoking Question 3
Answer: A

EDUCATIONAL OBJECTIVE: Choose most appropriate treatment of nicotine replacement for smoking cessation.

The best choice for this man is to negotiate a quit date on which he will quit smoking completely and start the nicotine patch in the strongest dosage available (21 mg/day). By agreeing on the actual quit date in the coming weeks, a patient can prepare for the date by identifying triggers for smoking and avoiding activities during which he might be tempted to smoke. Using the nicotine patch at 14 mg/day is not adequate to prevent withdrawal symptoms in someone who smokes two and a half packs per day. It is not safe to use the nicotine patch while the patient continues to smoke. There have been many case reports of myocardial infarction in patients who smoke more than five cigarettes a day while wearing the patch.

Nicotine gum is a less expensive alternative to the patch. It may be used on an as-needed basis or on a regular schedule. Efficacy in treating nicotine withdrawal, however, has not been shown in doses less than six pieces a day. The patient should not exceed 20 pieces per day for the 4-mg gum or 30 per day for the 2-mg gum.

Bibliography
1. **Fiore MC, Jorenby DE, Baker TB, Kenford SL.** Tobacco dependence and the nicotine patch. Clinical guidelines for effective use. JAMA. 1992;268:2687-94.
2. **Milan FB.** Smoking cessation. In: Wachtel TJ, Stein MD, eds. Practical Guide to the Care of the Ambulatory Patient. St. Louis: Mosby-Year Book, Inc; 1995.
3. **Fiore MC, Bailey WC, Cohen SJ, Dorfman SF, Goldstein MG, Gritz ER, et al.** Smoking Cessation. Clinical Practice Guideline No. 18. Rockville, Maryland: US Department of Health and Human Services, Public Health Service, Agency for Health Care Policy and Research. AHCPR Publication No. 96-0692. April 1996.

Smoking Question 4
Answer: D

EDUCATIONAL OBJECTIVE: Choose the most appropriate strategy for smoking cessation counseling.

This patient is in precontemplation and has not yet recognized her smoking habit as a problem. The goal is to educate her about her own health risks from smoking as well as to explore the pros and cons of smoking. In this patient, it would be necessary to address the role of smoking as a tension moderator and try to find a substitute. Until this patient is convinced that smoking is a problem and has the desire to quit, making plans for a quit attempt (with or without the nicotine patch) or referral to a smoking cessation program would be futile. In addition, the nicotine patch should be used only with complete cessation. She may be willing to cut down on her smoking but even that would be more successful if she was more motivated to make that change.

Bibliography
1. **Burns DM.** Overview of office-based smoking cessation assistance. In: Burns DM, Cohen SJ, Kottke TE, Gritz ER, eds. Tobacco and the Clinician: Interventions for Medical and Dental Practice. Monograph 5, NIH Publication NO. 94-3693, US Department of Health and Human Services, January 1994.
2. **Milan FB.** Smoking cessation. In: Wachtel TJ, Stein MD, eds. Practical Guide to The Care of the Ambulatory Patient. St. Louis: Mosby-Year Book, Inc; 1995.
3. **Goldstein MG, Ruggiero L, Guise BJ, Abrams DB.** Behavioral medicine strategies for medical patients. In: Stoudemire A, ed. Clinical Psychiatry for Medical Students. 2nd ed. Philadelphia: JB Lippincott Company; 1994.
4. **Fiore MC, Bailey WC, Cohen SJ, Dorfman SF, Goldstein MG, Gritz ER, et al.** Smoking Cessation. Clinical Practice Guideline No. 18. Rockville, Maryland: US Department of Health and Human Services, Public Health Service, Agency for Health Care Policy and Research. AHCPR Publication No. 96-0692. April 1996.

Smoking Question 5
Answer: B

EDUCATIONAL OBJECTIVE: Select the appropriate diagnostic evaluation for a suspected obstructing endobronchial mass.

The patient presents with his second episode of pneumonia in the same location over a 2-month period. The chest radiograph now shows upward displacement of the minor fissure, indicating volume loss in the right upper lobe. This finding, along with decreased breath sounds in the right upper anterior lung field (as opposed to bronchial breath sounds), suggests that there is an endobronchial obstruction proximal to the pneumonia.

The combination of recurrent pneumonia in the same location and volume loss is suspicious enough for endobronchial obstruction, particularly lung cancer in this heavy smoker, to justify further evaluation. The best procedure for visualization of bronchial anatomy and detection of a proximal endobronchial mass is fiberoptic bronchoscopy. Samples for cytologic and histologic analysis can also be obtained by washing, brushing, and endobronchial biopsy through the bronchoscope.

Needle aspiration of the right upper lobe might recover organisms from the postobstructive pneumonia but would not likely yield malignant cells from a more proximal endobronchial mass. Computed tomography is extremely useful for staging once a lung cancer is diagnosed, and it also provides valuable information about nodules or masses in the pulmonary parenchyma. However, it is inferior to bronchoscopy for evaluation of endobronchial masses, and it does not afford the opportunity to sample a lesion for cytologic and histologic analysis.

Wedge biopsy of the right upper lobe via thoracoscopy also would yield material for microbiologic diagnosis of the agent(s) causing pneumonia, but would not yield information about a central endobronchial mass. The clinical suspicion of an obstructing endobronchial lesion is high enough so that failure to pursue further evaluation would not be appropriate.

Bibliography

1. **Karsell PR, McDougall JC.** Diagnostic tests for lung cancer. Mayo Clin Proc. 1993;68:288-96.

2. **Patel AM, Peters SG.** Clinical manifestations of lung cancer. Mayo Clin Proc. 1993;68:273-7.

3. **Mack MJ, Aronoff RJ, Acuff TE, Douthit MB, Bowman RT, Ryan WH.** Present role of thoracoscopy in the diagnosis and treatment of diseases of the chest. Ann Thorac Surg. 1992;54:403-9.

4. **Arroliga AC, Matthay RA.** The role of bronchoscopy in lung cancer. Clin Chest Med. 1993;14:87-98.

SUBSTANCE ABUSE

Substance Abuse Question 1
Answer: A

EDUCATIONAL OBJECTIVE: Understand the principles of management of patients at risk for alcohol withdrawal seizures.

This patient presents with the alcohol-related complication of alcoholic hepatitis and is now at risk for symptoms of alcohol withdrawal, including alcohol withdrawal seizures. Long-acting benzodiazepines (chlordiazepoxide) are preferable to shorter-acting benzodiazepines (alprazolam) because of a lower risk of withdrawal seizures in patients treated with longer-acting drugs. Phenothiazines such as chlorpromazine have been used for treatment of withdrawal symptoms but increase the risk of seizures. Ethyl alcohol should be avoided because of the patient's alcoholic hepatitis. β-blockers can decrease some of the symptoms of alcohol withdrawal (for example, hypertension and tachycardia) but would not change the risk of seizures.

Bibliography

1. **Mayo-Smith MF.** Pharmacologic management of alcohol withdrawal: a meta-analysis and evidence based practice guideline. American Society of Addiction Medicine Working Group on Pharmacological Management of Alcohol Withdrawal. JAMA. 1997;278:144-51.

Substance Abuse Question 2
Answer: E

EDUCATIONAL OBJECTIVE: Recognize and manage heroin-induced pulmonary edema.

This patient presents with hypotension, hypoxia, and pulmonary infiltrates in the setting of injection drug use. This clinical picture is most consistent with heroin-induced pulmonary edema. Patients with heroin-induced pulmonary edema do not have increased central venous pressure. The onset of pulmonary edema can be up to 6 to 10 hours after the heroin is injected. Affected patients can have a rapid improvement following administration of naloxone (a narcotic antagonist) and oxygen. These patients have a low intravascular volume and hypovolemia, and therefore, diuretics are not beneficial and can lead to vascular collapse. A minority of such patients do not respond to supportive therapy and die.

Dopamine might be useful in supporting the blood pressure but would not be the first treatment of heroin-induced pulmonary edema. Treatment of the underlying hypotension would be more appropriate.

Digitalis administration would be appropriate for treatment of cardiogenic pulmonary edema; however, there is no evidence of cardiac failure, as demonstrated by the lack of a gallop and a normal cardiac silhouette. Flumazenil is used to reverse the respiratory suppression caused by benzodiazepines but would have no effect on heroin overdosage.

Bibliography

1. **Cherubin CE, Sapira JD.** The medical complications of drug addiction and the medical assessment of the intravenous drug user: 25 years later. Ann Intern Med. 1993;119:1017-28.
2. **Stein MD.** Medical complications of intravenous drug use. J Gen Intern Med. 1990;5:249-57.

Substance Abuse Question 3
Answer: B

EDUCATIONAL OBJECTIVE: Recognize and initiate proper therapy for alcoholic ketoacidosis.

This patient presents with abdominal pain, nausea, and vomiting. Physical examination and laboratory testing suggest alcoholic hepatitis. Alcoholic ketoacidosis is usually seen in the setting of binge drinking, with cessation of food intake for an extended period and vomiting. It appears to be more common in women than in men. Hyperglycemia is inconsistent and may be present in diabetics or mildly present in nondiabetics. This patient's slightly elevated glucose level makes diabetic ketoacidosis unlikely, and insulin therapy is not appropriate.

In a patient such as this, ingestion of other alcohols (ethylene glycol and methanol) should be considered, and it would be worthwhile to test for these alcohols.

Treatment of alcoholic ketoacidosis consists of rehydration with normal saline and intravenous administration of glucose. The ketosis will clear rapidly with therapy, and sodium bicarbonate usually is not indicated unless the acidosis is very severe. β-blockers have no place in this situation. Corticosteroids seem to benefit patients with severe alcoholic hepatitis but will not treat the acidosis.

Bibliography

1. **Fulop M.** Alcoholic ketoacidosis. Endocrinol Metab Clin North Am. 1993;22:209-19.
2. **Hooper RJ.** Alcoholic ketoacidosis: the late presentation of acidosis in an alcoholic. Ann Clin Biochem. 1994;31:579-82.

Substance Abuse Question 4
Answer: A

EDUCATIONAL OBJECTIVE: Evaluate abnormal isolated aminotransferase elevation.

This patient with a recently detected isolated aminotransferase elevation and moderate alcohol use has no evidence of chronic liver disease on physical examination. A substantial number of patients with an isolated aminotransferase elevation have normal values on follow-up testing and have no chronic hepatobiliary disease. It is appropriate to discontinue alcohol, which may be responsible, and to recheck laboratory tests again in 1 to 2 months. More detailed testing should be done only if follow-up chemistry tests suggest persisting liver injury, if information from the history or physical examination suggests a specific chronic liver disease (such as family history of hemochromatosis or presence of risk factors for viral hepatitis), or if indicators on physical examination suggests chronic liver disease.

When an enlarged liver is detected, an abdominal ultrasound would be appropriate to rule out an hepatic mass or to seek evidence of liver disease. The liver origin of isolated aspartate aminotransferase (AST) elevations should be confirmed by documenting simultaneous ALT elevation because AST may be from extrahepatic sites (muscle, kidney, heart). In the absence of evidence of liver disease or hepatomegaly on the physical examination, liver biopsy and ultrasound should be considered only after transient, nonspecific ALT elevation has been ruled out with repeat testing and an initial etiologic evaluation has been pursued.

A presumptive diagnosis of fatty liver is reasonable when: (1) risk factors for hepatic steatosis such as diabetes, steroid use, or marked obesity are present; (2) other etiologic evaluation for viral, autoimmune, and metabolic causes of chronic liver disease have been unrevealing; and (3) focal hepatic lesions have been ruled out. In this situation, weight reduction of 10% to 15% will often result in normalization of aminotransferases and support a presumptive diagnosis of fatty liver without need for liver biopsy.

Bibliography

1. **Fregia A, Jensen DM.** Evaluation of abnormal liver tests. Compr Ther. 1994;20:50-4.
2. **Palmer M, Schaffner F.** Effect of weight reduction on hepatic abnormalities in overweight patients. Gastroenterology. 1990;99:1408-13.

Substance Abuse Question 5
Answer: D

EDUCATIONAL OBJECTIVE: Recognize the findings on urinalysis characteristic of rhabdomyolysis.

This 21-year-old man has myoglobinuria, resulting from rhabdomyolysis. Myoglobinuria is one cause of discrepancies in urinalysis results. The urine dipstick test is positive for blood, but the microscopic examination is negative for erythrocytes. Other causes for similar discrepancies between dipstick and microscopic examination include hemoglobinuria as a result of intravascular hemolysis, hemolysis of urine erythrocytes most likely to occur in very dilute urine (specific gravity < 1.006), and contamination of urine with betadine. A further clue to the presence of rhabdomyolysis is the blood urea nitrogen:serum creatinine ratio, which is significantly less than the normal value of 10:1 to 15:1. This is due to the increased muscle breakdown of rhabdomyolysis, which causes increased release of creatinine into the circulation.

Brown pigmented casts containing myoglobin may also be seen in the urine of patients with rhabdomyolysis. Prerenal azotemia is usually associated with a bland urine sediment. The urinalyses in chronic glomerulonephritis and HIV nephropathy usually have significantly elevated amounts of protein. Acute interstitial nephritis is associated with both hematuria and pyuria.

Bibliography

1. **Roth D, Alarcon FJ, Fernandez JA, Preston RA, Bourgoignie JJ.** Acute rhabdomyolysis associated with cocaine intoxication. N Engl J Med. 1988;319:673-7.

Substance Abuse Question 6
Answer: E

EDUCATIONAL OBJECTIVE: Diagnose chronic pancreatitis in an alcoholic patient.

The diagnosis of chronic pancreatitis usually is suggested by history and confirmed by imaging studies or laboratory tests. The demonstration of diffuse, speckled calcification of the pancreas on a plain film of the abdomen is diagnostic of chronic pancreatitis. Although the sensitivity of this finding is only approximately 30%, a plain film of the abdomen should be the first diagnostic test because it is simple, not expensive, and specific.

The secretin stimulation test and ERCP are much more sensitive, but they are not more specific. The secretin stimulation test is available only in specialized centers, whereas ERCP is an expensive procedure associated with a significant rate of complications. ERCP should be reserved for patients in whom the diagnosis cannot be clearly established by other imaging techniques or for patients with recurrent acute pancreatitis without an obvious cause. The NBT-PABA test is an indirect pancreatic function test, which has a sensitivity of about 50%.

Bibliography

1. **Owyang C, Levitt M.** Chronic pancreatitis. In: Yamada T, ed. Textbook of Gastroenterology. Philadelphia: J.B. Lippincott Co.; 1991:1874-92.

Substance Abuse Question 7
Answer: B

EDUCATIONAL OBJECTIVE: Identify complications of habitual cocaine smoking.

There are several pulmonary effects of cocaine. When cocaine is smoked, these complications include cough productive of black sputum, hemoptysis, chest pain, cardiac palpitations, and impairment in the diffusing capacity of the lung (DL_{CO}).

Atelectasis, emphysema, eosinophilic pneumonitis, and pulmonary embolism are not recognized complications of cocaine smoking.

Bibliography

1. **Tashkin DP, Khalsa ME, Gorelick D, Chang P, Simmons MS, Coulson AH.** Pulmonary status of habitual cocaine smokers. Am Rev Respir Dis. 1992;145:92-100.

Substance Abuse Question 8
Answer: C

EDUCATIONAL OBJECTIVE: Evaluate and follow-up a patient with an alcohol use disorder.

This patient's history contains enough information for the diagnosis of alcohol abuse. He needs help preparing to stop his alcohol use. He will require both a well-designed program for primary medical care and treatment for his addiction. Treatment in a special program will consist of some form of psychosocial therapy to prevent relapse and may include the use of naltrexone (assuming he does not have severe hepatic dysfunction). You cannot force the patient to begin treatment or to enter Alcoholics Anonymous, but you should be direct and encourage him to enter a program. Although naltrexone is now available as pharmacotherapy (to reduce days spent drinking and the cravings for alcohol), there is no evidence to support its use without involvement in some type of psychosocial program. The brief intervention of explaining that there is a problem with excessive alcohol use can help some patients, but the patient's difficulties at work and driving while intoxicated indicate a more serious substance use disorder.

The atrial fibrillation appears to be from his recent heavy alcohol use (referred to as the *holiday heart syndrome*). He is younger than 60 years and does not have any obvious cardiovascular disease. The digoxin therapy can be safely discontinued. He should not require anticoagulation therapy, but if such therapy were required for a short period, the INR should be 2.0 to 3.0.

Bibliography

1. **Greenspon AJ, Schaal SF.** The "holiday heart": electrophysiologic studies of alcohol effects in alcoholics. Ann Intern Med. 1983;98:135-9.
2. **Pritchett EL.** Management of atrial fibrillation. N Engl J Med. 1992;326:1264-71.
3. **Volpicelli JR, Alterman AI, Hayashida M, O'Brien CP.** Naltrexone in the treatment of alcohol dependence. Arch Gen Psychiatry. 1992;49:876-80.

Substance Abuse Question 9
Answer: D

EDUCATIONAL OBJECTIVE: Manage infective endocarditis in injection drug users.

Injection drug users constitute a special risk group for infective endocarditis. Whereas streptococci are the most common microbes associated with native valve infective endocarditis in the general population, staphylococci account for most cases of infective endocarditis in injection drug users. *Pseudomonas aeruginosa* and enterococci are the next most common pathogens associated with infective endocarditis in injection drug users. Transesophageal echocardiography offers significant advantages over 2-dimension transthoracic echocardiography in injection drug users, just as it does in other patients. Transesophageal echocardiography has improved the sensitivity for detecting vegetations to 90% to 95% from the 30% to 80% recorded by transthoracic echocardiography. Transesophageal echocardiography is especially valuable in patients with aortic valve involvement, because perivalvular extension of infection that would mandate surgical correction is much more easily seen. The transesophageal echocardiography shows tricuspid valve vegetation. Unless there are specific contraindications, transesophageal echocardiography should be done in all patients in whom infective endocarditis is clinically suspected but transthoracic echocardiography is negative. Septic pulmonary embolization occurs in up to 75% of injection drug users with right-sided endocarditis. Pleuritic pain and abnormal chest radiographs may be the first clues to the diagnosis of endocarditis, because tricuspid murmurs are frequently difficult to discern.

The expense and inconvenience of 4- to 6-week intravenous antibiotic regimens coupled with the unsuitability of home intravenous therapy for some injection drug users have led to study of short (2-week) courses of intravenous therapy and exclusively oral therapies. Treatment of injection drug users with right-sided endocarditis due to methicillin-susceptible *Staphylococcus aureus* with a 2-week course of nafcillin and gentamicin was associated with an acceptable cure rate (over 90%) in two nonrandomized studies. Substitution of vancomycin for nafcillin resulted in substantially poorer outcome. Injection drug users with right-sided endocarditis should not be considered for the short-course therapy if left-sided endocarditis, signs of systemic embolization (for example, splinter hemorrhages), or an associated systemic focus of infection such as osteomyelitis is present. Frustrated by the noncompliance of some injection drug users, some authors have reported successful treatment of right-sided endocarditis due to *Staphylococcus aureus* with a 4-week course of ciprofloxacin and rifampin. However, there are no data with regard to 2-week courses of therapy for infective endocarditis caused by enterococci. Injection drug users with enterococcal endocarditis should be treated with a penicillin or vancomycin and gentamicin for 4 to 6 weeks.

A single randomized study showed equivalence of a 2-week course of cloxacillin to cloxacillin plus gentamicin (>90% cure rate).

Bibliography

1. **DiNubile MJ.** Short-course antibiotic therapy for right-sided endocarditis caused by *Staphylococcus aureus* in injection drug users. Ann Intern Med. 1994;121:873-6.

2. **Chambers HF.** Short-course combination and oral therapies of *Staphylococcus aureus* endocarditis. Infect Dis Clin North Am. 1993;7:69-80.

3. **Daniel WG, Mugge A.** Transesophageal echocardiography. N Engl J Med. 1995;332:1268-79.

4. **Wilson WR, Karchmer AW, Dajani AS, Taubert KA, Bayer A, Kaye D, et al.** Antibiotic treatment of adults with infective endocarditis due to streptococci, enterococci, staphylococci, and HACEK microorganisms. American Heart Association. JAMA. 1995;274:1706-13.

Normal Laboratory Values

U.S. traditional units are followed in parentheses by equivalent values expressed in S.I. units.

Blood, Plasma, and Serum Chemistries

Acetoacetate, plasma — Less than 3 mg/dL (0.3 mmol/L)
Alpha-fetoprotein, serum — 0-20 ng/mL (0-20 µg/L)
Aminotransferase, alanine (ALT, SGPT) — 0-35 U/L (0-0.58 µkat/L)
Aminotransferase, aspartate (AST, SGOT) — 0-35 U/L (0-0.58 µkat/L)
Ammonia, serum — 0-80 µg/dL (0-46.9 µmol/L)
Ammonium, blood — 40-70 mg/dL (23.5-41.1 µmol/L)
Amylase, serum — 0-130 U/L (0-2.17 µkat/L)
Antinuclear antibody agglutination — less than 1:80 titer
Antistreptolysin O titer — Less than 150 Todd units
Arterial studies, blood (room air)
    Po_2 - 70-100 mm Hg
    Pco_2 - 35-45 mm Hg
    pH - 7.38-7.44
    (H^+) - 40 nmol/L
Ascorbic acid (vitamin C), blood — 0.4-1.5 mg/dL (23-86 µmol/L)
    leukocyte - 16.5 ± 5.1 mg/dL of leukocytes
Bicarbonate, serum — 23-28 meq/L (23-28 mmol/L)
Bilirubin, serum
    Total — 0.3-1 mg/dL (5.1-17 µmol/L)
    Direct — 0.1-0.3 mg/dL (1.7-5.1 µmol/L)
Calcium, serum — 9-10.5 mg/dL (2.25-2.62 mmol/L)
Carbon dioxide content, serum — 23-28 meq/L (23-28 mmol/L)
Carotene, serum — 75-300 µg/dL (1.4-5.6 µmol/L)
Carcinoembryonic antigen — Less than 2 ng/mL (2 µg/L)
Ceruloplasmin, serum — 25-43 mg/dL (250-430 mg/L)
Chloride, serum — 98-106 meq/L (98-106 mmol/L)
Cholesterol, plasma — 150-199 mg/dL (3.88-5.15 mmol/L), desirable; 200-239 mg/dL (5.17-6.18 mmol/L), borderline high; 240 mg/dL (6.2 mmol/L) and above, high
Cholesterol, low-density lipoprotein (LDL), plasma — Less than or equal to 130 mg/dL (3.36 mmol/L), desirable; 131-159 mg/dL (3.36-4.11 mmol/L), borderline; greater than 160 mg/dL (4.14 mmol/L), high
Cholesterol, high-density lipoprotein (HDL), plasma — Greater than or equal to 40 mg/dL (1.03 mmol/L), desirable; 35-39 mg/dL (0.90-1.0 mmol/L), borderline; less than 35 mg/dL (0.90 mmol/L), high
Complement, serum
    C3 - 55-120 mg/dL (0.55-1.2 g/L)
    CH_{50} - 37-55 CH_{50}U/mL
Copper, serum — 70-155 µg/dL (11-24.3 µmol/L)
Creatine kinase, serum — 30-170 U/L
Creatinine, serum — 0.7-1.5 mg/dL (61.9-133 µmol/L)
Delta-aminolevulinic acid, serum — Less than 20 µg/dL (1.5 µmol/L)
Ethanol, blood — Less than 0.005% (coma level, more than 0.5%)
Fibrinogen, plasma — 150-350 mg/dL (1.5-3.5 g/L)
Folate, red cell — 160-855 ng/mL
Folate, serum — 2.5-20 ng/mL
Glucose, plasma — Fasting, 70-105 mg/dL (3.9-5.8 mmol/L); 2 hours postprandial greater than 140 mg/dL (7.8 mmol/L), abnormal
Homocysteine, serum — Male: 4-16 µmol/L; female: 3-14 µmol/L
Immunoglobulins
    IgG - 640-1430 mg/dL (6.4-14.3 g/L)
        IgG_1 - 280-1020 mg/dL (2.8-10.2 g/L)
        IgG_2 - 60-790 mg/dL (0.6-7.9 g/L)
        IgG_3 - 14-240 mg/dL (0.1-2.4 g/L)
        IgG_4 - 11-330 mg/dL (0.1-3.3 g/L)
    IgA - 70-300 mg/dL (0.7-3.0 g/L)
    IgM - 20-140 mg/dL (0.2-1.4 g/L)
    IgD - Less than 8 mg/dL (80 mg/L)
    IgE - 0.01-0.04 mg/dL (0.1-0.4 mg/L)
Iron, serum — 60-160 µg/dL (11-29 µmol/L); higher in males
Iron binding capacity, serum — 250-460 µg/dL (45-72 µmol/L)
Lactate dehydrogenase, serum — 60-100 U/L
Lactic acid, venous blood — 6-16 mg/dL (0.67-1.8 mmol/L)
Lead, blood — Less than 40 µg/dL (1.9 µmol/L)
Lipase, serum — Less than 95 U/L

Magnesium, serum — 1.5-2.4 mg/dL (0.62-0.99 mmol/L)
Manganese, serum — 0.15 µg/mL
Methylmalonic acid, serum — 150-370 nmol/L
Osmolality, plasma — 275-295 mosm/kg H_2O
Phosphatase (acid), serum — 0.5-5.5 U/L
Phosphatase (alkaline), serum — 36-92 U/L
Phosphorus (inorganic), serum — 3-4.5 mg/dL (0.97-1.45 mmol/L)
Potassium, serum — 3.5-5 meq/L (3.5-5 mmol/L)
Protein, serum
    Albumin - 3.5-5.5 g/dL (35-55 g/L)
    Globulin - 2.0-3.5 g/dL (20-35 g/L)
    $Alpha_1$ - 0.2-0.4 g/dL (2-4 g/L)
    $Alpha_2$ - 0.5-0.9 g/dL (5-9 g/L)
    Beta - 0.6-1.1 g/dL (6-11 g/L)
    Gamma - 0.7-1.7 g/dL (7-17 g/L)
Rheumatoid factor — less than 40 IU/mL
Sodium, serum — 136-145 meq/L (136-145 mmol/L)
Triglycerides — Less than 250 mg/dL (2.82 mmol/L), desirable; 250-500 mg/dL (2.82-5.65 mmol/L), borderline; greater than 500 mg/dL (5.65 mmol/L), elevated
Trypsinogen, serum — 10-85 ng/mL
Urea nitrogen, serum — 8-20 mg/dL (2.9-7.1 mmol/L)
Uric acid, serum — 2.5-8 mg/dL (0.15-0.48 mmol/L)
Vitamin B_{12}, serum — 200-800 pg/mL (148-590 pmol/L)

Cerebrospinal Fluid

Cell count — 0-5 cells/µL (0-5 x 10^6 cells/L)
Glucose — 40-80 mg/dL (2.5-4.4 mmol/L); greater than 30% of simultaneous plasma concentration in hypercalcemia
Protein — 15-60 mg/dL (150-600 mg/L)
Pressure (initial) — 70-200 cm H_2O

Endocrine

Adrenocorticotropin (ACTH) — 9-52 pg/mL (7-27 pmol/L)
Aldosterone, serum (normal sodium intake)
    Supine - 2-5 ng/dL (60-140 pmol/L)
    Standing - 7-20 ng/dL (194-555 pmol/L)
Aldosterone, urine — 5-19 µg/24 h (13.9-52.7 nmol/24 h)
Catecholamines — Epinephrine (supine): less than 75 ng/L (340 pmol/L); norepinephrine (supine): 50-440 ng/L (300-2600 pmol/L)
Catecholamines, 24-hour, urine — Less than 100 µg/d (591 nmol/d)
Cortisol
    Serum - 8 am: 8-20 µg/dL (138-662 nmol/L); 5 pm: 3-13 µg/dL (83-359 nmol/L);
    1 h after cosyntropin; 18; usually 8 or more above baseline overnight suppression test: less than 0.14 µmol/L (15 µg/dL) (138 nmol/L)
    Urine free cortisol: less than 90 µg/dL
Dehydroepiandrosterone sulfate, plasma — Male: 1300-5500 ng/mL (3.4-14.3 µmol/L); female: 600-3300 ng/mL (1.6-8.8 µmol/L)
11-deoxycortisol, serum — Basal: less than 1 µg/dL (30 nmol/L); after metyrapone: greater than 7 µg/dL (210 nmol/L)
Estradiol, serum — Male: 10-30 pg/mL (37-110 pmol/L); female: day 1-10, 184-370 pmol/L; day 11-20, 184-740 pmol/L; day 21-30, 259-550 pmol/L
Estriol, urine — Greater than 12 mg/24 h (42 µmol/d)
Follicle-stimulating hormone, serum — Male (adult): 3-15 mIU/mL (5-15 U/L); female: follicular or luteal phase, 5-20 mIU/mL (5-20 U/L); midcycle peak, 30-50 mIU/mL (30-50 U/L); postmenopausal, greater than 35 mIU/mL (50 U/L)
Growth hormone, plasma — After oral glucose, less than 2 ng/mL (2 µg/L); response to provocative stimuli: greater than 7 ng/mL (7 µg/L)
Insulin, serum (fasting) — 5-20 mU/L
17-hydroxycorticosteroids, urine (Porter-Silber) — Male: 3-10 mg/24 h (8.3-28 µmol/d); female: 2-8 mg/24 h (5.5-22.1 µmol/d)
17-ketosteroids, urine — Male: 8-22 mg/24 h (28-77 µmol/d); female: up to 15 µg/24 h

Luteinizing hormone, serum — Male: 3-15 mIU/mL (5-15 IU/L); female: follicular or luteal phase, 5-22 mIU/mL (5-22 IU/L); midcycle peak, 30-250 mIU/mL (30-250 IU/L); postmenopausal, greater than 30 mIU/mL (30 IU/L)

Metanephrine, urine — Less than 1.2 mg/24 h

Parathyroid hormone, serum — 10-65 pg/mL (normal range varies among laboratories)

Progesterone
Luteal — 3-30 ng/mL
Follicular — less than 1 ng/mL

Prolactin, serum — Male: less than 15 ng/mL (690 pmol/L); female: less than 20 ng/mL (920 pmol/L)

Renin activity (angiotensin-I radioimmunoassay)
Peripheral plasma
Normal diet: supine, 0.3-1.9 ng/mL per h (0.3-1.9 μg/L per h); upright, 0.2-3.6 ng/mL per h (0.2-3.6 μg/L per h)
Low-sodium diet: supine, 0.9-4.5 ng/mL per h (0.9-4.5 μg/L per h); upright, 4.1-9.1 ng/mL per h (4.1-9.1 μg/L per h)
Diuretics and low-sodium diet: 6.3-13.5 ng/mL per h (6.3-13.5 μg/L per h)

Sperm concentration — 20-150 million/mL

Sweat test for sodium and chloride — Less than 60 meq/L (60 mmol/L)

Testosterone, serum — Adult male: 400-1000 ng/dL (10-35 nmol/L); male: greater than 100 ng/dL (3.5 nmol/L); female: less than 100 ng/dL (3.5 nmol/L)

Thyroid function tests (normal ranges vary)
Thyroid iodine (^{131}I) uptake - 10% to 30% of administered dose at 24 h
Thyroid-stimulating hormone (TSH) - 0.5-4.5 μU/mL
Thyroxine (T_4), serum
Total - 5-12 μg/dL (64-154 nmol/L)
Free - 0.9-2.4 ng/dL (12-31 pmol/L)
Free T_4 index - 4-11
Triiodothyronine, resin (T_3) - 25%-35% uptake
Triiodothyronine, serum (T_3) - 70-195 ng/dL (1.2-2.7 nmol/L)

Vanillylmandelic acid, urine — Less than 8 mg/24 h (40.4 μmol/d)

Vitamin D
1,25-dihydroxy, serum - 25-65 pg/mL (60-156 pmol/L)
25-hydroxy, serum - 15-80 ng/mL (12.5-200 nmol/L)

Gastrointestinal

D-xylose absorption (after ingestion of 25 g of D-xylose) — Urine excretion: 5-8 g at 5 h (33-53 mmol); serum D-xylose: greater than 20 mg/dL at 2 h

Fecal urobilinogen — 40-280 mg/24 h (67-472 μmol/d)

Gastric secretion — Basal secretion: male: 4.0 ± 0.2 meq of HCl/h (4.0 ± 0.2 mmol/h); female: 2.1 ± 0.2 meq of HCl/h (2.1 ± 0.2 mmol/h); peak acid secretion: male: 37.4 ± 0.8 meq of HCl/h (37.4 ± 0.8 mmol/h); female: 24.9 ± 1.0 meq of HCl/h (24.9 ± 1.0 mmol/h)

Gastrin, serum — 0-180 pg/mL (0-180 ng/L)

Lactose tolerance test — Increase in plasma glucose: greater than 15 mg/dL (0.83 mmol/L)

Lipase, ascitic fluid — Less than 200 U/L

Secretin-cholecystokinin pancreatic function — Greater than 80 meq/L of HCO_3 in at least 1 specimen collected over 1 h

Stool fat — Less than 5 g/d on a 100-g fat diet

Stool nitrogen — Less than 2 g/d

Stool weight — Less than 200 g/d

Hematology

Activated partial thromboplastin time — Less than 25-35 s

Bleeding time — Less than 10 min

Coagulation factors, plasma
Factor I - 150-350 mg/dL (1.5-3.5 g/L)
Factor II - 60%-150% of normal
Factor V - 60%-150% of normal
Factor VII - 60%-150% of normal
Factor VIII - 60%-150% of normal
Factor IX - 60%-150% of normal
Factor X - 60%-150% of normal
Factor XI - 60%-150% of normal
Factor XII - 60%-150% of normal

Erythrocyte count — 4.2-5.9 million cells/μL (4.2-5.9 x 10^{12} cells/L)

Erythrocyte survival rate (^{51}Cr) — T ½ = 28 days

Erythropoietin — < 30 mU/mL

D-dimer — < 0.5 μg/mL

Ferritin — 15-200 μg/mL

Glucose-6-phosphate dehydrogenase — 5-15 U

Haptoglobin, serum (hemoglobin-binding capacity) — 50-150 mg/dL

Hematocrit — Male: 41%-51%; female: 36%-47%

Hemoglobin, blood — Male: 14-17 g/dL; female: 12-16 g/dL

Hemoglobin, plasma — 0.5-5 mg/dL (0.08-0.8 μmol/L)

Leukocyte alkaline phosphatase — 15-40 mg of phosphorus liberated/h per 10^{10} cells; score = 13-130/100 polymorphonuclear neutrophils and band forms

Leukocyte count — Nonblacks: 4000-10,000/μL (4.0-10 x 10^9/L); Blacks: 3500-10,000/μL (2.8-10 x 10^9/L)

Lymphocytes
CD4$^+$ cell count — 640-1175/μL
CD8$^+$ cell count — 335-875/μL
CD4: CD8 ratio — 1.0-4.0

Mean corpuscular hemoglobin (MCH) — 28-32 pg

Mean corpuscular hemoglobin concentration (MCHC) — 32-36 g/dL (320-360 g/L)

Mean corpuscular volume (MCV) — 80-100 fL

Osmotic fragility of erythrocytes — Increased if hemolysis occurs in over 0.5% NaCl, decreased if hemolysis is incomplete in 0.3% NaCl

Platelet count — 150,000-350,000/μL (150-350 x 10^9/L)

Platelet life span (^{51}Cr) — 8-12 days

Protein C activity — 67%-131%

Protein C resistance — 2.2-2.6

Protein S activity — 82%-144%

Prothrombin time — 11-13 s

Reticulocyte count — 0.5%-1.5% of erythrocytes; absolute: 23,000-90,000 cells/μL

Schilling test (oral administration of radioactive cobalamin labeled vitamin B$_{12}$) — 8.5%-28% excreted in urine per 24-48 h

Sedimentation rate, erythrocyte (Westergren) — Male: 0-15 mm/h; female: 0-20 mm/h

Volume, blood
Plasma - Male: 44 mL/kg body weight; female: 43 mL/kg body weight
Erythrocyte - Male: 25-35 mL/kg body weight; female: 20-30 mL/kg body weight

Pulmonary

Forced expiratory volume in 1 second (FEV$_1$) — Greater than 80% predicted

Forced vital capacity (FVC) — Greater than 80% predicted

FEV$_1$/FVC — Greater than 75%

Urine

Amino acids — 200-400 mg/24 h

Amylase — 6.5-48.1 U/h

Calcium — 100-300 mg/d (2.5-7.49 mmol/d) on unrestricted diet

Chloride — 80-250 meq/d (80-250 mmol/d) (varies with intake)

Copper — 0-100 μg/24 h (0-1.6 μmol/d)

Coproporphyrin — 50-250 μg/24 h (76-382 mmol/d)

Creatine — Male: 4-40 mg/24 h (0-0.3 mmol/d); female: 0-100 mg/24 h (0-0.76 mmol/d)

Creatinine — 15-25 mg/kg per 24 h (0.13-0.22 mmol/kg per d)

Creatinine clearance — 90-140 mL/min

5-hydroxyindoleacetic acid (5-HIAA) — 2-9 mg/24 h (10.5-47.1 μmol/d)

Osmolality — 38-1400 mosm/kg H_2O

Phosphate, tubular resorption — 79%-94% (0.79-0.94) of filtered load

Potassium — 25-100 meq/24 h (25-100 mmol/d) (varies with intake)

Protein — Less than 100 mg/24 h

Sodium — 100-260 meq/24 h (100-260 mmol/d) (varies with intake)

Uric acid — 250-750 mg/24 h (1.48-4.43 mmol/d) (varies with intake)

Urobilinogen — 0.05-2.5 mg/24 h (0.09-4.23 μmol/d)

American College of Physicians–American Society of Internal Medicine

190 North Independence Mall West, Philadelphia, PA 19106-1572